A Celebration of Sex

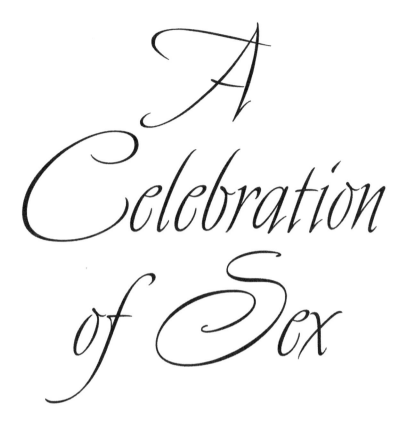

A Celebration of Sex

DR. DOUGLAS E. ROSENAU

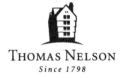

THOMAS NELSON
Since 1798

NASHVILLE   DALLAS   MEXICO CITY   RIO DE JANEIRO   BEIJING

Published in Nashville, Tennessee, by Thomas Nelson, Inc.

PUBLISHER'S NOTE: This book is intended for general information only and is not intended to supplant advice, diagnosis, treatment, or therapy by a personal physician or professional counselor.

Scripture quotations noted NKJV are taken from THE NEW KING JAMES VERSION. Copyright © 1979, 1980, 1982, Thomas Nelson, Inc., Publishers.

Scripture quotations marked NIV are taken from the HOLY BIBLE: NEW INTERNATIONAL VERSION®, copyright © 1973, 1978, 1984 by the International Bible Society, used by permission of Zondervan Publishing House. All rights reserved.

Illustrations by Alan Tiegreen.

Library of Congress Cataloging-in-Publication Data

Rosenau, Douglas.
    A celebration of sex / Douglas E. Rosenau.
      p. cm.
    Includes bibliographical references and index.
    ISBN 10: 0-7852-6467-1
    ISBN 13: 978-0-7852-6467-5
  1. Sex in marriage. 2. Sex—Religious aspects. I. Title.
HQ31.R8425 1994   93-32904
306.7—dc20   CIP

Printed in the United States of America
07 08 09 10 11 VIC 15 14 13 12

To my wife,
CATHERINE

How affirming to be adored
How invaluable to be supported
How healing to be unconditionally loved
How awesome to be erotically intimate

Without her this book could never have been created.

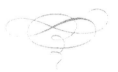

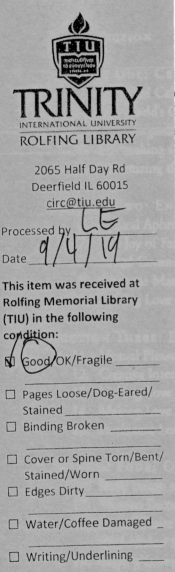

ix

Introduction

EVERYONE WANTS TO LOVE and be loved, to create passionate love relationships that reach deep into the soul and totally transform the individuals involved. Hollywood makes billions on this theme, but actually God is the author of this intimate desire. God is Love and humans are created in His very image to love. Nowhere is this more clearly revealed than through God's grand metaphor for intimacy, that picture window into the heart of the Almighty—sexuality.

God created sexuality to reveal Himself, how He operates, and the value He places on intimate relating—a wonderful picture into the Almighty, who desires His human creation to understand what love is all about. "So God created man in His own image; in the image of God He created him; male and female He created them" (Gen. 1:27 NKJV). With sexuality, God made two different types of relationships: the family and gender with brothers and sisters, fathers, mothers and children; and romantic marriage with erotic enjoyment and becoming one flesh. In both the gender and romantic modes, sexuality unveils God's excitement over committed relationships and loving connection.

God has a fantastic formula for your sex life:

AN INTIMATE MARRIAGE + MATURE LOVERS = A FULFILLING SEX LIFE

If you want powerful techniques and easy answers, you may be disappointed in this book. God's plan often involves time, effort, and difficult changes. It can be a wonderful journey if you are willing to take on this fun challenge of growing up into a skilled lover and learning to be truly intimate. You'll discover that sex is more about an exciting process and way of life than it is a simple acquisition of techniques.

In God's design, sexual fulfillment and an intimate marriage can never be separated. He wove sexuality intricately into the fabric of marital companionship and created the concept of two becoming, literally, one flesh. A fun, trusting friendship precedes fulfilling sexual inter-action. A great sex life will not ensure a great marriage because a loving companionship and a right relationship with God are the essentials. But, a great marital companionship can pro-vide the foundation for fantastic lovemaking.

ESSENTIALS FOR AN INTIMATE MARRIAGE AND A GREAT SEX LIFE

If a good sex life is built on an intimate marital companionship, what are the vital factors of this companionship and how is it built? What are reasonable expectations of an intimate rela-tionship, marriage, and a fulfilling sexual union?

A Dynamic, Covenant Partnership Must Be Formed

The Bible describes the beauty and complexity of the marital companionship that creates the context for lovemaking. The loving, intimate relationship of you and your spouse is mod-eled after the relationship of God and His chosen people. A mature marital partnership truly fashions itself after *redemption,* in that you die to yourself and let go of any self-protectiveness. A covenant is formed. Marriage is not a simple contract but a deep vow and promise.

You create a bonded partnership in which you submit your will for the good of your mate. You become naked, nurturing, and safe with each other. "Love is patient . . . It is not rude, it is not self-seeking . . . It always protects, always trusts, always hopes, always perseveres" (1 Cor. 13:4–5, 7 NIV). Your union is based on love, humility, gentleness, and trust.

Your trust is well founded because each of you reaches out and lovingly nurtures the other as carefully as you would watch out for your own body. In this union, you look honestly at your own rough edges and shortcomings and humbly try to change them. You choose to give as precious gifts the things that your mate desires and needs. It is a marvelous atmosphere for fun sexual relating and intimate connecting when this kind of tenderness, trust, genuine empathy, and cooperation abound.

I love the words *nurture* and *connected,* and I use them many times in this book. Great examples of nurturing are parents lovingly caring for their children or gardeners carefully watering and tending their plants. Mates lovingly nurture each other as well. You are con-nected with your mate in a way far more profound than the splicing together of two electric wires or the tying of two ropes. You are connected in a partnership that grows ever richer and deeper but takes constant attention and renewal. This is the concept of soul mates and of lovers cleaving together. Like steel being refined, a unique synthesis is created, and a profound connection is formed.

A wonderful synergistic dynamic can occur in marriage. The whole is much greater than the sum of its parts. Individuality, personal pleasure, and separate responsibility are not lost. In dying to self and becoming a one-flesh companion, each partner becomes stronger and achieves things that could not be accomplished alone. The two have the best of both worlds: they are a nurturing couple, and each flourishes as an individual. A totally unique and powerful partnership is created. From this unique relationship of marriage can come sexual enjoyment for both individuals, and as a couple. It will seem like one plus one equals four.

Reasonable, Biblical Expectations Must Be Incorporated

Most couples enter marriage with a variety of expectations about how it should be. Which of the following expectations did you bring into your marriage?

- You would never fight.
- The husband would automatically take the garbage out and vacuum.
- Your partner would never be attracted to anyone else.
- You would eat dinner together at the table most nights.
- Christmas Eve would be spent with your family—or with neither family.
- Money would be handled wisely, and there would be a joint checking account.
- Sex would fall into place easily.

I can remember the couple who told me that if they could only let go of all their expectations, they would have a happy marriage. I asked them, "Why get married if you don't expect anything from the relationship and your mate?" The task you face is not getting rid of all your expectations, but basing them realistically on biblical principles.

Here are ten reasonable desires based on God's economy for intimate companionship. May He give you wisdom and courage to make the changes you need within your partnership, because great sex flows from a great marriage. It may seem like strange advice, but the quality of your sex life may depend on turning off the television, picking a good fight, becoming independent of your parents, setting up a budget, or taking regular vacations.

1. Each of us will become a partner and soul mate offering unconditional love, understanding, and support. We will be best friends.

> The LORD God said, "It is not good that man should be alone." (Gen. 2:18 NKJV)

> Husbands . . . dwell with them with understanding, giving honor to the wife . . .
> All of you be of one mind. (1 Peter 3:7–8 NKJV)

> Husbands ought to love their wives as their own bodies . . . No one ever hated his own
> body, but he feeds and cares for it . . . And the two will become one flesh. (Eph.
> 5:28–29, 31 NIV)

> A friend loves at all times,
> And a brother [mate] is born for adversity . . .
> But there is a friend who sticks closer than a brother.
> (Prov. 17:17; 18:24 NIV)

In a boxing match, the boxer has in his corner a manager who is unconditionally committed to helping the fighter use his best shots, encouraging him, correcting mistakes, taking care of any wounds, and preparing him for maximum efficiency. Mates are each other's managers. Marriage is a safe retreat from the fight of daily living. You have an ally in your corner who will kiss your boo-boos and persist in supporting you. Someone who knows you better than anyone else in the world and still loves you.

An important part of cleaving together and becoming one flesh is being intimate companions. You become soul mates and best friends in marriage as you share your needs, your innermost feelings and desires, and your future goals. It is important to have a same-sex best friend, but your partner should also be a best friend. Both mates, and especially husbands, struggle with this—at times being too private and not disclosing needs and feelings to another. (Later on in the book, you'll learn the art of connecting conversation.)

2. Neither of us will expect the other to meet all of our needs or take sole responsibility for our personal happiness. We will give each other space to breathe and have a life.

> Work out your own salvation with fear and trembling; for it is God who works in
> you both to will and to do for His good pleasure. (Phil. 2:12–13 NKJV)

> Each one should test his own actions. Then he can take pride in himself, without comparing himself to somebody else, for each one should carry his own load.
> (Gal. 6:4–5 NIV)

Each of you must build support networks consisting of helpful friends and the Lord. Ultimately, you must rely on God because He is the only unfailing source of peace, purpose, and happiness. I remember the single person who came up to me after a conference and told me, "Dr. Rosenau, you are lucky to be married because you are never lonely and have instantly available sex." I reassured him that married people get lonely because we can't always be there for each other. I also told him I wasn't aware of that rule in marriage of instantly available sex, and I would have to tell my wife.

Your mate can meet your sexual needs, but you have many other needs that are impossible for one person to meet. You need a best friend of the same sex, supporting couple friendships, and fellowship groups. You will perhaps need tennis buddies, kindred political souls, good baby-sitters, efficient accountants, or surrogate grandparents.

You must also learn to nurture yourself and work out your own salvation as you become self-aware and confident. If you are insecure and possessive, you can smother your mate. Real love is free of fearful demands and gives breathing room for you and your mate to grow and experience life. You must work on your own happiness as you take responsibility to grow and experience contentment.

3. We will leave our fathers and mothers and create a new, independent, special family unit.

> For this reason a man will leave his father and mother and be united to his wife,
> and the two will become one flesh. (Eph. 5:31 NIV)

Disentangling yourself financially and emotionally from your parents and family is important. Together, you and your mate are creating a new partnership and family. You cannot hold on to the need to run back to your parents for constant nurturing. You need to make a definite, symbolic statement that your spouse is your first priority. It is the husband who is specifically commanded to leave father and mother. It's difficult to learn the wisdom and maturity of gently separating from parents and making your marriage a special unit.

Sometimes this process of becoming independent and separate is called individuating. This needs to happen individually before it can happen as a couple. Sometimes with age and maturity comes the ability to do this more effectively. It does not mean either disrespecting your parents or never leaning on them for support. The act of leaving your parents makes your mate feel special and protected—a priority as you meet your mate's needs. It creates that new and unique partnership. If you are having trouble individuating from your parents, you will probably need to move away from them geographically. You may also need to stay in a motel when you visit parents to give your partner a chance to regroup, to tell your parents you don't want to hear your mate put down, or to expand your group of wise counselors and "sounding boards" beyond the scope of them alone.

4. We will have one healthy fight or disagreement a week. Confrontation concerning our unmet personal needs will be believed and not dismissed.

> Correct, rebuke and encourage—with great patience and careful instruction. (2 Tim. 4:2 NIV)

> Speaking the truth in love . . . Therefore, putting away lying, "Let each one of you speak truth with his neighbor" . . . Do not let the sun go down on your wrath. (Eph. 4:15, 25–26 NKJV)

XIV   A CELEBRATION OF SEX

> For even if I made you sorry with my letter, I do not regret it. (2 Cor. 7:8 NKJV)

> Now no chastening seems to be joyful for the present, but painful; nevertheless, afterward it yields the peaceable fruit of righteousness to those who have been trained by it. (Heb. 12:11 NKJV)

> Exhort one another daily . . . lest any of you be hardened through the deceitfulness of sin. (Heb. 3:13 NKJV)

> Make straight paths for your feet, so that what is lame may not be dislocated, but rather be healed . . . [Look] carefully lest anyone fall short of the grace of God; lest any root of bitterness springing up cause trouble, and by this many become defiled. (Heb. 12:13, 15 NKJV)

Disappointed expectations, frustrated needs, stored hurt, and retained anger create bitterness and distance and destroy intimacy. You as a couple have to have the courage for healthy conflict and confrontation. Learn conflict-resolution skills (see Chapter 8), practice forgiveness, and let go of hurt as you resolve differences.

Mates are unique individuals who will be incompatible in certain ways. Each of you is a strong person with a distinct personality, gender, and family. These differences can actually enhance your marriage. With good communication skills and the resolution to not let the sun go down on your anger, you will be able to work through these differences. Frequent confrontation and conflict resolve issues, whereas drawn-out disagreements or sitting on issues is more likely to create resentment and bitterness.

Courage and honesty are needed to deal immediately with disagreements. Healthy conflict that resolves issues and clears the air is an important discipline within intimate companionship. You should be humble and loving enough to hear your partner and *believe what is being said*, and your mate should be willing to do the same for you. Learn the skills to resolve issues so that you don't repeat your fights over and over until someone leaves in frustration.

Don't attempt to use submission as an agent of change in your spouse's life. Loving rebuke and exhortation are God's method for correcting harmful behaviors—not attempts to enforce submission. Work out a patient, logical, and kind plan of correction (and perhaps to your surprise) your spouse may humbly listen, agree, and make needed changes. Have at least one good disagreement or confrontation a week.

5. We will take regular vacations and "honeymoons" throughout our marriage as we mend and enhance our intimacy.

> There is a time for everything,
> and a season for every activity under heaven . . .
> a time to tear down and a time to build . . .
> a time to mourn and a time to dance . . .
> a time to search and a time to give up . . .
> a time to tear and a time to mend. (Eccl. 3:1, 3–4, 6–7 NIV)

> When a man has taken a new wife, he shall not go out to war or be charged with
> any business; he shall be free at home one year, and bring happiness to his wife.
> (Deut. 24:5 NKJV)

There should be some special time set aside for a honeymoon and more concentrated, focused time in that first year together. It is a time of adjusting and getting to know each other. Getting away is a great principle for all married couples, no matter how long they have been married. In Chapter 6, I will explain the importance of couples taking vacations and rejuvenating their companionship and sex life. They need time away from home and free of duties as they concentrate on bringing happiness to each other and renewing their friendship.

The marital plague of the twenty-first century will be overinvolvement and busyness. Trust me, as busy as you are, if you do not plan in vacations and spend money to revive your companionship, you will never have the intimacy you desire. You may need to plan for a babysitter and a date night every week or two, an overnight trip away from home, or a complete second honeymoon. Give yourself permission to budget time and money for your partnership. Reasonable expectation of your marriage makes for a fun friendship and quality playtime together.

6. We will use credit carefully as we become wise stewards of our finances.

> Owe no one anything except to love one another. (Rom. 13:8 NKJV)

> Then he who had received the five talents went and traded with them, and made
> another five talents . . . His lord said to him, "Well done, good and faithful servant;
> you were faithful over a few things, I will make you ruler over many things. Enter
> into the joy of your lord." (Matt. 25:16, 21 NKJV)

A great sex life is closely dependent on staying out of debt and learning to handle finances wisely. It makes sense that any stressors in a marriage will weaken intimacy and the desire to make love.

Christian financial counselor Ron Blue has this marvelously simple principle for couples who want to avoid financial stress: Spend less than you make. Financial counselors especially advise against spending excessive money on depreciating items like a car, clothes, or furniture. Not borrowing money certainly means not using credit cards as you create sound spending and budgeting habits. Learn to be self-disciplined in this realm, for effective stewardship of your finances *will indeed help your sex life.*

God requires of Christians sound thinking and self-discipline in all important areas of life that can tend to the destructiveness of excess: "For God has not given us a spirit of fear, but of power and of love and of a sound mind" (2 Tim. 1:7 NKJV). Do a quick reality check in your marriage. Are you being undisciplined and blocking a deeper intimacy in some area other than finances? Television? Children? Work? Parents? Friends? Hobbies? Sports? Get your act together or, like financial trouble, the stress will begin to have an impact on your marriage and your love life. It is amazing how couples improve their marriages simply by turning off the television or going to bed together.

7. My mate will be faithful and committed to me.

> You shall not commit adultery. (Ex. 20:14 NKJV)

A great marital partnership has room for only two people in it. Commitment is vital to intimate companionship, and the creation of good boundaries is irreplaceable for a fantastic marriage and sex life. Feeling safe and trusting are critical for being "naked and unashamed," and these qualities are built on commitment.

Adulterate means "to contaminate by adding a foreign substance or watering down a product." You can adulterate your marital companionship in many ways other than by having a sexual affair. You can adulterate your marriage by overcommitting to work, children, or church. It is a valid desire and decision that mates avoid adulterating their marriage.

God's injunction of "you shall not commit adultery" is often portrayed in terms of a protective fence that guards the beautiful marital and sexual garden. So often we look at fences as something to jump so we can get to greener grass. Actually, the no-adultery fence is there so you can have the intimacy to create an unbelievable relationship within that enclosure—a deeper level of emotional and sexual connecting that can occur and flourish only in an intimate marriage. This barrier protects you from contaminating elements that can threaten the quality of your companionship.

Faithfulness and commitment are interesting concepts. They are processes that create an exclusive partnership with your mate. Some of the choices in mating are highly visible and are special and easily remembered symbols of commitment. The wedding vows are one, similar to the pillar Jacob erected in Bethel to serve as a reminder of God's promise and blessing (Gen. 28:18). Other obvious choices are children, a home, a mortgage, and retirement planning.

Probably more important but less obvious are commitments to your mate that come in a series of daily choices. Every day when you say to yourself, "I have my mate" and refuse to entertain thoughts about someone else, you are reaffirming your commitment. You are allowing sex to be rational and setting good boundaries as you choose to control your sexual impulses and preserve sexual integrity.

These little commitment choices to preserve and deepen intimacy pop up in all areas of marriage. It could mean calling off a lunch with a colleague, deciding whether to have that third child, going to a bed-and-breakfast for a weekend renewal, leaving work early, or buying that funny card and leaving it in the car for your spouse. It can be going to that marriage seminar, reading a book on sexual technique, apologizing for that unkind remark, or working harder to correct a personal character defect.

These choices are not always huge and obvious, but they create the glue that keeps a marriage and sexual relationship together. Daily you have to choose not to adulterate and water down your companionship. Daily you take those little steps that create the fences protecting your garden of fantastic intimacy and sexual pleasure. This is a reasonable expectation for a healthy marital relationship.

8. Either of us will be able to initiate marriage counseling, and the other will be willing to go. Our marriage will be constantly growing with individual and relational changes and improvements.

> The heart of him who has understanding seeks knowledge,
> But the mouth of fools feeds on foolishness. (Prov. 15:14 NKJV)

> He who heeds the word wisely will find good. (Prov. 16:20 NKJV)

> The sweetness of a man's friend gives delight by hearty counsel. (Prov. 27:9 NKJV)

> And this is my prayer: that your love may abound more and more in knowledge and depth of insight, so that you may be able to discern what is best. (Phil. 1:9–10 NIV)

> Speaking the truth in love, we will in all things grow up into him who is the Head, that is, Christ. (Eph. 4:15 NIV)

In a humble, loving marital partnership, you want your mate to be happy and fulfilled. Wise counsel can be so critical. If an impasse occurs, either mate will be able and encouraged to initiate counseling with the appropriate wise person.

We don't marry someone to change him or her, but it is a reasonable expectation that we will continue to grow up together as we rub off our rough edges and overcome our skill and character deficits. A great marriage and sex life is constantly growing and deepening.

Wise counsel is a fantastic source of marital enrichment. It may be a marriage counselor to

CHAPTER ONE

A Biblical Celebration

ISN'T IT FASCINATING that making love reached its peak expression in the Garden of Eden with Adam and Eve before the Fall? That is still the model for the twenty-first century. And in this chapter we'll develop a theology of sexuality from Genesis on. Since the Fall, sex has been in a downhill spiral of immaturity and distortion. As Christians, we have a responsibility to redeem and reclaim God's wonderful gift of sexual union as we experience making love in its Garden-of-Eden fullness: naked and unashamed.

GOD'S IMAGE

Genesis 1:27 states, "So God created man in His own image; in the image of God He created him; male and female He created them" (NKJV). Wow! God's image is reflected in both maleness and femaleness and the way they interrelate. As we better understand the Creator of man and woman and the interaction of the Trinity, we gain an intimate glance into the nature of gender and sexuality: differences and similarities within a complementary partnership and the needs for intimate relationship, excitement, and nurturing procreation and recreation. God wanted to reveal Himself and the value He places on intimate loving relationships, so He created sexuality.

In exploring these concepts, we must be careful not to anthropomorphize God. (*Anthropomorphize* is a five-syllable word that simply means "to make human.") We as human beings are limited to our experiences, and they do not give us enough vocabulary and concepts to truly understand God. We as Christians should also be careful not to keep God so far away from sexuality and marriage that we lose our Creator's insights into the importance of gender and becoming one flesh.

We can gain helpful understanding of gender differences by observing the different relational qualities of the persons of God. God the Father is an excellent model for the male role.

God wanted to be respected by and to be a loving Father to the Israelites as He led and provided. God the Son is an excellent model for the female role. Jesus said He wanted to protect and nurture "as a hen gathers her chicks under her wings" (Matt. 23:37 NIV). At Lazarus's death, Jesus wept and showed His emotions (John 11:35). Jesus gave us insights into femininity with His enjoyment of nurturing, intimate relating, and maternal protectiveness of people important to Him. He appreciated the nourishing wholeness of valuing emotions and disclosing Himself within intimate friendships, embodying the concept of femaleness He created.

Another fascinating aspect in God's creation is that there is as much similarity in two-gender humanness as there is in the three-person Godhead. Males and females have more common emotions, needs, and attributes than they have differences. Each human being contains aspects of both genders. Carl Jung called these two principles *anima* and *animus*. I, Doug, am male but also have a female side to me that I can acknowledge and maximize. I can be a mother hen as I hover protectively; I will sometimes gently hold someone's hand as we cry together. Each of us, whether male or female, has both genders' traits interacting in us in a way that brings a richness to personality and meaning to relationships, along with an awareness and appreciation of difference.

This idea of course leads into perplexing speculation about what exactly are the differences between maleness and femaleness, between husband and wife. The physical differences are readily apparent. There are other God-created differences, but it is easy to confuse them with prejudice, stereotypes, and power struggles. This is not God's design, for in Christ men and women are different but equal (Gal. 3:28; Col. 3:5–13).

We need to understand that some of these differences are not God-given distinctions but learned behaviors. For example, you have probably heard the saying that "men give affection to get sex and women give sex to get affection." This is not part of God's gender and sexual design. As a society, we have squelched female sexuality while allowing males to diminish the importance of emotions and intimate relating. These attitudes and actions should be disputed and changed by Christians.

We cannot deny that there are definite differences, and we can learn from each other as we incorporate the best of both gender worlds. What if men are more sexually immediate and women do value romance more? What if men do want challenge and adventure and women do desire security? Then our goal should be to combine the best of both genders, with men becoming more sensually romantic and women more assertively sexual.

Some gender differences will always be a mystery, much as is the image of our wonderfully complex God. However, recognizing basic differences is important because these differences directly affect your understanding and ability to please your mate, create an intimate marriage, and be a great lover. Here are some common generalizations. They may or may not apply to your situation, so be careful not to panic because your spouse does not conform to the universal concepts of masculinity and femininity. Most people blend characteristics from both lists.

CHARACTERISTICS OF MEN:

- Need to feel significant, admired, and respected, with sense of self-worth reinforced by affirmation and achievement; gain greater identity from what they do

- Take risks more easily (for example, no disability insurance)

- Are "one-track" and can be very focused on the opportunity of the moment (great strength and potential weakness, e.g., ballgame, completing a project, making love)

- Value self-sufficiency and can see life as a challenge and competition

- Desire to be competent and strong (can create defensiveness)

- Enjoy leading and providing (can lack flexibility and sensitivity to mate's desires)

- Less driven by feelings—can hold them in or lack the skills to express them; more left-brain and analytical, focused on a task

- Usually more hormonally driven (higher testosterone); tune in more visually to specific erotic cues and body parts—enjoy seeing their wife's body

- The eternal adolescent—childlike with curiosity and more immediate, playful enjoyment of sexuality (more prone to obsessive sexual behaviors)

- Are more predictable in what arouses them sexually

CHARACTERISTICS OF WOMEN:

- Need to feel secure and have a comfortable nest as their safety and emotional needs are met; need to be attended to and made to feel special and adored

- Do not take risks as readily

- Can multitask easier and use both left and right brain (prone to distractions)

- Want to feel connected and included; gain greater identity from relationships

- See life as more of an interactive, cooperative community and desire connecting conversation and emotional connection

- Are better at asking connecting questions (can feel like interrogation to husband) and engaging in conversation

- Want to nurture and protect (strength and potential weakness with the mother hen syndrome)

- Are freer in tuning in to and expressing emotions (can expect husband to understand or sense her feelings without communicating them)

- Enjoy sensuality and tune in visually to the whole person as well as erogenous zones

- Desire romance and emotional affiliation in lovemaking

- Are unpredictable in sexual arousal, both mentally and physically

ONE FLESH

God stated in the beginning of creation, "It is not good that man should be alone; I will make him a helper comparable to him" (Gen. 2:18 NKJV). Not only did God create the genders, but He designed a special, unique mating relationship. The scriptural account details, "A man shall leave his father and mother and be joined to his wife, and they shall become one flesh. And they were both naked, the man and his wife, and were not ashamed" (Gen. 2:24–25 NKJV).

It is tremendously moving to think of God's original one-flesh companionship. Adam and Eve, before the fall of Eden, had the marvelous capacity of being totally naked, physically and emotionally, with no shame or fear. They reveled in a childlike trust and curiosity—laughing, exploring, giving and receiving love. Sex was a glorious, innocent celebration lived out with instinctual honesty, respect, and zest for life. It was naked and unashamed with no performance anxiety, inhibitions, pain, or selfish skill deficits. What a relationship and sex life they were able to have as they truly "knew" each other, inside and out!

Being God's special creation gives us the power to control nature and ourselves, and to make choices in a way different from animal sexuality. We can decide when we want to have children and how many we can lovingly provide for. We can love and enjoy our children and families for a lifetime of purpose and intimacy. Unlike the animal kingdom, we can choose to have loveplay and lovemaking for intimate bonding and fun. We can purposefully create orgasms and enjoy the whole sexual process for recreation and the enhancement of intimacy.

Unfortunately, sex has not always been regarded so positively. Within Christianity, sex has often been portrayed as sinful or dangerous. Not too long ago, sex was justified only as a means of procreation. God was considered distant and mildly opposed to marital sexual pleasure. Some of this type of thinking dates back to St. Augustine and his conversion from a completely undisciplined and salacious sexuality. He and other church fathers created a restrictive, legalistic sexual economy because of their own struggles and fears, and in so doing they incorporated a theology that strayed from Scripture. Church prohibitions robbed couples, and especially women, of the ability to enjoy God's intended pleasure.

One-flesh unity is an exciting concept, replete with ideas of sexual uniting and recreating. It is indeed God's plan for men and women to appreciate sexual fun and recreation, and we as Christians need to claim, sanctify, and celebrate the wonder and enjoyment of our sexuality.

However, with greater freedom and grace in our sexuality comes the ability to make both constructive and destructive choices, and that is scary. The early church fathers dealt with this challenge legalistically, requiring less thought and energy on the part of Christians. Sexuality is indeed a powerful force in our lives, with tremendous potential for intimate bonding or harmful behaviors. We must constantly make the choices that will enhance our one-flesh partnership.

First Corinthians tells about the importance of keeping sexually connected in marriage: "Let the husband render to his wife the affection due her, and likewise also the wife to her husband . . . Do not deprive one another except with consent for a time . . . and come together again so that Satan does not tempt you because of your lack of self-control" (7:3, 5 NKJV). In a loving partnership, enjoying sexuality and connecting with a mate are gifts each brings to the other willingly—*not by demands or coercion.*

Please don't use God's loving guidelines as weapons against each other. Some husbands and wives club their mates with this passage and say things like, "If you don't have sex with me tonight, you are sinning." The real sin is theirs because they usually have never taken the time, loving-kindness, and energy to make changes needed to appeal to their mates romantically. Becoming one flesh has ceased to be the loving gift of meeting each other's needs and uniting. Remember, making love is about giving—not demanding.

On the other hand, are you too fatigued or busy or inhibited to have sexual relations regularly? You too are missing God's plan for marriage and the enjoyment of one of His avenues for increasing intimacy. Failing to structure frequent sexual activity into your companionship may open you up for Satan's temptations. Please hear my heart: get counseling and do whatever God calls you to do to get sex back into your marriage! As I tell Christian couples, "A meaningful sex life in your marriage is one hill worth dying on. This is not optional in God's eyes."

Satan tempts and destroys many marriages by extreme inhibitions, extramarital affairs, and other sexual distortions. Often it is a subtle drifting apart and a lack of warm, connecting companionship. God has given spouses something precious in the ability as husband and wife to share a physical intimacy that cannot be matched in any other relationship. There is no replacement for what God intended sex to be for intimate marriages. It is the framework for expressing many powerful and exciting emotions, like joy, love, trust, and playfulness. Making love also helps dissipate and defuse negative emotions and behaviors, such as hostility, nit-picking, and defensive distancing. Spouses who frequently play together sexually stay together in warm, bonded ways and keep at bay many of the dragons that can haunt intimate companionship.

GODLY SUBMISSION AND SELFISHNESS

Christians need to be able to practice both submission and a righteous selfishness. Sometimes I call it "selfness" because being selfish appears to be in direct conflict with the traditional Christian teachings of putting others first. We as Christians are indeed encouraged to be submissive. That is, we are encouraged to place our partners' needs and feelings ahead of our own. And submission is a significant part of a great sex life. Through submission, we honor our mates and nurture them unselfishly in ways they truly enjoy. We give as gifts sexual expressions they desire that are not as important to us.

But fulfilling sex also requires being selfish. If we are always other-focused and if we always repress or ignore our own needs, we forfeit complete sexual fulfillment. Intimate lovemaking is a partnership with both selfishness and unselfishness. Great lovers know their own bodies and enjoy their sexual feelings.

The Bible often develops two principles that seem conflicting but actually are two balancing parts of a paradoxical concept. Some examples are law/grace, masculinity/femininity, bear your own burdens/bear one another's burdens, and unselfishness/selfishness. When we emphasize only *one* half of these balanced concepts, their effectiveness is diminished. We must add to submissiveness and unselfishness the complementary principles of self-esteem and selfishness.

Selfishness doesn't seem to get equal time in practical Christian training. Self-awareness and the assumption of personal responsibility are crucial to building a fun sexuality. The Bible commands us to "love your neighbor as yourself" (Mark 12:31 NKJV), and it states that "husbands ought to love their own wives as their own bodies" (Eph. 5:28 NKJV). These teachings are based on the idea of a healthy self-concept.

As Christians, we are accountable to God for creating a good sexual self-image and accepting ourselves without comparing ourselves to others. We are answerable individually to build a vibrant self-awareness and to learn to love and appreciate our bodies' potential for sensuality. As individuals, we are responsible for developing our own sexuality and celebrating love. We need to understand our own sexual needs and assertively fulfill them. God encourages personal responsibility for our lives, our bodies, and our sexuality.

Orgasms are an excellent example of healthy sexual selfishness. Your mate does not experience your orgasm. You focus on your sexual feelings and allow them to build to a climax. This is an intensely personal pleasure within *your* mind and body, and you selfishly let your mind enjoy the intensity of your excitement.

As so often happens in God's complementary principles, selfishness and unselfishness balance each other and create a more complete wholeness. You selfishly enjoy your orgasm but unselfishly allow your mate to observe how much pleasure your mate brings to you. Your partner is aroused by your personal excitement and intense experiencing of erotic release. This selfishness creates a mutual intimacy that is fun and bonding. Selfishness is indeed a great turn-on to you and your mate.

The question may be hovering in your mind: Isn't there a destructive, sinful way of misusing submission and selfishness? Any principle can be distorted and become destructive when not appropriately applied. Godly submission does not imply that you allow your mate to take advantage of you sexually while you passively build resentment. Putting the other's needs ahead of your own does not mean discounting your needs or ignoring them. Submission does not prevent a mate from being assertive and confronting behaviors or desires that are personally or relationally counterproductive, damaging, or unromantic.

The downside of selfishness is being egocentric and thinking the world revolves around your needs. This creates an unwillingness to empathize with another person's needs and lovingly satisfy them. Greed, insecurity, false pride, and laziness create a negative self-centeredness and play havoc with sexual intimacy. This destructive selfishness may be quite subtle and come under the guise of caretaking so you don't have to face dealing with your needs, or you may allow your mate to nurture you ("No, let me stroke you; don't worry about me"). Or you may be a martyr and manipulate with guilt ("I've got a headache—but if you need to"). Or you may be fragile or supersensitive ("I don't think I can ever be as sexy as you need," or "I know it's been ten days, but you really hurt my feelings").

Here are two suggestions for minimizing destructive selfishness and submission:

1. Keep a godly balance of healthy selfishness and unselfishness as you practice both. You must ask for your needs to be met and relish your sexual pleasure. You must submit your needs and give as loving gifts the things that your spouse needs. Opposites need to be balanced out, and you can make a mental note when the ledger is starting to get uneven. Be evenly selfish and submissive.

2. Work on your personal spiritual growth as you humbly become Christlike. God's Spirit can help you become mature with playfulness, love, honesty, gentleness, and positive assertiveness. He can grant you a positive, sexy self-image (see Chapter 16) with fun sensuality and a warm, nurturing spirit.

A SPIRITUAL AND EMOTIONAL UNION

Commenting on the beauty and depth of marital companionship, Paul wrote, "'For this reason a man will leave his father and mother and be united to his wife, and the two will become one flesh.' This is a profound mystery—but I am talking about Christ and the church" (Eph. 5:31–32 NIV). Making love and creating a one-flesh partnership is a profound, mysterious, and dynamic process.

As we launch into our exploration of sexuality, we must remember that we lose something if we treat making love as simply physical excitement, intercourse, and techniques. Making love offers insight into Christ's relationship and *modus operandi* with His beloved followers, the church. It includes joy, excitement, trust, commitment, unselfish nurturing, self-esteem, and a mutually fulfilling, playful companionship. It is truly intimate, and we will never completely understand this mystery.

The apostle Paul dealt more with the fuller meaning of sexual interaction and intercourse in the sixth chapter of 1 Corinthians, as he talked about the temple prostitutes in the pagan worship of Aphrodite. Some of the Corinthian Christians were getting sexual excitement and release by visiting the temple prostitutes. He wrote, "Foods for the stomach and the stomach for foods . . . The body is not for sexual immorality but for the Lord . . . Do you not know that he who is joined to a harlot is one body with her? For 'the two,' He says, 'shall become one flesh' . . . Do you not know that your body is the temple of the Holy Spirit?" (1 Cor. 6:13, 16, 19 NKJV). Paul emphasized that sexual union has an emotional and a spiritual dimension to it; it is not like eating a meal or casually satisfying a bodily desire. Sexuality is truly three-dimensional, involving body, soul, and spirit (see Chapter 28 on sexual integrity and remaining three-dimensional).

Making love needs to be based on an intimate marital partnership. Without the playful, loving companionship, sex becomes another buzz or rush that loses its perspective and has increasingly diminishing returns. Going on a roller coaster or eating a big steak is fun, but we wouldn't want to do that two or three times a week for the rest of our lives. A one-flesh marriage—that is, the *spiritual and emotional* merger of wife and husband—allows sex to be ever new and exciting. Sex is a means to an end and never an end in itself. Making love unites and excites, but the relationship gives the context and meaning. Without the intimate relationship, we find that sex becomes an activity (like eating steak or shooting white-water rapids) that rapidly loses its dynamic appeal.

Making love in a special and meaningful way is modeled after Christ's relationship with the church. We need to understand Christ's deep commitment, gentleness and humility, and His ability to lead and serve and to speak the truth with love. He demonstrated the basis for true spiritual and emotional union.

A WELL OF WATER

My favorite scriptural passage as a sex therapist is Proverbs 5:15–19:

> Drink water from your own cistern,
>   running water from your own well.
> Should your springs overflow in the streets,
>   your streams of water in the public squares?
> Let them be yours alone,
>   never to be shared with strangers.
> May your fountain be blessed,
>   and may you rejoice in the wife of your youth.
> A loving doe, a graceful deer—
>   may her breasts satisfy you always,
>   may you ever be captivated by her love. (NIV)

We could paraphrase this for wives:

> Rejoice in the husband of your youth.
> A gentle stag, a strong deer—
>   may his hands and mouth satisfy you always,
>   may you ever be captivated by his love.

The Bible often uses water as a very powerful and fitting metaphor for cleansing, healing, and rejuvenating. There are beautiful images like "streams in the desert," "water of life," and "beside the still waters." What a tremendous portrayal of the dynamic nature of lovemaking: to compare it to a cistern, a well, a stream, and a fountain. It is like a cool, refreshing drink from your own safe supply.

In one way, your marital sex life is like a cistern in which you have stored many amorous, erotic memories and a sexy repertoire of arousing activities. You can dip into it again and again in your fantasy life and lovemaking for excitement and fun. In another way, making love is like a stream or spring of water. Sex in marriage has an ever-changing, renewing quality to it. Just as the ancient Greek philosopher Heracleitus gazed into the river and realized life was a dynamic process that never stayed the same, so you can anticipate infinite variety and newness in making love.

A routine sex life is not God's design. Read this book, renew your minds and attitudes, and get sexy and playful. You can make love four times a week for the next fifty years and still never plumb the surprising depths of this mysterious sexual "stream" of becoming one flesh.

I appreciate the words *rejoice*, *satisfy*, and *captivated* in the Proverbs passage. Pleasure and fun are an intended part of making love. Our creativity, imagination, and love allow us to rejoice and remain ever enthralled sexually with the lover of our youth, continually satisfied and captivated for a lifetime.

I really appreciate this saying from the Talmud, the Jewish teachings on the first five books of the Bible: "God will hold us accountable for every permitted pleasure that we forfeit." We as Christian couples and individuals may need to adjust our attitudes on rejoicing, being satisfied and enthralled, and enjoying sexual pleasure. You can experience tremendous joy, excitement, and fulfillment if you allow God to bless your lovemaking and you follow His design of being a fresh spring of water to your partner.

AN EROTIC CELEBRATION

In my earlier years, before I had listened to so much sexual tragedy, I used to think the Christian emphasis on sex as a spiritual and emotional union was a cop-out. I was tired of hearing about the importance of having a committed relationship and building good fences. I wanted more solid information and explicit discussion about sexual arousal and behaviors. I often thought that we spiritualized sex because we were afraid to talk about bodies, positions of intercourse, erotic fantasies, and the excitement of making love. We were afraid to face the concepts of pleasure and sexual techniques and erotic arousal.

As a sex therapist, I now realize how many problems are created by spiritual and soul deficits (for example, lack of honesty, a poor body image, or an inability to play or experience pleasure). I now understand better the need for relational skills, deeper commitment, and emotional bonding. Yet I still think the church has been reluctant to talk openly and honestly about sex, especially the erotic pleasure of it.

Sex is an erotic celebration! Not the shallow Hollywood recreational concept of eroticism with no depth or values. *Eros*, the Greek work for sexual love, includes the idea of fusion, passion, attraction, and bonding. Erotic love is getting lost in someone's eyes. Erotic love is mental imagery, anticipation, playfulness, ambiance, and lovers physically enjoying each other. The Song of Solomon contains many beautiful images of erotic love:

> Let him kiss me with the kisses of his mouth—
> For your love is better than wine. (1:2 NKJV)

> My lover is mine and I am his;
>   he browses among the lilies. (2:16 NIV)

> Your two breasts are like two fawns . . .
> Your plants are an orchard of pomegranates
>   with choice fruits . . .
> You are a garden fountain,
>   a well of flowing water . . .
> Let my lover come into his garden
>   and taste its choice fruits. (4:5, 13, 15–16 NIV)

> But my own vineyard is mine to give . . .
> Thus I have become . . . like one bringing contentment. (8:12, 10 NIV)

These passages so beautifully and poetically describe with erotic passion the fusion of body, emotion, fantasy, and soul. Sex is the curious and excited exploration of each other's erogenous zones to create pleasure. We as lovers are to entrust our private parts to our mates, for indeed "my own vineyard is mine to give," and we should learn to have no shame or inhibitions with the genital area. We can create stimulating atmospheres and frolic in each other's garden, sharing choice fruit, and drinking until contented from the flowing water of our sexual relationship.

Bring God's Love and Values into Your Marriage and Lovemaking

There have been many different interpretations about what is permissible for a Christian as you " browse among the lilies" and "taste the choice fruits" of your sexual garden. An example of this would be the different views about oral sex. Though the Song of Solomon seems to imply oral sex, the Christian community has often been skeptical of this behavior, sometimes for unworthy reasons, like thinking that the genital area is "dirty" or "too private" or thinking that Christians should be cautious about overindulging in playful sexual pleasure that doesn't lead to procreation.

When the Bible does not directly deal with a behavior like oral sex or masturbation, we turn to other scriptural values to help govern our sexual behaviors. Whether oral sex, using a vibrator, or trying new positions, we are called to be lovingly considerate and wise; never should we do anything that violates our mate's sensibilities or offends our mate sexually. Our bodies are God's temple and should be treated respectfully and not damaged. We are told to be self-disciplined and balanced, with oral sex or any erotic stimulation never becoming the focus of our whole lovemaking and intimate connecting. Making love is a celebration of our one-flesh companionship and should never be associated simply with orgasm, intercourse, or genital pleasuring.

With biblically neutral behaviors, such as oral sex, Christians will disagree about whether they are productive or counterproductive to married lovemaking. It is proper here for some to participate and some to abstain. God promises in Philippians 3:15–16 that if we act on the truth we do understand, He will help each of us mature and come to an understanding of His will and way. A purpose of this book is to encourage each of us to think carefully and bring our sexuality and lovemaking into accord with God's truth and sexual economy (*eco* meaning "a system," and *nomos* meaning "regulating guidelines"). This book is humble, based on God's truth. Together we as Christians need to carefully reclaim from distorted worldly values God's precious gift of sexuality. Let's create a practical and accurate sexual theology and practice.

Making love is intimate connecting and a breaking down of walls so that "my lover is mine and I am his [hers]." You are willingly naked and vulnerable. Lovers are able to experience freedom and abandonment together, based on love, trust, and commitment. It is a unique companionship and so exciting to be naked and not ashamed. The next chapter will develop further the importance of this loving partnership, and the need to be a mature lover.

CHAPTER TWO

The World's Greatest Lover

EVERYONE WANTS SOME POWERFUL TECHNIQUE to make them stand out as a lover. Unfortunately, or actually fortunately, fantastic lovemaking is based upon who you are as a person, not what you do. Attitudes and character are what count. True sexiness and an awesome sex life depend primarily on being a mature, sexy person.

So you want to be the world's greatest lover? Build into your mind and heart the following character traits possessed by all great lovers: playfulness, love, knowledge, honesty, forgiveness, creative romance, and discipline. These characteristics, gleaned from the Bible, will lead to great sex. Their effective use will show you how to truly arouse your mate's desire. Success is practically guaranteed, but it will take some real effort to incorporate them into your heart and life.

PLAYFULNESS

We as adults so easily forget the art of playfulness. It is the ability to let go of control and to frolic and be silly. It's the feeling that you deserve to have fun and being able to anticipate it. Then you have to learn to truly go along with the fun once you've created it. Remember that our Creator plays and knows we need this important skill to enjoy Him and participate fully in intimacy: "I was filled with delight day after day, rejoicing [*playing* and *laughing*] always in his presence, rejoicing [*playing*] in his whole world and delighting in mankind" (Prov. 8:30–31 NIV).

Making love is certainly built on the foundation of play. I am reminded of Christ's teaching that to truly experience the kingdom of God, we need to become like little children. Great sex takes place in the child state of the ego. An important part of being childlike is reveling in the awe of the moment and exhibiting uninhibited excitement or curiosity. Children love to ask about the nature of things, and they like to try them out in a playful manner. They are great teachers of amusement, as I learn every time my granddaughter and I spend time together. She squeals and claps her hands and is awed by something as simple as a flower.

I've taken the liberty of paraphrasing Christ's advice: "Unless you become childlike and learn to be playful, you will never experience God's kingdom of unbelievable intimacy." Learn from children's playfulness. They can be self-directed and demand pleasure. In their childlike mentality, life is a big playground, and they expect to have fun. Oh, how children love to sing at the top of their voices and big grins come so easily! Children can be excited a whole day about an anticipated ice-cream cone. Adults, however, sometimes have to be on vacation for two days before getting relaxed and starting to have fun. Playfulness is perhaps best described by the terms *joyful excitement, eager curiosity, lighthearted fun,* and *spontaneous frolicking.* Playfulness is the ability to be unpretentious and candid as you demand things with enthusiasm and laughter—expecting your needs to be met.

You cannot *work* at creating better lovemaking; you and your mate have to *play* at it. This character trait can be practiced in other areas of your life and then lessons learned may be brought over into your sex life. Get silly; anticipate an event for a week or more; risk a new behavior; laugh until you have tears in your eyes or roll on the floor; tickle and chase each other around the whole house; get wide-eyed with awe and wonder about something. In this, you are becoming a great lover.

Playing has a way of connecting people. Gentle teasing, shared games, and mutual laughter can be bonding experiences. Even sexual mistakes can create playful memories. So often in making love, partners do things that are silly or embarrassing. As playful partners, you can laugh rather than be awkward. You each have this childlike playfulness that is longing to be unleashed.

Time Out: Take time when you are out this week to stop and buy yourself a toy or two that would encourage you to play. You may want some that you and your mate can enjoy together, such as water pistols, jump ropes, rub-on tattoos, or Tinkertoy building blocks.

LOVE

The Bible says you are to love your neighbor or your mate just as you love yourself. Fun sex depends on husbands and wives who have learned to love themselves. This means that you take care of your health and exercise your body to keep it in shape. You should also enjoy and accept the body God gave you. Self-acceptance, self-esteem, and a good body image are healthy parts of sexiness and Christian self-love (see Chapter 16). Think of how difficult it is to sexually focus on your mate when you are embarrassed, inhibited, or self-conscious.

Wives, our society really does a number on women in what is accepted as sexually appealing.

I remember my female colleague who stated she was so frustrated that women's breasts seemed to come in only two sizes: too big or too small. "Sexy" in a God-given sense is a state of mind and not the shape of our bodies or our weight. If you learn to accept your body and revel in your sexual feelings, your husband will follow suit and be tremendously turned on by you.

Psychological research has shown us that the people and things we are more familiar with, we tend to like more. People who live in the same apartment complex or go to church together seem to grow to like one another just by being in proximity with one another and sharing common things. As you get more comfortable with seeing your body nude and allowing it to be in your thoughts without negative criticism, you will start to like it more.

Time Out: Stand nude in front of a full-length mirror. Now observe yourself and resist making any judgments. After observing a few minutes, start with your hair and proceed down to your feet, accepting and describing every one of your body parts with no negative judgments, such as: "This is my hair, and it is brown with a cowlick."

Sometimes when you are in front of the mirror, you may want to dispute some of the negative messages going around in your head. Start by looking at a part of your body that you appreciate, and truly affirm that part: "My eyes are big and brown and quite striking." Now observe more closely parts you don't like and verbally make yourself accept them and say something affirming about them: "God gave me these thighs, and they are strong and support me in many things I enjoy doing." "My shoulders have changed at age forty-eight, but I still hit the softball well."

An important part of love is respecting and unconditionally accepting your mate. If you want to find and focus on flaws, you will put a damper on your partner's sexiness and the whole lovemaking process. Allowing your mind to become preoccupied with the size of body parts or sags is very destructive. You reap the benefit (or destructiveness if you stay obsessive) of nurturing and helping your lover revel in sexual appeal. Every time you affirm some particular aspect of masculinity or femininity that you admire and enjoy, you lovingly increase your mate's sex appeal.

It is such a growth-producing process when you are unconditionally committed to accepting your own sexiness and affirming the sexiness of your partner. It creates the environment for a comfortable, safe, sexual-greenhouse, where playfulness and risk-taking blossom. Unconditional love and acceptance and affirmation set the temperature for some fantastic sex.

I like the word *lover* to describe your sexual partner. This is an important part of God's boundary and provision for great sex—one who loves within the commitment of an intimate marriage. Love creates trust so you can try new behaviors and risk appearing silly. Love produces warm excitement and fun companionship. Love helps you to remember and desire to meet your mate's needs. Learn to be a lover! The best sex is long-term, and love is the oil that keeps this type of lovemaking running smoothly.

Love is also gentle, kind, and forgiving as mates nurture each other. Mature love doesn't pout or harbor grudges and is able to reach out beyond your own needs—all vital for great sex. A great love life depends on allowing your mate to apologize and change. We will all do dumb things that can damage our lovemaking, and we need to be able to let go and move on. Mature love incorporates loving gestures that are nonsexual as well as sexual. Wives especially value hugs and caresses outside the bedroom, which build a loving ambiance and lay the groundwork for fun romance.

Practicing loving behaviors (unconditional acceptance, gentleness, forgiveness, meeting your mate's needs) produces strong, warm feelings of being in love. As you learn to love, your sexiness will increase.

KNOWLEDGE

There are two parts of being a wise and knowledgeable lover. First, become a student of your mate and yourself. The apostle Peter tells husbands: "Be considerate as you live with your wives" (1 Peter 3:7 NIV). An integral aspect of true consideration is constantly trying to know and understand your partner better. They often know what makes them smile or turns them on; do you?

In the language of the King James Version of the Bible, the word *know* is used to describe intercourse. For example, Isaac knew his wife, Rebekah, and they conceived a son. I used to think this wording was due to the reluctance of those times to deal with sex openly. Now, I like this word *know* in our era of casual sexual encounters. Lovemaking should be "knowing" what your mate enjoys and needs. This knowledge takes time, curiosity, a good memory, and the willingness to be a student.

Time Out: Take a moment to do a quick personal inventory. Which areas of your sex life can benefit from greater knowledge? Which do you hope to improve by reading this book? How are you going to implement change?

Study your mate's responses to know what is most enjoyable. No book can give you that information. Women, even more than men, vary about what feels good—even the strokes and rhythms that are most pleasurable. Be a lifelong student of your partner's body and reactions.

Acquire a reservoir of knowledge of what excites your partner physically and mentally. Set the romantic ambiance, practice the right moves, and reap the exciting benefits of being a wise lover.

Another aspect of being an informed and sexy lover is knowing your own body and sexual responses. You are the teacher of your mate. Do you know what turns you on and increases your desire? It will be difficult teaching your erotic needs to your partner if you are not aware of them. Tune in to your sexuality, and keep expanding your repertoire of sensual delights. A healthy, selfish focusing on your sexual feelings not only allows you to get excited but also turns your mate on. Knowledge of yourself and your mate is crucial to great sex.

The second part of being a knowledgeable lover is your technical knowledge of sexuality. Sexual technique is not the be-all and end-all of a great sexual relationship, but *its importance cannot be underestimated.* Wives often tell me they wish their husbands knew how to "take them." They aren't talking about selfish using, but a wise leader that is confident sexually and can assertively take the lead in producing pleasure.

Many chapters of this book are about technique. The couple with their act together sexually knows how to create ambiance and be uninhibitedly sensual and playful. They understand various positions of intercourse, and they have built a comfortable, exciting repertoire of sexual moves. The wife understands how to "ring her husband's chimes." The husband knows how to orchestrate his wife's responses to produce exciting, sexual music together. Each is wise and skillful, sexually speaking.

SEXINESS = A KNOWLEDGEABLE, TOGETHER PERSON + A GREAT RELATIONSHIP!

HONESTY

In making love, dishonesty destroys trust, allows boredom, and creates confusion and hostility. It may take the form of the dishonest husband who lacks skills but can't admit to himself he is a nonromantic sexual illiterate. He may think, *She says sex isn't very fun, but she reaches a climax most of the time.* A wife may play manipulative sexual games. Instead of confronting issues, she angrily (in passive aggressive fashion) vows to herself, "If he forgets our anniversary again, he won't get any sex for six months." Both may also be unaware of their sexual needs and feelings—a more subtle form of dishonesty. It is not easy to be self-aware and truly transparent with our needs and feelings. It takes a real maturity to achieve this level of "naked and unashamed."

Many couples find it uncomfortable to initiate sexual conversations and openly discuss individual needs and desires. The wife may be upset because her husband gets defensive or pouts if she openly refuses sex or makes a small suggestion. The husband may be angry because his wife turns him down after he enacts the romantic rituals like taking a quick shower or rubbing her back. These are great times for clearing the air, honest discussion, and confrontation to openly express feelings and needs (see Chapter 8).

Time Out: Do you have any dishonest sexual games you need to eliminate from your sex life? Do you sulk or pout rather than talk through your needs? Have you asked your mate what he or she needs? Do you avoid becoming passionate because you are afraid to let go of control, but you rationalize it by saying your partner is too pushy? Do you fear confrontation and settle for mediocrity? Do you fake orgasms? Do you neglect to share your feelings? When your needs are satisfied, do you know this and feel fulfilled?

God's guidelines are very explicit for relationships. He tells us to speak "the truth in love" and put away lying (Eph. 4:15, 25 NKJV). But even in love, the truth is sometimes tough to take, and even little sexual communications during lovemaking—"That doesn't feel good tonight," or "Please rub harder"—are occasionally difficult to express and can create defensiveness. Great sex is based on mature lovers who can be honest with themselves and their mates. They are self-aware and can assertively communicate.

Before leaving the character trait of honesty, let's acknowledge the ultimate dishonest kiss of death to a great sex life: the extramarital affair. Nothing can sabotage trust and the special quality of a love life more thoroughly than adultery. Sneaking, keeping secrets, broken promises, and divided loyalties rob a couple of sexual celebration in their marriage. An affair is a powerful negative illustration of the importance of honesty for sexual love to flourish.

FORGIVENESS

It is a messy and broken world that we live in. Each of us is only human and capable of so many hurtful, immature behaviors. The psalmist describes our loving Father and His gently forgiving way as He compassionately operates in a fallen world, "The LORD is compassionate and gracious, slow to anger, abounding in love . . . He does not treat us as our sins deserve or repay us according to our iniquities . . . for he knows how we are formed, he remembers that we are dust [human]" (Ps. 103:8, 10, 14 NIV).

We are fallible and must cut each other slack, because we know even the people most committed to our well-being will let us down. "Bearing with one another, and forgiving" (Col. 3:13 NKJV), God calls us to follow His example as we build intimate relationships in this sinful, imperfect world: "And be kind to one another, tenderhearted, forgiving one another, even as God in Christ forgave you" (Eph. 4:32 NKJV).

The depth of the marital and sexual relationship over a lifetime brings out feelings and hurts that the individuals did not know could be experienced. Our mate can feel like the enemy many times, and forgiveness becomes huge in maintaining passionate intimacy. Being gracious and letting go of hurts is not an easy discipline.

Time Out: What do you need to forgive and let go of to increase the passion of your sex life? What do you need to forgive yourself for so that you can grow into a better lover?

A genuine part of maturity is learning to live with all the ambiguity of human error and disappointed expectations. It is not by accident that Scripture encourages people to lovingly give each other the benefit of the doubt and learn to live the gentle life: "Therefore as God's chosen people, holy and dearly loved, clothe yourselves with compassion, kindness, humility, gentleness and patience. *Bear with each other and forgive*" (Col. 3:12–13 NIV, emphasis added).

So many love lives are compromised and sabotaged by a lack of forgiveness. Sexual lovemaking is fraught with potential messes and hurt feelings. Bear with each other, cut slack, let go of hurt and resentment. Life is never perfect, but it is amazing how our positive and mature approach to it can make a difference. Mates won't always climax at the right times and places, or have matching desires and never hurt each other's feelings. It's about living forgiveness.

CREATIVE ROMANCE

Sexy lovers take the time to develop the sensual, romantic part of their minds and personalities. Every person has an exciting romantic side, but few take the time and energy to unleash their passionate capacities. Mates can be surprised at how talented and creative they are in planning sexy surprises for each other—yes, even husbands, who can be more "romantically challenged." They easily come up with exciting, unique ideas as they focus on the importance of sensuality and setting a mood—anticipation builds, and fresh attitudes pervade the whole sexual scene.

Time Out: How would you define *romantic?* Creating moods, being sexy, mysterious, spontaneous, passionate, sentimental? Many wives and husbands wish their spouses would be more romantic. Make a brief list of behaviors that you consider romantic and do one or two this week.

Couples always enjoy letting their romantic side out. This may include surprise gifts, foot and leg massages, verbal demonstrativeness, mutual showers, or dinners with candlelight and soft glances. Of course, romantic lovemaking doesn't always involve completely new techniques and experiences. There are certain positions, ways of caressing, places, rhythms, restaurants, moods, and vocabulary that remain enjoyable favorites.

Being creatively romantic is such an important quality to incorporate. Why then do you think it is so easy to fall into ruts and forget to employ this character trait for a great sex life? Here are a few barriers to healthy romance, and possible ways to break them down:

1. *Problem:* too busy; a modern plague demonstrated by an inability to say no and scale down as priorities are constantly violated

Solution: create date nights and time together

2. *Problem:* no plan

Solution: mobilize willpower and create goals while structuring a varied, exciting sex life; plan optimal times for dates and intimacy

3. *Problem:* inhibitions and ignorance; a lack of time and energy invested in changing attitudes and increasing sexual knowledge

Solution: read, go to workshops, talk, and attempt new behaviors; get some sex therapy

4. *Problem:* tension, conflict in the relationship with unresolved traumas, hurt, and anger

Solution: learn to communicate and resolve conflict; get counseling

5. *Problem:* demands of child rearing on time and energy

Solution: structure and set careful boundaries; create a baby-sitting network (see Chapter 19)

6. *Problem:* procrastination

Solution: start making love at 9:30 P.M.; enjoy quickies once in a while; turn off the television; ignore fatigue, and just do it

Time Out: They are making a movie of your sex life. What would its title be? What type of movie? What about its length? Do this exercise twice: (1) the way your love life is presently, and (2) the way you would like it to be.

You want to be a great, sexy lover? Become a creative romantic. You as an individual and couple breathe life and excitement into the material of this book with your imagination and relationship and character traits. Sexiness comes from your imaginative creativity and romantic inspirations that can be God-given—but they require the discipline (and time and energy) to carry them out.

DISCIPLINE

Discipline may seem an odd character trait to include for a lover, and may appear to be the opposite of spontaneity, playfulness, and creativity. The truth of the matter is that an undisciplined lifestyle will end up with very infrequent sex. Discipline doesn't have to destroy the fun and spontaneity of sex or put pressure on you. The truth is that if you don't plan sex into your schedules and take advantage of optimal times, you will never make love with any frequency! The ambiance, activity, place, timing, and technique are up to your romantic creativity. Just keep a time sacredly reserved for sex.

Time Out: Put your heads together and plan when and how often you are going to make love each week as you allow time for spontaneous sex into your intimate companionship.

One of my supervisors in my sex therapy training, Dr. Domeena Renshaw, said she was always amazed by couples. Both would heartily agree that the activity of lovemaking was fun, relaxing, and important to them. Then they placed it around number twenty-five on their list of priorities and wrote it in pencil so they could move it lower if something else came up.

There are few couples whose sex life has not been seriously sabotaged by lack of discipline and priority. They may start making love at 11:00 P.M., when one or both have already turned into pumpkins—physically and emotionally spent. They may try to get all the chores done first or not plan carefully enough around the children's needs. They may make love only when the mood and circumstances are perfect—averaging about once every two months.

A few disciplined adjustments create more sexiness: go to bed at the same time, teach the children to respect a locked door, and agree to schedule lovemaking so many times a week regardless of distractions or fatigue as you find those optimal times. Let's face it, if you have to schedule for church and grocery shopping, lovemaking may need to be scheduled in also.

A fundamental aspect of discipline in relation to a quality sex life is developing in a healthy, godly way the emotions of shame and guilt. These emotions play a crucial part in keeping your sex life pleasurable. Paul, when he wrote to the Corinthians, did not try to distinguish between guilt and shame but called those emotions "godly sorrow." He explained the importance of godly sorrow in the Christian's life as a motivational feeling to protect and mold a productive life: "Godly sorrow brings repentance that leads to salvation and leaves no regret . . . See what this godly sorrow has produced in you: what earnestness, what eagerness to clear yourselves, what indignation, what alarm, what longing, what concern, what readiness to see justice done" (2 Cor. 7:10–11 NIV). God does not want you to feel shame for having sexual feelings. But there should be healthy shame and guilt in your sex life throughout your marriage.

Godly sorrow might come because you neglect lovemaking as a wonderful avenue for bonding or are complacent in not incorporating variety and new skills. You may feel guilty for choices that hurt your intimacy. You may feel true, godly sorrow because you avoid love-making and your mate is withering away because of it. As long as shame and guilt drive you to seek out God's best, your love life will thrive, and you will maintain healthy discipline.

You have the promise of being a great lover. Incorporate the character traits of being loving, honest, playful, forgiving, knowledgeable, and disciplined. Build real commitment. Tune in to God's emotional signals of shame and guilt and make necessary changes. As you become more disciplined, you actually will become more spontaneous and will have a more intimate, comfortable, sexual fulfillment.

In a world of new techniques, bigger-is-better beliefs, and instant answers, it is difficult but truly rewarding to take the time and energy to improve yourself and your relationship. May you have wisdom and courage as you appreciate and conform to God's guidelines for great lovemaking.

An Intimate Marriage + A Mature Lover = A Fulfilling Sex Life!

CHAPTER THREE

Your Erogenous Zones

WHAT AN EROTIC CONCEPT, erogenous zones. They are parts of the body that have a concentration of sensory nerve endings, which can be stimulated to cause sexual arousal. But discovering and enjoying these spots is not always that simple. Let's consider Jim and Susan, who enjoy making love but need some education. Sometimes both are a little lazy in searching out new areas of arousal or in letting the other know what feels particularly good. Neither is completely comfortable letting the other explore the genital area intimately.

Jim wishes Susan would be more active in pleasuring all of his erogenous zones. He appreciates her enjoyment of his penis and its key role in arousing him, but he wishes she would also caress other parts of his body sometimes. He enjoys giving her pleasure and it is very stimulating to him, but recently, he has felt a little neglected. He isn't sure exactly what he needs, but his worry and dissatisfaction are starting to get in the way. He doesn't want to lose the tremendous enjoyment they experience in making love.

Susan gets upset because she wishes Jim would give her greater variety in caressing and loveplay. He seldom focuses on her stomach or face, and they are very special areas for her. She has told him a couple of times, but he seems to forget. If anyone were making a list of the attributes for a great lover, she would want it to include an excellent memory. It isn't enough for her to tell him; he has to remember what she likes when they make love.

If you asked Jim and Susan, they would say they have a good sex life overall. They do. They are great companions and have fun playing together as friends and lovers. Their bed is a fun sexual playground, and they try to take the time to create a romantic atmosphere. Overall, both like their bodies and trust that the other will enjoy what is seen and touched. They may never need sex therapy for a specific problem, but they could profit tremendously from education about sexual reflexes and erogenous zones.

SEXUAL REFLEXES

Your body's mechanisms for sexual arousal demonstrate a beautifully complex relationship among hormones, nerves, blood vessels, and muscles. Yet all you have to do is simply relax and tune in to your God-given erogenous zones and responses. The sexual parts of your mind and body may be repressed or lying dormant, but they are there. Making love and stimulating erogenous zones is the essence of simplicity, but it is important to first understand your sexual reflexes and how arousal occurs. This is the foundation for enjoying erogenous zones. Many couples short-circuit their lovemaking by sometimes worrying too much about sexual arousal and not enjoying their reflexive sexual reactions enough.

Hormones and the Autonomic Nervous System

Why do we experience a sexual touch and begin to get an erection or vaginal lubrication? God has designed our bodies so that our hormones, nerve endings, and minds can create sexual arousal. It is a cooperative process of hormones and the nervous system. The hormones activate the process in our bodies and bloodstreams, and then our nerves relay sexual information from our senses to our brains and back to our genitals to create physical arousal. Without getting too technical, the autonomic, or involuntary, nervous system is involved in the sexual arousal cycle. I was referring to it when I said that both Jim and Susan in the opening example were worrying too much and getting upset and, in the process, sabotaging their natural, reflexive sexual responses. They needed to get out of the way of God's automatic arousal patterns and enjoy their bodies and erogenous zones more.

The autonomic nervous system has two branches, one called the sympathetic nervous system (SNS) and the other called the parasympathetic nervous system (PNS). The PNS and the SNS operate in opposite manners. The parasympathetic is operative when we are relaxed, and it has a creative, building effect on the body. The sympathetic springs into action when we are intensely aroused (to trigger orgasm) or when we are threatened (to shut down the PNS). Both arousal and orgasm are involuntary, reflexive actions. You simply have to relax and enjoy erogenous zones.

Sabotaging Arousal and Erogenous Zones

So Jim, and in some ways Susan too, were short-circuiting God's design of relaxing with their erogenous zones and allowing pleasurable sensations (PNS) to build. He was anxious about not getting enough attention from his wife. Anxiety, anger, boredom, and resentment trigger SNS reactions and are great saboteurs of having stimulating times making love. Jim was not going with his automatic parasympathetic system to allow arousal to mount. He was too worried about having his body caressed, while wondering whether they were having fun yet. Susan was not that much different because she built some resentment about the way he stimulated her clitoris. Both could experience some sabotaging results from blocking their PNS unless they begin to relax and enjoy.

This couple was blocking their enjoyment of erogenous zones with resentment and worry and lack of variety. Other people have never allowed their erogenous zones to be sensitized and create sexual arousal. They are inexperienced at tuning in to sexual feelings and identifying how sexual arousal happens. All of us have nerve endings that can produce sexual feelings, but they do have to be activated by allowing our hormones to create sexual arousal and our minds to interpret these sensations as sexual.

Because of a conservative Christian background, natural shyness, or discomfort with their bodies, some mates have never explored their physical sexual responses. The hormones and nervous system are obviously in place, so they enjoy some types of arousal. But the parasympathetic system needs to be turned loose, tuning in to sexual feelings without intense exertion.

Too many couples are guilty of sabotaging their erogenous zones and sexual enjoyment with ignorance, anxiety, and sheer effort. Intimate marital companions have usually never developed their sexual awareness to include even half of the erogenous zones on their bodies, and they often short-circuit their sexual reflexes. But the encouraging thing is that mates who have fallen into a rut still can break their patterns and make many fun sexual discoveries in their erogenous zones.

EROGENOUS ZONES

Sensuality and sensitivity to touch have to be developed and connected to your sexual lovemaking. Overall, our erogenous zones are more alike than different, whether we are male or female, experienced or inexperienced, overweight or underweight, active or inactive. But some individuals will experience more sensitivity and arousal from certain erogenous spots than from others. These may also change over time and, for women, after having children. In the last section of this chapter we will explore how some of this can be a product of sensual erotic conditioning. There can be individual differences, though, which is why you must continually be a student of your mate and learn every inch of the other's body—remembering what is arousing but not locking into boring patterns of stimulation.

The erogenous areas can be divided into three levels according to their sensitivity in producing sexual arousal. Level-three areas are less sexual in nature but capable of producing sensual arousal and sexual excitement. Level-two areas contain a greater concentration of the nerve endings and can be more sexual. Mucous membranes (for example, the mouth and surrounding tissue) and tissue in the areas around the genitals are very sensitive and sexually aroused. Level-one areas are the nipples and the genitals. These are the most sensitive areas and are capable of building greater sexual tension—with the most crucial organs for triggering the orgasmic response being the penis and the clitoris.

Level Three

This level includes the entire body, with its skin and nerve endings. You may be asking, "Why is the whole skin area considered erogenous? When I rub my arm, I don't get turned on." The skin is the most extensive area of sensuality. A whole chapter on sensual massage is included in this book for that very reason. If you want to become a sensual lover, learn to revel in and appreciate your whole body being caressed. Lie back, close your eyes, and discover the erogenous zone God has created with your skin.

You don't have to have special training or expensive equipment to enjoy a massage. The object is to pleasure your mate's skin by touching and caressing. The experience can be enhanced by warming some oil and letting the other rest comfortably on a towel or something that can be easily washed, as you sensuously stroke in smooth, continuous motions—moving from one area of the body to another. You can give so much enjoyment as you use your hands and fingers to create pleasure and intimate bonding.

Massage and caress your lover's arms, shoulders, outer ears and earlobes, scalp, upper chest, buttocks, and calves. They may not have the concentration of sensory nerve endings as other parts of the body, but they are still very sensual and can contribute to a delightfully sensual experience.

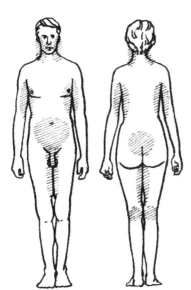

Fig. 3.1. Level two erogenous zones
[silhouette of front of male and back of female]

Level Two

This level includes parts of the body that are normally stimulated during foreplay. If you desire to be a great lover, become familiar with these areas of your partner's body. Have your mate take fingertips or mouth and tongue and explore the level-two erogenous zones. Communicate with each other and determine if you do or do not feel greater sensitivity in these areas than level-three parts of the body. If you can focus your mind on enjoying the sensual feelings, you will find your ticklishness is less. You can also ask your partner to apply firmer pressure.

Take time and do some prospecting in these sensual areas on your mate's body. Stimulate the sensory nerve endings as you experience the pleasurable feelings of (1) the back of the knees; (2) the inner thighs; (3) the armpits and breast area; (4) the abdomen area and the navel; (5) the small of the back and buttocks; (6) the neck from back to front; (7) the palms of the hands and bottoms of the feet; (8) the face, especially the (9) eyelids, (10) the edges of the nose over the sinus cavities, (11) the temples, and (12) the mouth and tongue. These areas are rich in sensory nerve endings. Allow these gentle touches and nuzzling to be a sensual treat and to become arousing sexually, too.

Sensate focus or sensual massage is an exercise developed by Masters and Johnson and other sex therapists as they helped couples overcome performance anxiety and become sensual lovers. As you play with your mate and focus on sensual feelings, you relax, and a sense of companionship emerges. You experience a connection and stimulate your sensory nerve endings for more fulfilling sexual arousal.

Time Out: Set aside at least a half hour. One partner will be the passive receiver and the other will be the active giver for fifteen minutes; then exchange roles. Both partners should be nude for this experience. If you are the active giver, touch and caress your mate in ways that bring pleasure to you. There is no right way to do this because you are touching for your own pleasure. If your mate does not like to be touched in certain areas, refrain out of love and respect. The passive partner will enjoy receiving pleasurable massage and pleasing you. The passive receiver is learning what touch feels best personally and what kind of active touch you like to give. This exercise focuses on level-three and level-two erogenous zones. There should be no touching of the genital area and nipples. Do not go on to making love during this session.

It is fun to incorporate sensate focus into your companionship as a relaxing, educational, and bonding exercise. You may want to be more active and coach with feedback as you help each other give the kind of touches that feel best to you. You can incorporate aspects of this sensual massage into your lovemaking, but it is important to be able to touch and not always have the activity progress into intercourse and orgasm. This is a great way to learn about level-two erogenous zones.

Level One

The most sensitive and sexually stimulating erogenous zones are the nipples and the genitals. The genitals most directly stimulate sexual arousal, and the third section of this chapter carefully explores this aspect of lovemaking. The nipples are a favorite spot of both men and women for stimulating sexual excitement. The nerve endings are especially sensitive and connected to sexual arousal. The nipples show sexual arousal by becoming erect, and the center portion (papilla) hardens.

Remember! Level-one erogenous zones should not be the immediate focus of loveplay. Tease and caress the areas around the nipples and genitals before turning attention to the nipples, penis, or clitoris. Both men and women will enjoy a quickie occasionally. They will want their mates to stimulate the genitals with the goal of achieving a rapid orgasm. This is fun and exciting but often fails to achieve the same level of arousal as taking time to tease and play.

Men especially need to learn to go from general arousal to specific locations. Be mysterious, surprising, and tantalizing. Great lovers practice the sexual process of amplifying tension by gradually increasing stimulation in a teasing and slow manner.

Men and women often differ in their preferences regarding the pace of stimulation and intensity. Generally, a man doesn't seem to mind immediate and direct, firm stimulation of the penis and even the nipples. This quick approach is often not to his wife's advantage if she wishes to prolong the lovemaking process. A woman seems to prefer a slower and more teasing approach with more firm and rapid stimulation when approaching climax. A woman also seems to need more varied stroking and techniques. She appreciates her husband's being an expert lover and having many alternatives to caressing and arousing her body and stimulating her erogenous zones.

THE GENITALS

Male and female genitals conform to the same general pattern but vary uniquely in shape, color, angles, and size. Variations have nothing to do with the ability to be a great lover and experience or give sexual pleasure. The following figures will help you develop an understanding of genital erogenous zones so you can better pleasure your mate.

The Male Genitals

The male genitals are more visible to the eye and familiar to the man because he has contact with his penis every time he urinates. Yet many men have never taken the time to truly examine the penis.

At birth the penis is uncircumcised, with the foreskin covering the glans, or head. The foreskin can be removed surgically for hygienic reasons. There is no truth to the myth that the uncircumcised penis is much more sensitive to touch.

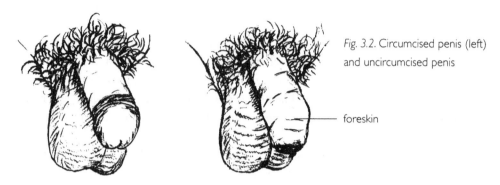

Fig. 3.2. Circumcised penis (left) and uncircumcised penis

foreskin

The penis. The penis is composed of three columns of spongy tissue with the urethra running through the bottom column (corpus spongiosum). These spongy tissues fill with blood in a type of "hydraulic system" that creates the erection. The whole penis is an intricate network of blood vessels and nerves, with the glans of the penis being especially sensitive. The skin of the penis is loosely attached to allow for easier stimulation. Penises can vary in the angle of erection, shape of the head, length, and color. This has nothing to do with the ability to give and receive pleasure. The myth of the importance of penis size in making love must forever be put to rest. When flaccid, the size of the penis will vary greatly; when erect, the size for most men falls into the range of six inches, plus or minus an inch or so. The outer third of the vagina is the most sensitive, and it would take a penis only three inches or less in length to create great pleasure. Men, quit being obsessed with penis size—it is not on the list of needed qualities for being a great lover.

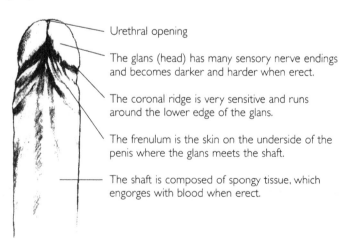

Urethral opening

The glans (head) has many sensory nerve endings and becomes darker and harder when erect.

The coronal ridge is very sensitive and runs around the lower edge of the glans.

The frenulum is the skin on the underside of the penis where the glans meets the shaft.

The shaft is composed of spongy tissue, which engorges with blood when erect.

Fig. 3.3. The penis

The scrotum and testes. The scrotum is a sac of skin enclosing the testes. Under the skin is a muscle that can contract in response to cold or during sexual arousal, causing the scrotum to hang lower or get tighter to the body. The scrotum and the base of the penis contain hair follicles and sebaceous glands that can become ingrown and infected, much like pimples. Sometimes a varicocele occurs in the scrotum. It is a bundle of dilated veins of the spermatic cord, much like varicose veins. This condition can be painful and may require minor surgery to repair.

The testicles will hang with one lower than the other. The testes are outside the body and contract toward the body with cold because they produce sperm and hormones, and the sperm need to develop in a constant temperature that is several degrees lower than body temperature.

The epididymis is a coil of small tubes attached to a testis. The coil can sometimes get infected (epididymitis) and needs to be medically treated. The epididymis ends in the vas deferens, which is the tube that conducts sperm to the seminal vesicles and the ejaculatory duct. During a vasectomy, the vas is cut and tied off to prevent sperm from reaching the semen.

The seminal vesicles, bladder, prostate, and urethra. As you trace the vas deferens, it becomes a complex valve system with the seminal vesicles, the bladder, and the urethra, which passes through the prostate. The vas deferens brings sperm to the seminal vesicles and narrows to form the ejaculatory duct. This duct runs through and joins the urethra in the prostate. The prostate is about the size of a chestnut and produces fluid that forms part of the semen. The prostate can become infected (prostatitis) or cancerous, which necessitates medical treatment. Cancer may require a prostatectomy, which can create retrograde ejaculation: the ejaculate goes back into the bladder rather than out through the urethra and penis. (This condition does not have to affect sexual pleasure.) In an orgasm the muscles around the prostate and ejaculatory duct and the base of the penis contract, propelling the semen out through the urethra.

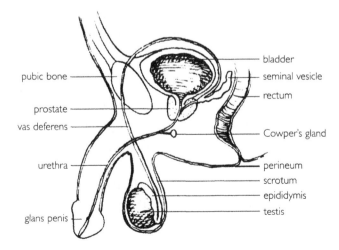

Fig. 3.4. The internal and external male organs

The Male Genital Erogenous Zones

Nipples. The male's nipples are sensitive to touch and create pleasurable feelings when stimulated orally or manually, often becoming hard just like the female's.

Penis. The wife will often need her husband to demonstrate the strokes he appreciates most on his penis. It usually is firmer with the whole hand encircling the organ and often more rapid, especially when approaching orgasm, than she might expect. The underside of the penis is often very sensitive and responds well to fingertip stroking. The greatest concentration of nerve endings is in the head of the penis. Oral stimulation, the hand (lubrication helps), or the vagina create arousal. Again, it will need to be firm stimulation, or it will not be felt or appreciated as much. A wife can place her hand over her husband's hand and learn the strokes and rhythms he enjoys the most.

Scrotum and testicles. The testicles are sensitive to being hit but can be touched quite firmly if done gently. These very erotic parts of a man's body create sensations with caressing or lightly tugging on the scrotal sac.

Perineum. This is the area between the scrotum and the anus. It is over the prostate gland as well as being at the base of the penis. It can be quite exciting to rub this area with moderate firmness—especially if done in conjunction with manually stroking the penis with the other hand. You, as partners, will have to explore and experiment, as you have done with level-three and level-two erogenous zones, while discovering what feels most exciting and pleasurable.

The Female Genitals

The vulva. The vulva comprises the external genitals of the female. The vulva varies greatly in shape and size of outer and inner lips and density of pubic hair. The vulva begins in front, with the pubic mound (mons pubis) covered with pubic hair, and extends down to the perineum above the anus. On either side are the outer labia and inner labia with the clitoris, followed by the urethral opening and the vagina.

The mons pubis and labia majora. The mons pubis is soft tissue over the pelvic bones. It is covered with hair and acts as a cushion during the thrusting of intercourse. The outer lips (labia majora) start down at the vagina and extend up to meet at the mons. They are soft folds of tissue that, with the hair on them, protect the inner organs and are often all that are visible as they come together over the inner lips. During sexual arousal, the outer lips become engorged with blood and become flatter.

The clitoris hood and labia minora. The inner lips (labia minora) are hairless and start at the vaginal opening and extend upward to meet at the clitoral hood. If the hood is pulled back, the external part of the clitoris can be seen, like a small pea in size. The inner lips vary greatly in size and shape among females. With some women they are larger and extend outside the outer lips. There is no perfect size, but each unique shape will become intensely erotic to the woman's husband. The inner labia become engorged during sexual arousal and change color and increase in thickness. They create a chute that the penis travels down to the vagina for penetration.

The clitoris and shaft. The clitoris is homologous to the penis and contains the most sensitive nerve endings. In a wonderful way, it is given to the female solely for sexual pleasure, and stimulating it is the key to tension buildup and climax. The clitoris doubles in size and becomes hard like the penis. The clitoral shaft is primarily beneath the surface of the skin under the clitoral hood. (See Figure 3.5.)

The urethral opening. The urethral opening is between the clitoris and vaginal opening but is small and sometimes difficult to detect. The urethra has nothing to do with sexual arousal but is located near the wall of the vagina and can become irritated with the thrusting of intercourse. Also with intercourse, bacteria can be pushed up into the urethra and can create infections. Urinating after lovemaking can help prevent this.

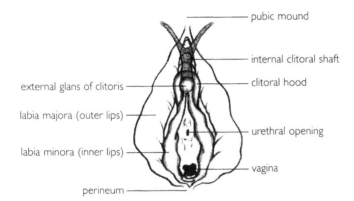

Fig. 3.5. The clitoris with labia

The hymen. At birth the opening to the vagina is covered by a thin perforated piece of skin called the hymen. It is often broken with the insertion of tampons or during physical activities. In rare cases it is so strong that a physician must perform a hymenectomy and surgically cut the hymen to allow intercourse. Usually, it is broken without intense pain and can be stretched by inserting the thumb or two fingers and gently pushing or pulling before first intercourse. For some couples it may be more painful with first intercourse, and going gently with plenty of artificial lubrication helps.

The vagina. The vagina is a shaft or tube of tissue with the sides touching. It is around three inches in length; it is muscular and expands so that it can accommodate any size of penis, especially with arousal. With arousal, the outer third of the vagina swells and creates the orgasmic platform, and the inner part balloons. After arousal, the greater penile stimulation will occur at the mouth, or outer third, of the vagina. The vagina has folds of skin and sweats out lubrication when sexually aroused, to allow intercourse. It is also delicately balanced with bacteria and acidic fluids to slow down bacterial growth. Be cautious with douches or placing a finger that has been near the bacteria of the anus within the vagina and upsetting the balance.

The cervix. The cervix is at the upper end of the vagina and opens into the uterus. It can be sensitive to the hard thrusting of intercourse, but there are front and rear fornices on either side of the cervix. The rear fornix takes most of the hard thrusts of vigorous intercourse and is designed to collect the semen and hold it near the cervix to increase the likelihood of insemination.

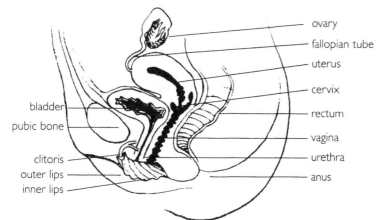

Fig. 3.6. The internal female organs

The Female Genital Erogenous Zones

The breasts and nipples. The breasts and nipples are very exciting to both husband and wife. The husband enjoys the unique femininity of his wife's breasts and sees the nipples becoming erect as a more obvious sign of sexual arousal. (Nipples can also become hard as a reaction to temperature change and do not always signal sexual arousal.) He needs to remember that his wife will not usually appreciate a direct attack on the nipples or genital area. A woman more often appreciates an indirect, teasing approach. It is also wise to understand that a woman more than a man will vary in what feels stimulating or irritating from one lovemaking session to another. Nipples, for instance, can be affected by hormonal fluctuations. Always be creative as you caress, nibble, lightly touch, or stroke more firmly. Vary the direction and types of stroking as you invite and remember suggestions. Husbands, circular or light-tease stroking around prime areas can keep you more varied and prevent always heading for the parts men seem to be drawn to immediately.

The labia. The outer and inner lips have many nerve endings and create sexual excitement. Again, vary the touch as you start with the outer lips and mons. Place the whole hand over the genital area; run a finger from bottom to top of outer labia; lightly rub the labia together over the clitoral area. Allow sexual tension to build. The penis is a marvelous wand for creating pleasure, especially its soft head. Use it to gently stimulate the inner labia and the clitoris. Let the tension begin to build before active stimulation of the clitoris.

The clitoris. The wife will have to discover the strokes and places that she prefers for clitoral stimulation and then teach her partner. She may have to tune in to and become aware herself of the fun sensations her clitoris can provide; she can suggest techniques for her husband to use that are helpful for arousing her. One wife had trouble showing her husband the place she preferred to be stimulated. She liked a firm, sideways stroke with his finger over the erect clitoral shaft right above the hood as she thrust up to meet the pressure. Eventually, she and her husband coordinated their movements, and it was tremendously arousing for her. The husband came to realize that the stimulation of his wife's clitoris was very similar to that of his penis. She desired rapid stroking as she approached her climax, with firmer and vigorous caressing. Your partner is unique; learn to nurture and excite her.

The vagina. The outer third of the vagina is the most sensitive. This sensitivity should be kept in mind with either manual or penile stimulation. Quick, shallow thrusts, as well as slow, sensual, longer motions, can be very arousing. Often there is greater sensation at twelve o'clock (toward the clitoris) and six o'clock (toward the anus) within the vagina. Positions that stimulate these areas create exciting sensations. (The G spot, which is located about an inch within the vagina at twelve o'clock and can be most easily located when the woman is aroused, will be discussed in a later chapter. With some women, the G spot creates particular pleasure and arousal.)

The perineum and areas adjacent to the vulva. The perineum, or tissue between the anus and vagina, is sensitive to touch. Any skin or tissues immediately surrounding the vulva can be categorized as level-two erogenous zones, which would include areas such as the inner thighs, bottom, and stomach. Though not the direct genital area, they are very sensitive to caresses, licking, and teasing strokes—almost becoming an extension of the vulva. Remain creative and varied as you enjoy level-one erogenous zones. Stimulating the genital area does not always lead to orgasm but can be done with nondemanding pleasuring. (See Chapter 11.)

SENSUAL EROTIC PAIRING

Our senses and hormones stimulate sexual feelings, and the nervous system communicates these to the brain. The brain then signals the muscles and blood system of the genitals and creates arousal. Your task is to be sensual and learn the erogenous zones so that you can caress your mate's body and both of you can experience the automatic sexual arousal that will occur as the hormones are released and the brain automatically sends signals through the nervous system. Your body and mind will cooperate, but you may need to be sensitized to enjoy a fuller range of sexual feelings as you stimulate erogenous zones and experience greater sexual arousal.

Another concept that can help you understand and enjoy the erogenous zones is a psychological principle that Russian psychologist Ivan Pavlov discovered. He taught dogs to salivate

Time Out: Let the husband get into a comfortable position lying on his
back. The wife is going to gently and carefully explore and touch the genital area
from perineum to the tip of the penis. Observe the penis both flaccid and erect.
Let him tell her what feels especially sensitive and arousing. Now let the wife lie on
her back and the husband do the same, taking time to explore what feels best in
the vagina as well as the labia and clitoris. Pull back the clitoral hood and notice
the clitoris—massage it to greater arousal and feel the clitoris become erect.
Become a student of your mate's body.

at a ringing bell by associating the bell with food. We call this classical conditioning. Perhaps
it is easier to understand this conditioning process by calling it pairing. The formula below
shows you how sexual pairing occurs. An unconditioned stimulus is paired with a conditioned
stimulus, and you get aroused in time simply with the conditioned stimulus.

UNCONDITIONED STIMULUS (HORMONES) = UNCONDITIONED RESPONSE
(EXCITEMENT)
CONDITIONED STIMULUS (KISS) = CONDITIONED RESPONSE (EXCITEMENT)

Pairing takes place in your mind as you stimulate the erogenous zones or sensually (touch,
sight, smell) notice them and associate (pair) these experiences with hormones and sexual
arousal. As you become more aroused, more hormones are released and you can continue to pair
various touches and visual experiences so that they become sexually arousing to you—like kissing or observing your mate's genitals. This is the beauty of a long-term intimate companionship:
the pairing/conditioning never ceases, and stored in your mind are many sexually arousing symbols that you can draw on to create or enhance sexual arousal. Stimulating the erogenous zones
can continually become charged with sensual and erotic pleasure over a lifetime of lovemaking.

Another beauty is that this bodily arousal is also complexly paired up with our hearts and
souls. We aren't just caressing a body; we are sensuously connecting with the special body of
the person we love. God takes the beauty of sexual touching out of the purely physical and
into the intimate place of the heart. We can simply have sex and learn to skillfully arouse—
or, we can learn to make love in the erogenous zones.

Relax, explore, caress, pair, discover, stroke, expand, touch, love, and sensuously feel as you
fully enjoy God's wonderful gift of sexual pleasure.

CHAPTER FOUR

Lovemaking Cycles

CREATING AND REVELING in a sexy atmosphere; the mounting excitement of the penis growing erect and the vagina lubricating in anticipation of intercourse; looking deeply into the eyes, the windows to the soul of our lover; and becoming playfully vulnerable and surrendering to orgasms—all stir up in each of us the passion and mystery of sexuality. God has designed a marvelously complex and intimate process to be set in motion when a couple makes love.

A *process* can be defined as "a continuous series of changes over time." This chapter will develop two models of lovemaking cycles, or processes, with their evolving changes. The first, with Masters and Johnson, looks at the physical and bodily changes, while the second model, with Christopher McCluskey and his Lovemaking Cycle, considers the increasing emotional and relational intimacy that builds during lovemaking.

THE FOUR-PHASE PHYSICAL PROCESS

A four-phase cycle sounds like part of a course in electrical engineering. Actually, it is the exciting way our physical bodies function in lovemaking. (See Figure 4.1.) Sex researchers Masters and Johnson developed from their research four separate phases of physical buildup and changes during sex: excitement, plateau, orgasm, and resolution. Understanding these phases can help couples enhance their arousal as they maximize each stage of the physical process.

1. The Excitement Phase

The husband's sexual excitement is a blend of physical friction in the erogenous zones and the mental and emotional arousal through sensual stimulation. The beginning of male arousal

Fig. 4.1. The four phases of arousal and satisfaction.

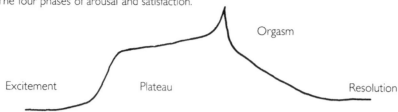

Orgasm

Excitement   Plateau   Resolution

can be observed by the penis becoming erect. Remember that erections and vaginal lubrication can be reflexive and are not always indications of complete arousal. Erections are almost taken for granted until there are difficulties, but all men will struggle with getting or maintaining an erection at some point. Fatigue, alcohol, medications, and performance anxiety are common causes. The key is not to panic because that will just compound the problem. Create plenty of erotic stimulation and realize it is temporary.

Often during the excitement and plateau phases, the erection becomes partial (softer) or completely subsides because the husband focuses on pleasuring his mate and has less direct penile stimulation. He also may get distracted and less focused and lose the erection. That is normal. As he enjoys the loveplay and erotic stimulation, the erection will return. The aging process may mean that erections become less firm and more direct stimulation of the penis will be needed to create an erection.

Female arousal in the excitement phase is demonstrated by vaginal lubrication, which is like beads of saliva that sweat through the outer walls of the vagina. This occurs within the first minute or two of arousal but can vary, especially with aging or distraction and an inability to focus on pleasure. The vaginal secretions have an odor much like saliva. Some foods (for example, asparagus) will affect the odor of the secretions. The mind is a wonderful tool as it can pair the odors of making love (semen, vaginal secretions, perspiration) with sexual excitement and pleasure, and they become exciting stimuli. The nipples of the female become erect in the central papillae area during sexual excitement. The nipples (male and female) are a fun part of sexual loveplay.

Within the vagina, the outer third becomes more engorged with blood (tumescent) during the excitement phase and is called the orgasmic platform. It is the most sensitive vaginal tissue and stimulating the orgasmic platform feels great for both partners.

During arousal, the outer lips flatten and the inner lips of the vulva enlarge, creating a chute for the penis to travel down to the vagina. The clitoris enlarges to two or three times its relaxed size, but this occurs under the skin at the clitoral hood and is not readily observable. It can be felt by rolling a finger over this area right above the clitoral hood, feeling much like a firm cord under the skin. Women vary immensely as to how they enjoy the clitoral stimulation and can change over the various phases. Keep coaching and communicating. The wife may need to demonstrate how she prefers the clitoris to be stimulated.

PHYSICAL CHANGES IN THE PHASES OF AROUSAL AND FULFILLMENT

Phase	Women	Men

Excitement	Nipples erect
	Breast enlargement
	Sex flush (75%)
	Clitoral tumescence
	Vaginal lubrication
	Outer lips flatten and enlarge
	Inner lips enlarge
	Heart rate and blood pressure
	    increase
		Nipples erect (60%)
		Sex flush (25%)
		Penis erect/tumescent
		Scrotum thickens and sac elevates
		Heart rate and blood pressure
		    increase

Plateau	Orgasmic platform with
	    ballooning
	Increased sex flush and
	    cardiorespiratory
	Involuntary muscle contractions
	Increased blood flow in breasts
	    and vulva; color changes
		Seepage from penis; prostate and
		    seminal vesicles contract
		Increased cardiorespiratory
		Involuntary muscle contractions
		Head of penis enlarges and color
		    deepens; testes rise and rotate

Orgasm	Muscle contractions at 0.8
	    second in orgasmic platform,
	    rectal sphincter, uterus
	Involuntary muscle spasm in
	    pelvis and entire body
	Heart rate and breathing
	    elevated
		Muscle contractions at 0.8 second
		    in prostate, seminal duct
		    system, base of penis/rectal
		    area produce ejaculation
		Involuntary muscle spasm in
		    pelvis and entire body
		Heart and breathing rate elevated

Resolution	Relief of vasocongestion and
	    enlargement of breasts and
	    genitals
	Muscles relax
	Skin flush disappears
	Heart rate, blood pressure, and
	    breathing return to normal
		Relief of vasocongestion and
		    enlargement of penis, scrotum,
		    and testes
		Muscles relax
		Skin flush disappears
		Heart rate, blood pressure, and
		    breathing return to normal

2. The Plateau Phase

This phase should be the longest and perhaps the most enjoyable one of the sexual cycle. The initial arousal is there, and the loveplay can build on this tension as it progresses from general stimulation to specific locations. The penis becomes fuller and the head a deeper color as it is further engorged. The orgasmic platform in the outer third of the vagina also becomes larger, giving firmer friction on the penis during intercourse. The inner two-thirds of the vagina expands, creating a receptacle for the semen, and the uterus elevates, giving greater comfort with thrusting because the cervix is pulled away.

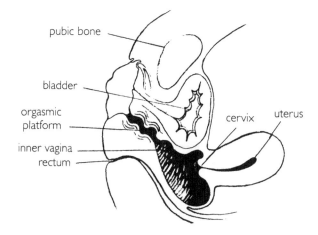

Fig. 4.2. Orgasmic platform with ballooning in inner vagina

In the male, preparation for ejaculation is taking place as the prostate and seminal vesicles contract. Some seepage from the penis occurs; it does contain sperm, so be cautious to have birth control in place if not desiring pregnancy. In an ejaculation there are approximately 300 million sperm, and it takes only one to create a baby. The seminal fluid is building in the urethra and area around the prostate, preparing for orgasm.

Both males and females experience increased heart rates, a rise in blood pressure, and intensified breathing. With some, there is a sex flush on the upper torso, neck, and face. Muscles involuntarily contract, and sexual excitement continues to build gradually during this plateau phase. The loveplay will increase in intensity with active intercourse and more vigorous direct stimulation of the erogenous zones.

Research has found that a man, if actively thrusting, will often climax in less than two minutes while a woman will take much longer to reach an orgasm. The wise couple intersperses intercourse throughout the plateau phase as the husband starts and stops and keeps his arousal on a plateau without peaking too soon. Both husband and wife can learn to approach an orgasm and then back off as they maintain the plateau phase for extended periods of pleasurable and sensuous lovemaking.

3. The Orgasm Phase

This phase focuses on producing an orgasm in one or both partners. The plateau phase is a time of increased excitement, and now both partners are ready to climb that last peak with focused stimulation.

In allowing the reflexive action of an orgasm to occur, you must focus on your body and the tension that is building. Allow your mind to give in to the increasing arousal and revel in the approaching climax. At orgasm, you become self-focused and trust your partner with grimaces and squeals and muscle contractions. You are oblivious to how you look as your mind is selfishly centered on your growing excitement.

Physically, both the male and female experience muscle contractions, eight-tenths of a second in duration, as the central part of the orgasmic response. For the female, the contractions center in the vaginal area in the orgasmic platform with the PC (pubococcygeal) muscle and the rectal sphincter (the circular muscle at the opening of the rectum). The uterus also contracts, much as in labor pains. The female experiences a series of spasms, four to twelve in duration depending on the intensity of the orgasm. The male experiences spasms during his ejaculation, which also vary in intensity depending on level of arousal and abandonment to the experience. His contractions occur around the prostate gland, anus, and his PC muscles, as the semen is propelled outward through the urethra and penis.

Ejaculation for the male occurs in two phases. In the first, preparatory stage, the prostate gland begins contractions and the sphincter muscle to the bladder closes off so semen does not back up into the bladder. (With prostate surgery, sometimes the sphincter does not close off and the ejaculate goes back into the bladder with the orgasm. This can decrease sensation, and it takes time to allow orgasms to achieve some of their original intensity.) The left testicle elevates and rotates, and semen gathers in the urethra at the base of the penis. In the second phase, which is unable to be interrupted, ejaculation inevitably takes place with muscle contraction. The semen that has collected in the upper urethra is propelled out of the penis.

With orgasm also come involuntary contractions of the muscles of the arms, legs, pelvis, and back. Breathing, blood pressure, and heart rate will increase. Sometimes deliberately simulating these physiological aspects of an orgasm, tensing muscles and breathing heavily, can trigger the climax.

Many men experience orgasm with an intense genital focus. Their descriptions are more of explosions, fireworks of release, and intense feelings that build and then come with a powerful rush. These feelings are often centered on the penis and, at the moment of release, include the muscle spasms in the genital area with intense emotional and physical release through the exploding of ejaculation. Men struggle as they age and ejaculations are less in quantity of semen and less intense in the propulsion of semen.

Women, too, can have intense orgasms with exciting explosions of feelings in the clitoral and vaginal area. They often describe their release as waves of pleasure and a flooding of feelings. These intense feelings, which are more than the vaginal and uterine contractions, may begin in the genital area but seem to diffuse throughout the body—through the abdomen, breasts, legs, and head. For both sexes, the mind is a fantastic tool for focusing and increasing the intensity of the climax.

One wife in the course of therapy was surprised to hear her husband say that sometimes orgasms felt like a volcano and at other times it was a mild, pleasurable fizzle of feelings. She thought that because males ejaculated, their orgasms were all strong and identical in nature. She was surprised to find herself similar to her husband, with orgasms varying in intensity depending on the particular lovemaking session.

There are interesting distinctions between male and female orgasmic capabilities. Males have a refractory period, or recuperative time, between orgasms. At age nineteen, this rest period may be a few minutes; with aging, it increases to a few hours or days. The second orgasm following close upon the first may take more stimulation and may be less intense.

Females, on the other hand, do not have a refractory period. They are capable of having repeated orgasms, and rather than diminish, succeeding orgasms may be more intense. Females, with this capability for multiple orgasms, may experience separate orgasms minutes apart, or during an intense lovemaking session with increasing arousal, they may experience an extended orgasm from seconds to a minute. Some women also experience a gushing of secretions almost like ejaculation, and a greater wetness. This is normal and is not urine but secretions much as the ejaculate in men.

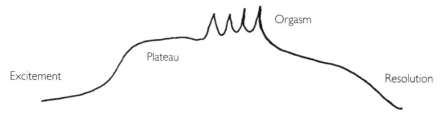

Fig. 4.3. The four phases of arousal and fulfillment in the multiorgasmic female

In the orgasm phase, a common concern is whether the wife should be able to climax during lovemaking by penile thrusting alone. No; almost two-thirds of women can't achieve an orgasm without direct stimulation of the clitoris. Most wives will need manual or oral stimulation of the clitoris to create arousal up to the point of climaxing. Climaxing through intercourse could be likened to the husband having an orgasm by stroking his testicles but not his penis.

Remember that an orgasm is a reflexive response; it is not an intentional act of the will. You cannot consciously will yourself to have an orgasm. Orgasms are a product of sufficient buildup of physical, mental, and emotional stimulation as the mind focuses on that increasing sexual tension. For most women, the stimulation needs to be in the clitoral area where there is a concentration of nerve endings.

This is where the husband has to allow the wife to coach him as to what touches stimulate her best and what rhythm she desires. He controls his orgasm and rhythm by being the one thrusting his penis in her vagina, fast, slow, intensely, gently—however he desires. She is dependent on his hand, mouth, or penis to create the friction and buildup with the right touch, tempo, and building intensity—an important leadership task for the husband.

Some women enjoy their orgasms with the penis in the vagina and experience greater intensity, while some prefer not to have the penis in the vagina as they focus on their own sensations. Some couples like orgasms close together, and others prefer allowing a woman to climax several times before the man. Create the patterns and rhythms that fit you as an individual and as a couple.

4. The Resolution Phase

After an orgasm, both men and women experience a release of tension as the body returns to its original state before sexual arousal. This is physically the final enjoyment of an orgasm as the muscles relax, blood vessels and tissue release the engorged blood, and the congestion abruptly eases. Sometimes, both with men and women, the genitals become very sensitive after an orgasm.

There is a feeling of tension release with an orgasm as the blood congestion leaves the genitals and pelvic area with a pleasant, perhaps tingling, sensation. In the woman, unlike the man, there is the potential to return quite quickly to an aroused state and experience multiple orgasms. The wife may learn to experience several orgasms as she then returns to the plateau phase with her husband. It can be fulfilling for both of them.

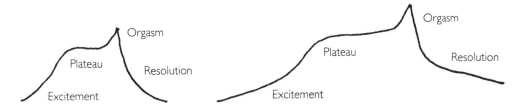

Fig. 4.4. The four phases: frustrated (left) and fulfilled (right)

Spend time allowing the body to enjoy each of the four phases as you cycle through the physical arousal with climax and resolution. In becoming an expert lover, the right-hand graph is more pleasurable, especially for the wife, than the one on the left. This should be more characteristic of a fun lovemaking session, with prolonged excitement, plateau, and resolution phases.

THE LOVEMAKING CYCLE

While Masters and Johnson focus on four phases of physical arousal, Christian sex therapist Christopher McCluskey has created a more relational and emotional Lovemaking Cycle. He insists that there is a great deal of difference between having sex and making love. True lovemaking (The Cycle) creates a growing intimacy and an increasing sexual passion based on two hearts who are becoming spiritually and emotionally one.

In McCluskey's model, each part of the cycle feeds into the next, creating an ever-deepening experience of vulnerability and intimacy with your mate and lover. He emphasizes that if one part is neglected, lovemaking will "clunk" every time it hits that weak spot and throw off the whole cycle, much like a wheel that is flat in one area and no longer round. Lovemaking will in time break down because each of the four parts represents a deep emotional and relational need that is critical for maintaining passionate lovemaking.

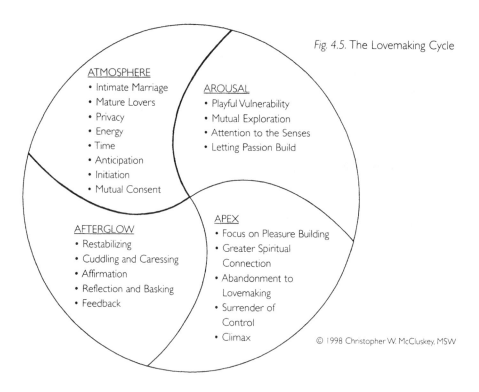

Fig. 4.5. The Lovemaking Cycle

ATMOSPHERE
• Intimate Marriage
• Mature Lovers
• Privacy
• Energy
• Time
• Anticipation
• Initiation
• Mutual Consent

AROUSAL
• Playful Vulnerability
• Mutual Exploration
• Attention to the Senses
• Letting Passion Build

AFTERGLOW
• Restabilizing
• Cuddling and Caressing
• Affirmation
• Reflection and Basking
• Feedback

APEX
• Focus on Pleasure Building
• Greater Spiritual Connection
• Abandonment to Lovemaking
• Surrender of Control
• Climax

© 1998 Christopher W. McCluskey, MSW

This model identifies many important factors that can facilitate progressively deeper levels of intimacy in lovemaking. Each will be briefly examined and explained, with an emphasis on the four key areas that are truly interactive and must flow from the heart: atmosphere, arousal, apex, and afterglow. (A brief disclaimer is in order. Though this is Christopher's model, much of the illustrations and descriptive manner are my own and may not reflect his style or values.)

1. Atmosphere

Mood setting can never be simply lighting a candle or creating a little ambiance. *The concept of atmosphere is much deeper.* It is lovingly building an intimate relationship with your covenant companion so that energy is reserved and time is devoted for sexuality. Time, energy, and anticipation are powerful aphrodisiacs. Desire is never just hormonal, especially for the wife. Sex begins with loving attention in the kitchen and flows into passion in the bedroom. Lovers anticipate each other and sexual passion permeates the relationship, regardless of place or circumstances.

Intimate marriage and mature lovers. This goes back to the formula for fulfilling and passionate sexual encounters. The foundation of fantastic lovemaking is an intimate, grown-up companionship that includes effective communication. This point could be paraphrased as "grow up and fall deeper in love." God has given us the capacity to accomplish both of these tasks. Remember,

AN INTIMATE MARRIAGE + MATURE LOVERS = A FULFILLING SEX LIFE

Privacy. God designed sexual intimacy to be a very special and private interaction between husband and wife. Though making love should not be confined to the bedroom, it will be the primary love nest because of the need for privacy as well as for comfort. Mood lighting or candles, sensuous linens, and the ability to control the temperature are sexual enhancements that can give the bedroom very private, sensual, and erotic qualities. You can also create an intimate privacy in other rooms of your home and in that hotel room on your vacations. It is just the two of you alone. You may need to make some special efforts to overcome the effect of children on privacy (see Chapter 19).

Energy. Whether you are newlyweds or married for years, you will have to reserve some energy for sex. You know how exhausted you get just keeping up with the demands of life. Think of what rest and a boost of energy can do. Putting some extra current into your love life will have a marvelous effect, and you can't always wait for a vacation to do this. An extra nap or making some personal time can be creatively arranged if it's a priority. Rest and recreation create energy.

Time. If ten minutes is great, then thirty minutes will be even more intimate. Time may be the most precious gift you bring to your sex life. It is the bottom line in creating the sexy, connected atmosphere as you get beyond quickies to luxuriating. Five-second hugs, lingering, deep kisses, and two-hour picnics in bed will do wonders.

Anticipation. Great lovers are childlike in their ability to anticipate pleasure with glee. Husbands and especially wives can enjoy their God-given imagination and think about love-making more—like a kid who has looked forward to an ice-cream cone all day. Anticipation also has a deeper quality of mentally preparing your bodies and spirits to be truly naked and vulnerable.

Wives and husbands seem to apply and appreciate this skill in different ways. Wives will often relate how in the busyness of life, sex gets put on the back burner. Thinking about and anticipating making love on that evening or weekend brings desire and interest that would not have been there without looking forward to it. Husbands tell how anticipation can help them discipline their sexual thoughts and urges during the day toward their wives, as well as make them very aroused by the time they get home. Then they need to work on their gentle, patient initiation skills.

Initiation. Lovemaking has to start somewhere, and a part of ambiance is both husband and wife initiating sexual activity. Remember, it does not have to lead to intercourse but can be that passionate kiss when coming home from work. Grow into verbal as well as nonverbal forms of initiating. The verbal can be even more intimate, though feeling more risky of rejection, than nonverbal.

A husband appreciates his wife initiating because it demonstrates her interest in lovemaking and in him. A wife appreciates initiating that includes emotional attention and not just heading for favorite parts—as well as the ability to hear her say "no" too. What a complex but invaluable skill to become assertive at initiating and graceful in hearing refusals.

Mutual consent. If you want to maintain a great mood for sex, be *assertive* and *empathetic* in your intimate communication. Lovemaking is about giving and not demanding. We aren't trying to service each other. The husband or the wife may not be in the mood and that's fine. What great fireworks happen when you do mutually engage.

It is important to remember this idea of *mutual consent.* If a person cannot refuse and say "no" then his or her yeses will have little meaning and be more out of duty. If a person cannot initiate passionately and say "yes" joyfully, then God's wonderful gift of consent to intimate lovemaking is also forfeited. Mutuality is not always easy.

2. Arousal

Sexual maturity helps us grow beyond the arousal of sexual rushes and buzzes. Deep, erotic arousal grows from a three-dimensional (body, soul, spirit) connection and bonding. When you and your mate learn to be aroused in a truly *intimate* way, you will be amazed at the feelings that occur. The physical and emotional interaction and fusion (God-given eros) create an unbeatable intimacy high.

Sexual arousal involves body, soul, and spirit. Allow yourself to focus on each one of these

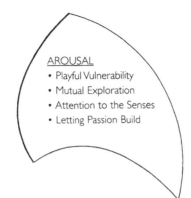

 AROUSAL
• Playful Vulnerability
• Mutual Exploration
• Attention to the Senses
• Letting Passion Build

Fig. 4.6. Arousal quadrant

three dimensions of your mate during this passion building process. Neglecting the body, soul, or spirit can lessen all that God intends in passionate intimacy. Remember that these are dimensions and not totally separate parts; they are complexly interactive and cooperative.

We are created in God's image with bodies and their hormones, nerve endings, and brain centers. Don't just focus in on sexual parts of the anatomy; the entire skin is erogenous. Go to those tender places, like the face, and the spots that your mate finds sexy.

Our minds and feelings may be the centers of sexual arousal. Use your imagination as you focus in on your mate and lovemaking. Become passionately emotional and very self-aware as you dwell in your child ego state. Know that to be human is to have a will that can choose to focus in and be present for your mate sexually. The eyes are often the windows of the soul— look deeply into each other's eyes with love and excitement during this arousal phase.

Every human being created in God's image longs for completion and deep intimacy. In arousal, remember that you are affirming your love in important ways. You are not simply making love to a body, you are making love to a special person that you have committed your life and well-being to. This is intimate covenant arousal.

Playful vulnerability. Fun and open lovemaking takes place in the child ego state. Each of us has that curious, silly, innocent, playful part of us that loves to romp. "Naked and unashamed" is a very vulnerable and powerful place to be. (See Chapter 2 and the discussion of playfulness.)

God gave us imaginations and the ability to be romantic to create and enjoy various means of enticing and playing with our mates. Flickering candlelight with soothing music in the background creates totally different feelings from that of bright sunlight employed in an afternoon delight with some jazz on the stereo. Pillows to lean against as you have intimate conversations or to use in positions of pleasuring and intercourse, satin sheets, and the ability to control the thermostat—all help make the bed the playground it should be. (See Chapter 6.)

Some couples worry about unleashing playful sensuality and wonder if sinful fleshly desires could enter in to sabotage lovemaking and their goal of being truly open to each other. Here are some practical suggestions to prevent that from happening: (1) remain playfully in perspective and don't focus in one thing as being needed in order to have fun; (2) never engage in activity that takes away from your trust and respect, or invites another person into your bedroom (sexual movies, for example)—this will kill vulnerability; and (3) enhance true three-dimensional (body, soul, and spirit) passion. Arousal is dependent on feeling safe and inviting vulnerability on all three dimensions of body, soul, and spirit. Couples will have to define some of what they find playful as they keep that openness to each other and lovemaking.

Mutual exploration. Many mates have never taken the time to examine each other's genitals and familiarize themselves with the hot spots. Take the time to truly be present with each other in curious, teasing, and exploratory ways. The Song of Solomon delightfully encourages lovers to "browse among the lilies" (2:16 NIV).

Learn the hot spots and the turn-offs. What delightful lovemaking when you can help your mate discover an arousing spot he or she wasn't aware of, or experience a new situation that gets the other excited. An attitude of exploration keeps lovemaking fresh and your mate truly attended to. It is God's plan that we "know" our mates and get our Ph.D.'s in them.

Attention to the senses. Every couple can wisely make two lists. The first list is of each of the five senses and how each sense can cue you in to sexual arousal—how you want that sense to be utilized. The second list is what turns you off with each sense and detracts from lovemaking. A sample list:

1. Sight. Turn-ons: show up naked; a couple holding hands; strategically placed mirrors; seductive dances; bright satin sheets; emerald boxers; soft peach teddies. Turn-offs: bright lights; a beer gut; the same nightgown; dirty sheets.

2. Smell. Turn-ons: perfumes, candles, incense, scented lotions; semen; bubble bath. Turn-offs: semen; body odor; dirty sheets; dragon breath.

3. Taste. Turn-ons: chocolate and strawberries; minty kisses; a favorite wine; Turn-offs: certain lubricants; garlic kisses.

4. Hearing. Turn-ons: "Bolero" or favorite songs; sexy talking; uninhibited groans and squeals. Turn-offs: squeals in ear; silence; television; slang.

5. Touch. Turn-ons: soaping each other up; ice cubes over sensitive areas; a fur rug; satin gloves (fabrics are sensual); lotions; sweaty bodies rubbing. Turn-offs: unshaven beards; rough hands; sweaty bodies; types of tickling.

Letting passion build. Arousal carries with it the idea of a crescendo and increasing excitement. In a mature way, you are responsible for your own passionate feelings. A healthy self-focus is important in letting passions build. Get into your private feelings and even risk sharing some of them with your mate—perhaps nonverbally with groans or squeals. It is not only focusing in on your arousal feelings, but also increasingly letting go of control and truly being in the moment.

What a powerful turn-on as you build towards the apex. You are excited and your mate is excited by your excitement, and arousal has become a connecting experience. You are truly making love.

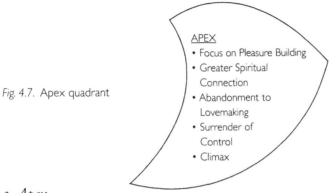

APEX
• Focus on Pleasure Building
• Greater Spiritual Connection
• Abandonment to Lovemaking
• Surrender of Control
• Climax

Fig. 4.7. Apex quadrant

3. *Apex*

It takes a mature person to understand that the emotional center of the apex is not orgasm, but a surrender to feelings and to each other. The term *apex* is purposefully used to de-emphasize chasing orgasms and to emphasize the deeper idea of abandonment and achieving a deeper oneness. Most often there will be that exciting climax, but there will be some times when an orgasm will not occur and yet an apex is achieved. Mature, older couples have often grown into this level of apex and enjoy its beauty. Souls have surrendered and joyful sexual-peak experiences are achieved, though no orgasm has occurred.

Focus on pleasure building. Remember that women vary more in what they find pleasurable, and the center of sensory nerves for them is the clitoris and not the vagina. Stay in the moment with a growing focus on accenting what each partner is experiencing and needing.

As has been stated, some of this focus will be a personal, inner attention to building feelings. This does not exclude the mate but almost like worship, our bodies and souls are reveling in the experience and taking in more and more. This is a special time of self as well as mutual sharing. Our mate is enjoying our growing arousal and his or her part in enhancing this pleasure building—what a fun part of apexing.

Greater spiritual connection. Look deeply into each other's eyes and get lost in the other and the sharing of passion. Lovemaking can make you more totally "naked" than any other mutual experience. Your emotions and your bodies are making heavenly music that is much more profound than the friction.

It is so meaningful in these moments of great arousal to tell your mate you love him or her or look lovingly at the other's body and face, as you pair up the physical, soul, and spiritual union with climax. God made us to desire being one with our mate and to have this loving spiritual union of two humans, male and female, in covenant intimacy.

Abandonment to lovemaking. Think of what the word *abandon* means emotionally and physically. Can you remember as a child when you would leap from an object into the arms of your parents with no fear for your safety? That's abandonment. Or, maybe like a roller-coaster ride, when we can throw our hands up and give in to powerful feelings, zooming down that steep incline. Or, maybe you've experienced lifting your hands in worship and just giving in to God's presence and joy.

Only with tremendous commitment and trust do you feel safe enough to truly abandon yourself to another person. Your covenant companionship provides that context. You no longer need to be self-conscious but can be passionate without any holding back. You are unconditionally loved and accepted. This is the private, secure place that allows us to romp and resonate in love and nakedness.

This facet of the apex, abandonment to lovemaking, correlates to the next step of individual surrender but is looking more at the overall *process* of lovemaking. Abandonment is the ongoing event of giving up feeling inhibited in any way as mates throw themselves into the experience totally. It includes a comfortable body image, acceptance of intense feelings, and a deep commitment as soul mates.

Surrender of control. This is the heart of the apex and, indeed, of becoming orgasmic. Orgasms are such beautiful metaphors of uninhibited worship and giving up control to Christ. You are allowing your bodies and souls to soar with surrender.

Apexes cannot be reached without letting go, which is built on a series of individual choices. I will choose to trust; I will choose to feel; I will choose to give up control in front of and to my mate. It is interesting that many couples can create orgasms but not an apex because there are too many fears and walls to deep intimacy and trust. Let God help you surrender to Him and to each other on important nonsexual levels. This can create the foundation for sexual surrender.

Climax. This is the time when you lose time and your body and feelings overwhelm the rational. What a precious gift to share with that lifetime lover—again and again with ever-increasing meaning and passion.

In stating that the apex is more than orgasms, it is not intended to diminish the importance of experiencing climaxes. For the wife who has not achieved this ability yet—work on it together. (See Chapter 17.) God created orgasms to be a special expression of feelings in a three-dimensional way. Experiencing and sharing climaxes is a fun and crucial part of this facet of lovemaking.

4. Afterglow

The lovemaking wheel will begin clunking if lovers neglect this important stage. It may be three to five minutes or an hour, but this time is critical for maintaining sexual passion. The

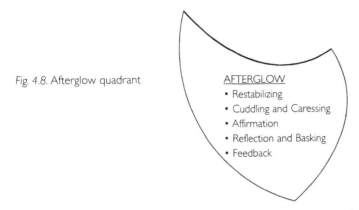

Fig. 4.8. Afterglow quadrant

AFTERGLOW
• Restabilizing
• Cuddling and Caressing
• Affirmation
• Reflection and Basking
• Feedback

afterglow, with regrouping, complimenting, evaluating, and an anticipation of future love-making, fuels the fire and greases the wheel for your next time of connection.

The afterglow may be even more important to the wife, who has chosen to be vulnerable in physical and emotional ways. This is a time of her being affirmed that this was meaningful and real and loving. The husband too can enjoy and link his intimate emotions with his physical feelings—and even communicate more in this fun part of lovemaking.

Restabilizing. After the apex you need to catch your breath and come down physically and emotionally. This is the afterglow that is warmly intimate but less intense. A time of recreating and affirming the recently shared intimate moment will be appreciated and is needed. Just as our bodies are physically returning to normal from their sexually aroused state, our emotions also are coming back into focus and restabilizing.

Cuddling and caressing. Wives are especially vulnerable after literally opening themselves up to their husbands. Rather than jumping out of bed to clean up, hold each other and bask in the afterglow of intense connecting and shared surrender. Or, clean up and come back to bed for a few more minutes.

Relax in the closeness and continue lovemaking in a more gentle and tender way. With your cuddling, include much eye contact and holding each other close. Allow yourself to feel your love and express it in different ways than arousal or apex. Your souls are connecting in this ongoing cycle of making love.

Affirmation. Husbands so want to please their wives and be great lovers. A "Wow, I can't believe what you just did" goes really far at this time. The wife wants to feel sexy and valued with compliments important to her too. They blossom when we as husbands affirm their femininity and sexiness. Not expressions like "Great butt!" but more along the lines of "It's awesome how your body makes me irrational." Mates, like all people, soak up praise and compliments.

This can be a time of lovemaking that encourages compliments that may not come as quickly in the ordinary rush of life. Lay back and talk and affirm. You'll be surprised how great it feels and what it can do to heat up the next time you're together.

Reflection and basking. Wives often comment how their husbands will engage in connecting conversation after lovemaking more than any other time. You have become vulnerably close at this phase of lovemaking. Reflect and bask in the relationship as well as in the events of the past moments.

It is like that Thanksgiving feast where we sit together as a family afterward and compliment and reflect. "Wow, you got creative with that dish—some new spices!" "I'll never get enough of that." "Can I take the leftovers home?" Lovemaking grows richer with the basking.

Feedback. Feedback can start the wheel rolling for the next lovemaking session. "Let's do that again," or "Could we make love Thursday morning?" This is indeed an ongoing party, and you are enriching and preparing for the next festivity.

It is better here to emphasize the positive, but some laughing over the slip-ups with some future planning is also in order. Suggestions for the future that might piggyback on some enjoyed pleasure can enhance this ongoing cycle.

Isn't lovemaking exciting?! You will be learning new pleasures fifty years from now. Keep tuning in to all four aspects of atmosphere, arousal, apex, and afterglow so that the wheel of your love life doesn't become unbalanced. Learn to include and experience the ever-increasing passion God designed.

(Note: Christopher McCluskey and his wife, Rachel, have written a forthcoming book on the Lovemaking Cycle with Baker/Revell Publishers. He also has an excellent videotape, *Coaching Couples into Passionate Intimacy*, that explains the model, and it can be ordered through his Web site, at www.christian-living.com.)

Time Out: 1. Discuss your turn-ons and turn-offs in each of your senses: sight, smell, taste, hearing, and touch.

2. What gets in the way of really surrendering to your climaxes? Discuss this together. While making love and the apex approaches, pretend you are on a roller-coaster ride and trust your mate as you truly surrender to this ride and its out-of-control feelings.

CHAPTER FIVE

Minimizing the Mess

HOW MANY LOVERS, as they are contemplating the joys of sex, think of lovemaking as being messy? The word *mess* can be defined as a condition or situation that is uncomfortable, confusing, unpleasant, or untidy. This certainly fits many aspects of sex. It is unfortunate, but many couples let the untidiness seriously dampen their sexual intimacy. Here is a sample of complaints from marriage partners:

- "He never wants to make love during the menstrual cycle even if the flow is very light."
- "She always jumps up and runs to the bathroom to clean up right after we make love."
- "We were using some lubrication and he squeezed the tube too hard and I became one gooey mess."
- "Life can get in the way of a good sex life—at first it was my pregnancy, then his bladder infection, and now the demands of the children."
- "He wants to make love at the most inopportune times—when I am dressed, have my hair done and my lipstick on, and am ready to leave the house."
- "He enjoys having sex on Saturdays after working in the yard when he is all sweaty and smelly—he also hasn't shaved and gives me beard burn."
- She says, "We're in the mood and fooling around, then we have to mess with inserting birth control and lose our spontaneity." He says, "I hate condoms. They don't feel natural and are such a nuisance."
- He says, "She and I both enjoy oral sex. But sometimes it's awkward for me if she didn't have time to bathe first." She says, "I love it when he climaxes. But I can't seem to get used to how sticky semen feels."

- "Sex is so embarrassing with all its noises and funny faces and awkward positions. The personal intensity of sex with its passion and perspiration intimidates me."

- She says, "I hate sex in the morning—I'm not a morning person, and then I seep semen all day." He says, "She turns into a pumpkin at nine at night, and that's just when I am getting going."

Your environment does not always cooperate, encourage, and support lovemaking. Time is difficult to come by, and children's many demands interfere. The physicalness of sex is not always stately and smooth, birth control can be a nuisance, and bodies are more real than romantic at times. Minimizing the mess and controlling the environment are integral parts of making love. You can learn to relax and handle the untidy in style, or you can let God's wonderful gift of sex be sabotaged. You may discover that what you thought was an unpleasant aspect of sex can actually be a fun part of mutual lovemaking.

The above complaints are organized into four separate categories that we will work through together. This is not an exciting or erotically arousing chapter, but very practical and important. Often the little things mess up a great sex life.

GETTING PHYSICAL

One woman felt that sex was animalistic. She was a romantic who much preferred her dating days. At that time, she and her husband-to-be were usually at their best (clean, rested, and dressed up), on their way out on a date. She enjoyed kissing and flirting and being feminine without the physicalness of their present sexuality. She detested his demands and the coarse thrusting of intercourse, and all the secretions seemed so uncouth. She was disappointed that sex involved the reality of bodies and could not remain more romantic and civilized.

Though this reaction may be a little unusual, all of us are sometimes put off by the reality of semen, vaginal secretions, the noises of the penis in the vagina or the vagina releasing trapped air, and the funny contortions of sexual ecstasy or intercourse. But these are all part of making love. They can actually create erotic arousal and playfulness or at least be minimized as they are dealt with matter-of-factly or humorously.

Physical Sexuality

A fundamental part of making love is that it is passionate, with physical arousal, active loveplay, and noise. If you are an emotional person who can go down a waterslide with your mouth wide open and screaming, the passionate part of sex won't seem that messy. If you enjoy sports and perspiring and don't worry about making a face and grunting when you hit a tennis ball, you probably won't be put off by the sheer physicalness of making love on a summer afternoon.

But you may not like to sweat or get too involved in feelings. You may have to give yourself permission to be erotically physical as you allow this activity to grow into being more romantic. As adults, we often forget how to be truly excited and let go of control. Being wildly abandoned as you revel in your body and the body of your mate can seem very untidy and uncontrolled. To be a great lover, you will have to be open to becoming passionate and be adaptable to change as you learn to enjoy new and exciting experiences.

You'll make funny noises and unsettling mistakes as you enjoy making love. At some point most husbands ejaculate all over their wives' tummies; or vocal excitement may render a wife nearly deaf if his mouth is too close to her ear; or the wife may dribble evidence of her husband's recently spent passion when she sits astride his body. The vagina will make noises as air escapes; the wife's body will be spread in gymnastic contortions. If you don't have a sense of humor or can't forgive yourself and your mate, sex won't be very much fun. Being sensual, passionate, and playful is never neat. Bodies and their functions are never totally romantic, but they can create some marvelous sexual connection.

It won't happen overnight, but active thrusting, sweat, semen, and vaginal secretions will become arousing stimulants of pleasure and sexual excitement as you associate them with your mate and fun times together. You and your mate can be open to each other's feelings. You both can make an effort to anticipate when the other may consider seepage or contact with the body's natural fluids to be unpleasant. The love you have for each other encourages you to control some activities (like climaxing in her mouth or dealing with menstrual flow) so that enjoyment is equal. A box of tissues is a smart thing to keep near the bed to help you minimize the messiness. Making love will slowly cease to seem as unpleasant or out of control as you take steps to lessen the interferences and to slowly change some attitudes.

Menstrual Cycle

What is a good rule of thumb for lovemaking when the wife is in her menstrual cycle? Like other types of sexual interaction, it depends on the sensibilities of the individuals and the couple. Please sort through this situation carefully. Many couples lose some opportune times for making love by completely avoiding intercourse or other loveplay during this time. God may also be instituting a break or encouragement to engage in sex play other than intercourse. There are some commonsense ideas that you will need to discuss together as sexual lovers and partners.

First, there is nothing dirty about the menstrual flow, and there is nothing wrong with having sex during this time if a couple wishes. Both mates may have negative attitudes they need to talk through and resolve.

Second, the vagina and genitals can be tender during the menstrual cycle, and during the heavy flow, many men and women prefer not to have intercourse. That does not negate making love—which you never want to associate solely with intercourse. There can still be mutual pleasuring through to orgasm and fun sex play. Because of aesthetics or tenderness, you may wish to avoid the days of heavy flow altogether.

Third, though not foolproof, during and immediately after the cycle are safe times to have sex with a very low risk of pregnancy. Many couples enjoy sex during the lighter flow at the end of the period. They may put a towel under them during intercourse and keep tissues or a washcloth handy for cleanup afterward. Some couples find it enjoyable to have intercourse regardless of flow and take a quick shower after or even make love in the shower. It depends on you or your mate's sensitivities.

If you have not taken the time to talk through this aspect of minimizing the mess, do it now. You may assume you know what your mate thinks and feels, but your assumptions could get you in trouble and rob you of many permitted pleasures. Let the wife tell of her growing-up experiences and how she has felt about her period over her developmental years. How does each of you feel aesthetically, and what would you feel comfortable trying sexually, during the menstrual cycle? Talk it through and come to some mutual understandings.

Pregnancy

The exciting time of conceiving or expecting a child is a hurdle that many couples face, along with the demands of children, in keeping their sex lives active and enjoyable. The issues of conceiving and infertility, with their impact on making love, will be covered in Chapter 25. Chapter 19 further develops lovemaking during the children years and discusses sex during pregnancy.

A final word about sex and pregnancy: Some couples have difficulty getting their sex lives started again after the baby comes. This is especially so if the pregnancy was difficult or surgery was necessary. You may wish to incorporate some of the ideas on sexual desire and making love discussed in Chapter 18 and get beyond the awkwardness. If it has been more than two months since you have made love, make a choice to do so this weekend or seek counseling.

BIRTH CONTROL AND LUBRICATION

The Genesis passage on being fruitful and multiplying is in the context of God's giving humankind control of the natural world. We are to be wise stewards of the children God places in our care. To choose to have one or two or five has to be a thoughtful and prayerful decision.

You as a couple will have to sort through which method of birth control best fits you as you consider personal sensitivities and values. Some of you may come from a Catholic back-

Time Out: Stop a minute and talk about the physical aspects of sex with your mate. What part of physical sex is tough for you or causes some misgivings? Don't simply hint around. Be specific in your comments and communicate your feelings in love.

ground and will have to sort through this whole concept. It is good for all of us to remember that God values family and procreation with the planting of seed and the possibility of conception. Thinking through birth control requires us to sort through our theology of procreation and life, and the deeper meaning of lovemaking in God's overall sexual economy.

Birth Control

Here are nine common methods of birth control. You as a couple will have to sort through which one is most applicable along lines of personal sensitivities, health, and who takes responsibility. Withdrawal of the penis before ejaculation is not included as a method of birth control because of its ineffectiveness. There are millions of sperm in one ejaculation, and it takes only one to cause fertilization. Sperm are present in the seepage before ejaculation as well, and it is difficult to time the withdrawal exactly. Recognize that *some of the failures of birth control are due to improper usage.* Putting on a condom after thrusting has begun is like practicing the withdrawal method with sperm already present in the vagina.

I have abbreviated this section knowing that you can get more information through your physician or the Internet as needed, but here are the common methods of birth control. Obviously, none of these methods will be effective *unless carefully followed.* Birth control can either dump on your sex life or you can learn to manage it gracefully. The different types are as follows:

1. Rhythm or natural method. This method is based on the fact that pregnancy occurs during ovulation, when the sperm meets the egg. If you are trying to keep from getting pregnant, you will not want to have intercourse during the time of ovulation. Sperm live approximately two days and the female egg one day unless fertilized. Four methods are used to predict ovulation and gauge a "safe" period of time for intercourse. The first uses the calendar and considers that ovulation occurs around fourteen days before the onset of the menstrual flow. The second way of determining ovulation is through the woman's charting her temperature upon awakening. The third method involves observing the cervical mucus and learning the natural changes in its consistency near the time of ovulation. The fourth involves the test that can chemically detect if ovulation is occurring.

The rhythm method poses no health risk and does not include apparatus to dampen spontaneity. It does put a damper on intercourse during a significant part of the month. Before excluding this method, take the time to read a little about it.

2. Hormonal interventions. Birth control pills contain the synthetic hormone estrogen or progestin or a combination of the two. The pills alter the body's hormone balance and (a) prevent the ovaries from ovulating, (b) change the consistency of the cervical mucus, and (c) change the consistency of the fallopian tubes and the uterus. An advantage of the pill is that it does not interfere with naturalness. A couple can make love as the mood strikes. The pill, if properly used, has a high success rate of preventing pregnancy, although nothing is foolproof. It also can have side effects of weight gain and *dampening of sexual desire*, so keep consulting with your physician. Progesterone is also utilized with Norplant, which is inserted under the skin and can last up to five years. The Nuva Ring is inserted in the vagina much as a diaphragm with progesterone for three weeks. It is taken out during the menstrual cycle. These last two methods absorb the progesterone into the body and by-pass the liver unlike oral contraception.

3. Condoms. Condom use is a method of birth control that the husband can take responsibility for. Here are some important instructions:

- Put the condom on before approaching the vagina, and be careful not to get seepage on the outside of the condom.

- Use a new condom for every ejaculation or act of intercourse—this prevents seepage or breakage with sperm in the condom.

- Withdraw the penis before the erection is fully lost, and above all, hold the condom as you withdraw the penis to prevent its slipping off.

An advantage of condoms is that they are easily available and effective if properly used, perhaps in conjunction with a spermicidal jelly. A disadvantage is that some men and women dislike the reduced sensation in the penis or the vagina. Condoms and other methods of birth control like a diaphragm can be incorporated into your lovemaking. The wife can help create a romantic mood by unrolling the condom on her husband's penis as part of the loveplay.

4. Female condom. Female condoms are not a new concept but have more recently been brought back on the market. Like the male condom, it is made of a thin, strong latex and is a sheath. The female variety has a flexible ring at each end and is inserted into the vagina before intercourse. The rings keep it in place and it creates a protective lining in the vagina to contain the penis and sperm. The instructions for the male condom apply also to the female condom. Any barrier method loses some of the spontaneity.

5. Diaphragm and cervical cap. A diaphragm and a cervical cap are round rubber devices with a covered metal rim. Each is inserted into the vagina with spermicidal jelly, foam, or suppository as a barrier against the sperm swimming into the cervix and uterus. The diaphragm is inserted in the vagina behind the pubic bone and holds the spermicide over the cervix. The cervical cap is a smaller version of the diaphragm and covers only the cervix. A diaphragm or a cap needs to be fitted and prescribed by a gynecologist. Its advantage (like the sponge) is that it is easy to use and can be inserted prior to making love.

6. Spermicidal sponge. Available over the counter, the spermicidal sponge is dampened with water before inserting it into the vagina. This action releases the spermicidal foam. The sponge acts as a barrier, and it has spermicide to counteract impregnation. Like any barrier method, it is still somewhat intrusive and has to be prepared for ahead of time.

7. Intrauterine devices. The intrauterine device is a small coil or loop inserted into the uterus. Once inserted, it can be left in place for a year or more. It works by causing the uterus to reject the fertilized egg, so for some couples, this might violate personal ethics. The IUD is long-term and effective and does not have the mess of the barrier methods. But some IUDs have caused infections in the uterus and must be used with caution. For some women, they are still effective when used under a physician's care.

8. Spermicidal foam, jelly, and suppository. These chemicals are inserted into the vagina and kill the sperm, but some women have to experiment to find ones that don't cause an allergic reaction. The spermicides can be used alone as a method of birth control, but this is not recommended. They are much more effective if used with a condom or a diaphragm.

9. Vasectomy or tubal ligation. A vasectomy is a fairly simple office procedure in which the physician makes a small incision in the scrotal sac and a portion of each vas deferens is cut off and the ends are tied. Sperm are prevented from swimming from the testicles to the seminal fluid. A vasectomy does not alter ejaculation or the presence of semen and does not interfere with hormones and sexual desire.

The procedure is nearly 100 percent effective—but only if done properly. Occasionally, a tube will come untied and heal back, but that is very rare. Vasectomy should be considered irreversible and be done only as a permanent form of birth control. Surgical procedures may reverse a vasectomy, but they are not always effective. After a vasectomy, at least two sperm counts in the following months are taken to be certain that all sperm is out of the system and intercourse is safe without risk of pregnancy.

A tubal ligation is a hospital procedure and more complex than a vasectomy. Like a vasectomy, this method should be seen as irreversible and done only when no more children are desired. In this procedure, the female tubes are tied or cut and sutured to prevent the egg from meeting with the sperm. This is accomplished through a small incision in the abdomen. The advantage of a vasectomy or tubal ligation is its permanence. It is perhaps as foolproof as any method in preventing pregnancy. There are occasional complications from the surgery, but they are rare.

Many failures of any method of birth control are due to the improper and careless application of that method. This is not something you can afford to get sloppy about or take chances with.

Pray that God will help you remain wise, careful, and disciplined in this area of your life. It's a necessary part of lovemaking and you can learn to gracefully adjust.

Types of Lubrication

In response to thrusting and other stimulation, our bodies produce lubrication to prepare for intercourse. The fact of the matter is that this will not always be adequate even if you are young and healthy. You may be taking a decongestant that is making you dry or prolonged lovemaking may need something extra. Every couple should have some artificial lubrication handy to use as needed as an aid to great lovemaking.

Many drugstores sell a variety of artificial lubricants in the same section as the condoms and spermicides. Vaseline is an old standby, but because it is not water soluble, it can be more difficult for the vagina to be self-cleansing and for cleanup in general. K-Y Jelly is another standby that works well. Some couples complain that K-Y dries out, and they prefer a different type such as Astroglide or Wet. These are more liquid and come in a small plastic dispenser. Wet also make its Fun Flavors lubricants that taste good if oral stimulation is also going to be enjoyed.

The type of lubrication that some women appreciate is a vaginal suppository. It is not a spermicidal suppository but a lubricant that slowly dissolves. One of these vaginal suppositories, called Lubrin, assists and mixes with the vaginal secretions. It can be inserted fifteen to thirty minutes before intercourse to allow it to dissolve.

Many couples find natural oils from coconut to olive oil appealing for smell and consistency. They are edible and don't interfere with oral stimulation of the genitals. Vegetable oils (corn or safflower) work fine if you have forgotten to get something you like better. Take some time to experiment and find out what works best for you.

Minimizing Birth Control and Lubrication

A theme of this chapter is minimizing the messy, or needed-but-nuisance, parts of sex. However, even better than minimizing the mess is taking these untidy aspects of sex and incorporating them in such a way that they enhance your lovemaking. You as lovers can make birth control and lubrication easier and more erotic.

Keep supplies readily available and easy to put into action. Getting up from bed and going to get them, not having them handy, or forgetting to purchase them puts a damper on spontaneity. Incorporate them into your loveplay and erotic arousal. Putting on the condom or inserting the diaphragm can be very stimulating. Lubrication can be slowly and sensuously applied.

Both of you take responsibility for birth control and lubrication. Don't make it the sole job of either mate. Share in the purchase and use of whatever method you choose, stay creative, and keep a fun variety. Try different kinds of lubrication. Sometimes don't include intercourse so you don't have to deal with birth control if you are using a barrier method. Keep as spontaneous, playful, and sensuous as you can.

PERSONAL AND ENVIRONMENTAL TIMING

As much as a couple might like it, spontaneous and exciting sex doesn't happen that often. Consider this normal couple with two children. The husband's job is demanding and requires some travel, and the wife works part-time at a dentist's office. She doesn't start functioning until three cups of coffee and after a time to slowly wake herself in the mornings. The husband turns into a pumpkin at ten o'clock every night. The two boys are very active and demand their share of attention.

It does not take a marriage and sex therapist to see some problems plaguing this couple's sex life. You also have to throw into this equation that the wife is a perfectionist who needs structure and routines in her life, and is given to worry. The husband flies by the seat of his pants, is always late, and has a penchant for procrastinating. She is not known for her flexibility, nor he for his sensitivity. With some work, they actually ended up with a very active and fulfilling sex life as they learned to minimize the messy distractions.

Children

Chapter 19 deals more in depth with this fun nuisance in every parent's love life. I have never met a parent who could truly understand how much kids affect a sex life until they are into the experience. From the fatigue of early infancy, to the demands of an active toddler, to the interruptions of elementary days, to the late nights of the teenager—parents must deal with the confusing variable that children present to their lovemaking.

Personality Differences

One husband had a good friend to whom he could talk about anything. He had great discussions with his friend, who had some of the same personality differences in his sex life. The friend was a morning person, too. They both loved vacations for the same reason. The friend said he had made an agreement with his wife that once a month she would surprise him with a quickie in the morning before work. He in turn agreed that they would, at least once a month, have a long, leisurely late-night session after a romantic date. Both men comiserated that PMS was a real obstacle and necessary to negotiate around.

The friend was fussy and could get stuck in sexual routines without much spontaneity and variety. He and his wife tried once a week to make love using variety as their theme. They would try different places, techniques, lengths of time, and loveplay. This challenged him and thrilled his wife, who grew weary of his need for controlled routine. With the first couple, it was interesting that though the wife was more controlled and structured, she could actually be more playful and adventurous in expressing feelings than her husband. He was the one who had to allow himself to truly enjoy the roller-coaster ride of feelings.

It helped this husband to talk to his friend. He got rid of some of his self-pity and help-lessness. He decided to become more proactive in minimizing personality differences with his wife; they were just a part of the sex life of any normal couple. He could become more passionate, and she could become more flexible. They could continue to seek compromises on issues, like being a night person versus a day person. He also fretted over basic gender differences and his need for more visual variety and her desire for erotic romanticism with extended loveplay. With creativity, they often came up with solutions that met the needs of both.

Timing

Any way she sliced it, however, the wife did not appreciate her husband's timing, and there were occasions she saw it as a big nuisance to take all of her clothes off again. Having sex without messing up her makeup and hair was very difficult. It wasn't that she minded getting sweaty and making love actively. But the mornings before work just weren't very convenient, and on weekends the boys interfered or the family was on the way to participate in some activity. As much as she enjoyed sex, she was surprised she thought that it was an inconvenience and how tough it was to increase the frequency.

The more you make love, the more you will make love. Busy couples don't have a choice but to structure times that they make sacred and reserve for lovemaking. This couple found a real solution with Saturday mornings, and they tried to seek out one weeknight that would work. They ended up having to plan a different night each week, but they decided on Sunday evenings which night it would be, when they knew their weekly schedules.

The husband found he could help his wife minimize the mess with more sensitive initiating, and he felt she became more adaptable. They sometimes made love without taking all their clothes off, or she would pleasure him to an orgasm and then take off on her errands. He learned to catch her earlier before she had taken her bath or was completely dressed. He helped her with chores and got her to come to bed earlier so they could make love before he conked out. It was a constant effort to work on timing and prioritizing sex in their busy schedules. Vacations really helped, and they did better in making quality time to connect and play sexually during the week.

Hygiene and Cleanup

The husband, in his hang-loose attitude toward life, did not always pay attention to whether he was shaved and showered. He slowly discovered that a freshly shaved face with cologne and a body smelling of soap made his wife feel romantic and special. He had to admit he associated many erotic memories with the smell of Irish Spring. Her favorite bubble bath was lilac scented, and she was much more open to sex after a leisurely soak. He never thought of her genital area as dirty in any way, but he appreciated its soft lilac fragrance after her bath.

Fortunately, they learned to talk and share openly with each other and express their needs concerning hygiene and personal sensitivities. She actually found active sex very stimulating, and perspiring with her man was exciting. She explained that in her mind, freshly brushed teeth and a quick shower showed respect and forethought to their lovemaking process. She also agreed that a spontaneous romp once in a while was fun.

The wife was on the pill and appreciated the freedom it gave her in making love. There was one time, though, when she envied her friend who used a diaphragm, and inserted it right before making love during her period. She thought about getting fitted for one just to make sex easier during that time of the month.

When they were first married, the wife had thought she would need to douche after sex or during her period to keep odors at a minimum. Her gynecologist told her that this would not be good for her vagina. It could upset the bacterial balance and make her prone to yeast infections; and it is actually unnecessary because the vagina is self-cleansing and some odors are just a part of sex and periods.

The biggest fight the couple had was over his irritating habit of jumping up immediately after ejaculation to run to the bathroom and wipe himself off. After he climaxed, she wanted him to lie there with her and feel close. Even after his erection went down, she did not want the afterglow interrupted. He said that he not only worried about dripping on the sheets but also assumed that she felt very uncomfortable. Usually, that would be true of his wife, but in reality very little semen leaked out. Basking in the warm, close connectedness overrode her need for tidiness, and she wanted her husband to lie still and hold her.

The compromise was really quite simple, and they felt a little silly later when thinking what a major issue it had become. They kept some tissues beside the bed. He could wipe off, and she could quickly place a couple between her legs without ruining the mood. She also bought some panty shields. After a quickie in the morning, she wore them as protection against any seepage during the day.

Often couples learn that minimizing the mess has many creative compromises and solutions. Keeping tissues or a washcloth by the bed, planning ahead on birth control and lubrication, and relaxing with the normal aspects of the human body and its functioning greatly help.

Consider these key qualities you need in dealing with the messiness of a great sex life:

- *Sense of humor*. Laughing together and not taking yourself so seriously are invaluable. Sex will be funny and full of mishaps and playfulness.
- *Flexibility*. Keep out of routines and let go of a strong need to always be in control. You

will enjoy yourself more in making love if you can go with the flow and are able to adapt.

- *Forgiveness.* Let each other make mistakes, and let go of resentment and hurt. Allow each other to change as both work through tough areas, and cut each other some slack as both focus on positive solutions. Forgiveness is the cleansing agent that helps create a great marriage and sex life.

- *Effective communication.* A couple must be able to assertively express needs and feelings and truly hear each other. No topic is off-limits, and with dialogue and compromise, solutions can be reached.

- *Love and trust.* If you like each other and believe your mate wants you to be happy and sexually fulfilled, it is easier to discuss and negotiate. An intimate relationship is vital in responsibly using birth control, creatively experimenting, and flexibly communicating.

- *Being disciplined.* This trait may seem in direct contrast to the final point, but minimizing the mess requires both. A couple must carefully follow the prescribed birth control's directions. Remembering ahead to have tissues or lubricants can make a real difference in spontaneity.

- *Being uninhibited.* Let yourself go as you enjoy your mate and God's gift of sex. Being uninhibited and sensual has a way of overcoming and transforming the mess of sex into an aphrodisiac.

You and your partner can ensure that the untidiness of sex never gets in the way of a thriving love life. Let God give you the wisdom to find those many creative compromises and solutions. You can also grow into that place of maturity where you live more easily with the messiness of life and lovemaking.

CHAPTER SIX

Natural Aphrodisiacs and Creating a Mood

THE QUESTION IS OFTEN ASKED and has been pursued down through the centuries: "Are there sexual aphrodisiacs?" Ginseng root, hormones, Viagra, special herbs or teas—nothing has been proven to work universally. If it seems to help, you may not want to discontinue it; however, some chemicals that can be harmful to physical or relational health should be avoided. Drugs like alcohol or marijuana may relax you or lower inhibitions, but they do nothing for sexual performance. If taken in excess, they dampen sexual arousal and the ability to enjoy making love.

Here's the good news. Our gracious Creator has provided us as couples many natural and revitalizing aphrodisiacs that we constantly neglect—to the detriment of our lovemaking. These aphrodisiacs can greatly enhance our love lives. The first section of this chapter identifies these natural aphrodisiacs. The second section discusses setting sexual goals for your relationship. Overcommitted couples (that's you) won't have much quantity or quality in lovemaking unless goals are set and a bonding sex life is given a priority. The third section explores further ideas for creating an ambiance for making love—focusing on the bedroom environment.

NATURAL APHRODISIACS

God has freely given you many natural ways to enhance your lovemaking. Discover them along with your mate.

Taking Time and Focusing on the Moment

Take time to enjoy each other sexually. Taking more time increases loveplay and, in a fun way, forces you into being more creative. One of the building blocks of a great sex life is taking sufficient time to enjoy each other, and both enjoy the extra attention and playfulness.

Taking time is a marvelous aphrodisiac because it allows a couple to create an ambiance and be more imaginatively sensual. If ten minutes of mood-setting and loveplay enhance sensuality, forty minutes may do four times as much for intimacy. Time gives you the luxury of thinking about and enjoying sexuality in old and new ways.

Another aphrodisiac with time is focusing in and enjoying truly being present with your mate. It isn't just time, but tuning in to the erotic and the three-dimensional love relationship while you have the time. There is an art, which wives have a more difficult time practicing, of leaving distractions and concerns while you enjoy this moment with your lover. You must learn to think, *This thirty minutes is totally for us and will be sacredly spent sexually connecting.*

Initiative and Frequency Versus Inertia

Vacations are an interesting time of discovering natural aphrodisiacs. On vacation couples expect to make love. Away from their many distractions, mates suddenly think about lovemaking and are unexpectedly frisky. They often make a mental note of things they have been avoiding in enhancing their sex lives and want to be sure to include while away. They take props, such as sexy outfits and books like this one. The mind and attitude are more sexually specific and expectant than when at home. Mates take time to hold hands and have connecting conversations, and they create initiative that is absent in the busyness of life.

So many things in life have a way of snowballing. The more you do them, the easier they become and the more you want to do them—like a snowball rolling downhill and picking up more snow as it goes. It is like the law of inertia, which states that a body in motion tends to stay in motion and a body at rest tends to stay at rest. If sex has become awkward or if it has been placed on the back burner, mates will consciously have to get the lovemaking started again. A sex life in motion tends to pick up speed, and the couple that makes love once a month will soon be making love once every three months.

Physical Fitness, Rest, and Affection

Good health and physical fitness are marvelous aphrodisiacs. Being rested vitalizes attitudes and gives added capacity for sex. Getting the body in shape with long walks or other forms of exercise enhances sex. Making vigorous love affirms your sense of physical well-being.

Rest and physical closeness have a marvelous effect on the mind and heart. Each of us has

Time Out: You don't have to wait for a vacation to enhance your sex life. Make love every day for five days in a row! Start on Thursday and have sexual activity every day through Monday. (The weekend times should be easier than weekdays.) Sex will become an expected part of each day's activity, and you will learn so much about initiative and making love as you overcome fatigue and other obstacles.

a skin hunger that is more a need for affirmation and comfort than erotic interaction. Tuning out the world and making time for relaxed touching may be tough in the busyness of life but is a great aphrodisiac. Somehow couples need to create their own insulated islands where they can retreat for long hugs as well as passionate lovemaking. You may need to deal with your environment better so it can encourage you in being rested and affectionate.

Adventure, Variety, and Uninhibited Feelings

God has created us with a desire for variety and adventure. Uninhibited and varied sex is arousing. Wives wearing see-through lingerie or the husband buying a special CD may sexually excite both partners. You may want to try some new positions. Or the wife may allow the husband to orally bring her to an orgasm for the first time.

Make sure you stay within God's economy in enjoying variety. Keep adventures within the love and respect each has for the other's feelings, and don't pressure each other. Let your creative minds and loving companionship produce the ultimate in electricity and adventure. Determine to be more experimental, curious, and adventuresome in lovemaking. Explore individual inspirations and risk being uncomfortable trying new things.

Adventure can be enhanced as you also find the energy and childlikeness to give way to uninhibited feelings. Getting excited, silly, truly alive and aroused has a marvelous aphrodisiac effect. Romp in the shower, groan in passionate ecstasy, and have long gourmet sessions of fun feelings.

Traditions

Here is another of those paradoxes, and we need both sides for exciting sexual intimacy. God is a God of adventure and variety but is also the same yesterday, today, and forever. Comfortable patterns and consistent enjoyment are also a part of aphrodisiacs. Couples will have positions of intercourse, special touches, and certain places they will return to again and again. Familiarity can breed joy and arousal.

Intimate Companionship

A fun companionship stimulates a great sex life. If you feel *in* love, you will be more likely to *make* love. Here are some ways to maintain sexual closeness:

Plan more regular vacations. Be creative. A vacation doesn't have to be a week in the Bahamas. But busy couples should plan at least two one-week vacations and six other overnights or long weekends in a year. It isn't an option if you are a busy couple wanting to revitalize your companionship and lovemaking.

Plan date nights for romantic companionship. Make a date night at least twice a month, and go out to enjoy each other. Find a window of time to talk each night, and keep in better touch with each other through phone and e-mail. Connection really helps both partners feel like making love more often.

Plan surprises for variety and routines for closeness. Try new sexual techniques. Make sure you've taken privacy precautions and then make love in every room of the house, in the shower, or in both cars. Plan surprises for each other from a romantic video to some fabulous-smelling body lotion. Be playful with each other.

Couples also need routines to foster that loving interaction. Concentrate more on simple, nurturing gestures like kissing each other when one or both leave or get home from work. Go to bed together and hug nude for a minute before putting on nightclothes. Talk for ten minutes after meals or hold hands in the car. Routines maintain closeness.

Set goals and prioritize. Commit to certain days to make love. Negotiate in structured time for sex. Make it a priority that you won't bump from your schedule.

SEXUAL GOAL SETTING

A Rose Parade float is an excellent analogy for a couple's sex life. The beauty, creativity, delightful movements, and sensuous appeal are awe-inspiring. All of this is made possible because of the inner framework, motors, and a driver. The beautiful flowers and motions of the float that are visible to the eye are anchored to and driven by an inner structure of steel, wood, and ingeniously programmed motors, all consciously guided by a human driver.

Does your float lack beauty, creativity, motion, and sensuality because its inner structure is defective? Begin working from the inside out. Consciously decide together that sex is going to be a priority.

Every busy couple needs a structured framework on which to create a beautiful love life. There are two separate tasks that comprise this framework: negotiating realistic goals and prioritizing them. Remember that sex is *not* the most important part of your marriage. You may need to take these goal-setting and prioritizing ideas and apply them to many other areas of your partnership in addition to your lovemaking. Do you pray together, have regular companionship time, enjoy family devotions, and budget your money? These are vital areas to set effective goals and may need to be implemented before your sex life can flourish.

Setting Effective Sexual Goals

Beginning goals may be to choose when during the week and when during the weekend you are going to make love, and then to set that time aside as sacred to each of you. As busy as your schedules are, if you don't find your optimal times and structure in making love, you will have sex about once a month. And you do not have to destroy your spontaneity. Goal setting is simply the inner structure and doesn't have to dampen excitement and creativity.

Sexual goals involve more than frequency. They should also deal with the quality of your lovemaking and the quality of your intimate companionship. Goals may include reading at least a chapter a month in a book on sex, each mate initiating one new technique or idea as a contribution to creativity and variety, scheduling regular vacation times, and planning new things for the lovemaking. Goals need to be:

1. Specific. "We will make love more often" is not an effective goal. It must be more specific and include behavioral steps so you can tell if you have accomplished it. "We will have the kids in bed by 9:00 P.M. on Tuesday and make love immediately before doing any chores" is specific and measurable. Having a quickie once in a while is not specific enough for the busy couple. You can allow for spontaneity and yet still be more specific: "Wednesday and Friday mornings I don't have to go to work as early. I would enjoy making love a couple of times a month on these days. If it's okay with you, since I am a morning person, I will initiate and get the birth control ready."

2. Realistic and attainable. Goals should take small steps as mates start to make changes so they won't be overwhelming. Goals that are not reasonable and do not consider time, energy, and money demands will quickly be sabotaged. "We will make love four times a week" or "Let's redecorate the bedroom" may be too optimistic. "Let's get some new sheets and some scented candles" or "Let's make love on Saturday mornings" may be more realistic.

3. Scheduled. If you don't give your goals specific time guidelines, you may not accomplish them. Scheduling includes not only when you will do something but also when you will begin doing it and how long you will try to keep doing it. "Let's try to be more creative in our lovemaking" is neither specific enough nor is it scheduled. This goal will probably never be accomplished, or it may be done sporadically. Effective scheduling would redefine this goal: "Each of us will read about and incorporate one new idea into our lovemaking each month, starting in September."

Goal setting takes negotiating and much thoughtful introspection and prayer. Each of you may want to think through what is important sexually and then discuss it. You may need to do this on a weekend away with time for discussion. In doing so, you are wisely committing to nurture your marital companionship and sex life.

Time Out: Negotiate together how many times a week you would like to make love. Be specific and realistic. Schedule definite days and hours. This internal structure will help you be spontaneous, creative, and playful. How might you both sabotage this scheduled time and not keep it sacred?

4. Prioritized. It is not enough to have goals that are specific, realistic, and scheduled. You as a couple will have to consciously choose to make them a priority and follow through on them. Some of you who are reading this book haven't had sex in months or years, or your lovemaking is the main point of conflict in an otherwise great marriage. Change won't be easy. Here are some ways to make your sexual goals a priority that will help you accomplish them over the long haul:

- Choose a limited number of goals and make them baby steps. (Example: "We will have sexual closeness once a week on Sunday afternoon.")
- Mutually explore and acknowledge the vital importance of your selected goals, and then covenant together to follow through on them. (Example: "I am sorry for our sexual deficits. I will pray daily, and we will lift up this request every time we say grace over meals.")
- Create individual and marital attitudes that will support your goals. (Example: "I will hug my mate three times every day and do one thing each day that might make him or her want to make love.")
- Establish a lifestyle conducive to accomplishing the goals. (Example: "We will create a great baby-sitting network.")
- Set up specific behaviors that you flag as warning signals when your goals are being sabotaged. (Example: "Neither of us can cancel a vacation without a long discussion and another time being agreed upon.")

CREATING A MOOD

Setting the mood is the backbone of being romantic and creating exciting variety in your love life, and it involves at least three different aspects of your lovemaking.

Mental Mood Setting

Mental mood setting includes using your mind and will to fantasize about sex and to choose to tune in to sexual cues as you structure making love into your marriage. As you tune in to sexual cues mentally, you can relax in your masculinity or femininity, fantasize about your mate, and set goals.

Wives, this will be especially important for you. During a busy day, you may need to stop and think about sex and allow yourself to feel sexual. I remember one wife who related in counseling that she wore a new teddy and somehow it felt different and reminded her all day of her sexuality. She jumped her husband when he came home, much to his delight. You may have to put "TS" on your calendar as you "Think Sex."

Emotional Atmosphere

Emotional mood setting means creating an atmosphere in which you can be rested, excited, and warmly intimate. Good sex is predicated on an emotional mood and atmosphere. It involves enjoying adventure, being stress-free, and feeling in love enough to focus on your sexual feelings. Creating this emotional atmosphere will be developed more in the section on becoming passionate lovers (in Chapter 15). Remember, great lovemaking is more about who you are rather than simply what you do.

Environmental Ambiance

Environmental mood setting encourages romantic ambiance by altering your surroundings. It involves creating an environment that enhances and stimulates sexual arousal and meaningful, exciting interaction.

To enhance environmental mood, consider mood setting in three categories: sensuality, the bedroom, and props. Some of the more playful ideas will not seem as softly romantic as candles and gentle background music. Making love to Sousa marches, squirting each other's genitals with water pistols, having a pillow fight, or finger painting each other can also set a playful ambiance and be arousing. Allow the ideas to stimulate your imagination and creativity. You, as lovers, can greatly expand on what's presented in the rest of this chapter.

Sensuality. Sight, smell, taste, hearing, and touch are the five senses to maximize as you explore creating and enjoying a romantic ambiance.

1. Sight: Male and female enjoyment of the visual may vary, but it is important to both. The husband may love to see his wife's body, and an afternoon delight with the sun shining in brightly can be very sensual. His wife may prefer gentle light that softens and dims the body while the other senses are enhanced. Experiment with lighting and find ways to add variety. Flickering candlelight gives ambiance and a pleasant scent, while leaving the bathroom door cracked may give just enough light to feel less exposed but visually connected. The partially covered is often more erotically stimulating than the fully exposed.

Couples often find strategically placed mirrors exciting, and can enjoy being aroused by all that is going on. Movement and choreography are fun turn-ons, as are seductive behavior and dances that you do for the viewing pleasure of your mate. In all of this lovemaking and sensuality, both of you need to both be yourselves and stretch yourselves. I remember a female friend of ours who related that her mom did not do that much in talking about sex, but said one thing that was very helpful: "Your husband is going to want to see you naked." We don't have to be sex maniacs, just open and playful.

Colors are visually sensual. It doesn't have to be the stereotypical red with black lace. One wife related in counseling that her husband only wanted red lingerie with black lace and it was scratchy to her. She much preferred satin in pastel colors that highlighted her skin tones and clung to her figure. Husband, don't dump on your wife's sensuality and sexuality with your narrow ideas of what is sexy. Wives, occasionally give as a gift something that your husband desires sensually. Bright satin sheets, emerald-green boxer shorts, soft peach teddies, a peacock feather—all contribute to the mood.

Go slow. Setting the mood is something you can enjoy without following through on making love. Tease and revel in your sexual feelings from the visual stimulation. Make the bedroom aesthetically appealing to the eyes and other senses. (The bedroom is important enough that we will take a separate section to discuss it.)

2. Smell: Scents are an exciting part of creating a sensual mood. The mind connects sensations such as the odor of perfume to erotic arousal and experiences. The wife's perfume may be paired in the husband's mind with her total person and especially her femininity and sexuality. Just a scent of it and he feels more in love and can become aroused. The lingering smell of suntan lotion after being on the beach can provoke it. Candles, incense, and scented lotions also add sensual pleasure and an ambiance to making love.

3. Taste: Taste is not always associated with creating sexual moods, but it is a stimulating form of sexuality. The mouth, tongue, and lips are erogenous zones with many nerve endings and a particular sensuality about them.

Lingering over a sumptuous meal is a very sensual experience. Candlelight and long conversations while having coffee and dessert are great mood setters. In the privacy of your own home, feeding each other food and placing favorite tastes in strategic places can be very erotic. There are also flavored lubricants that can be used in lovemaking and add an interesting sensuality.

4. Hearing: Soft music or your favorite song creates marvelous atmosphere. Slow-dance to songs that express the love and commitment you feel for each other. Play favorite music during sex and pair up some CDs with your arousal and excitement. You can then listen to them in the car and begin your lovemaking mentally before you arrive home. Take advantage of sexy talking and uninhibited groans and squeals of pleasure during sexual sessions.

5. Touch: Don't neglect to employ a wide variety of sensual touching experiences. Many women hate to be stimulated continuously in the same way. Try gently rubbing an ice cube over sensitive areas and revel in the sensations. Use a feather duster, satin gloves, a silk scarf, or some fur. Lotions add a different feel to the touching and caressing. Many couples find it very erotic and sensual to spread a covering out and get oily together.

Nerve endings and tactile senses can obviously involve more than touching with fingertips.

Lightly blowing can create marvelous sensations on the chest, stomach, or genital area. Breathing gently into the ear can be profoundly erotic. Taking the hair or beard and tickling or teasing sensitive areas produces great sensations. The tongue lightly licking or the mouth gently kissing like a butterfly flitting around can create delightful effects.

The bedroom. Romance and sexuality should pervade intimate companionship, and making love will be varied and should not be confined to the bedroom. Because of privacy and comfort, though, the bedroom will be the primary love nest. It is the place that can be made secluded and arousing, and it provides a place to store props like lotions and birth control. It can also have special mood-setting qualities.

Aesthetics is defined as "the art of making something beautiful or appealing to one's taste." The bedroom needs to be aesthetically appealing to you. Live flowers in a pretty vase, potpourri, mood lighting or candles, sensuous linens, and the ability to control the temperature are sexual enhancements. You are pairing in your mind the bedroom with fun, sensual, erotic experiences. Just walking into the bedroom should create a different mood.

It helps to have a bed that doesn't squeak and a comfortable mattress; these may be necessary expenditures for your love life. Make sure the room is secure against children, with a lock on the door, and train them to respect your privacy when they find it locked. The bedroom is the central environmental setting for making love and creating mood. It probably has been neglected, so do some brainstorming as you spice it up.

Props. Candles, music, and lingerie stimulate ambiance. Flickering candlelight with soothing music in the background creates a totally different mood from that established by mirrors employed in an afternoon delight with some jazz on the stereo. Clothing can be endlessly varied: garters and black hose, red boxers with hearts, T-shirts and cutoffs, bathing suits, a dress shirt with nothing else, a tank top, robes and peignoir sets, teddies, matching bra and panties, a tuxedo, and the list can keep going. The creativity is not just in the clothing but how you choose to slowly take it off in a sensual, seductive manner.

Couples sometimes worry that certain props (like sexy lingerie, strategically placed mirrors, or vibrators) create artificial or sinfully seductive arousal and will detract from their natural lovemaking. God gave imaginations and romantic abilities for us to create and enjoy various means of enticing and playing with our mates, and props can be the means to enhance experiences and sensations.

Remember that props should: (1) remain playfully in perspective and never become an obsessive fetish; (2) not detract from your vulnerability and respect, because arousal is dependent on feeling safe and inviting vulnerability on all three dimensions of body, soul, and spirit; (3) never invite anyone else into your bedroom, as pornography does; and (4) enhance true three-dimensional passion and connection. Remember that sexual connecting is God's gift for demonstrating intimate love. Props should be utilized by each couple, according to what each person finds playful and intimacy-enhancing. They are simply a means to an end: creating a sexy environment and providing the tools to enhance lovemaking. The relationship and personal romantic creativity remain the foundation of great sex.

A quick comment on vibrators is in order. Some husbands worry that a vibrator can create sensations that cannot be duplicated by him in creating orgasms, and that it may become addictive. I have not seen addiction but can understand the couple who does not wish to become dependent on a vibrator to create a climax for the wife. But for some women, a vibrator can enhance their ability to achieve an orgasm and seems very appropriate. I don't think there is any Christian prohibition, and for many couples it is simply a prop that gives pleasure and is used occasionally to enhance sensual feelings.

Couples worry that they can only buy vibrators at sex shops. There are many kinds of vibrators that can be bought in regular stores or over the Internet. Smaller ones with less intensity than the larger wands for deep-muscle back massage are better in lovemaking. There are a variety of vibrators that are battery operated for easy use, but finding sources of electricity isn't really a problem in today's world.

Pillows are great to lean against as you have intimate conversations or to use in positions of pleasuring and intercourse. They help make the bed the playground it should be. Purchase various shapes and sizes, and use them to keep backs, necks, and muscles from getting too tired. Pillows can be placed strategically to lie on and prop up the genital area for more accessibility. Pillows can also have certain appealing aesthetics in decorating the bed.

Keep handy items for loveplay, from feathers to fruit and lotions to satin gloves. Oils and scented lotions add sensuality to massage as you linger over skin and muscles and curves. Items like a feather duster or satin gloves give different and stimulating sensations. You are limited only by your imagination and creativity. A certain enticing perfume sprayed lightly over hair or after-shave applied after a quick shave can become quite erotic. You may need to get a locking carrying case for your love paraphernalia that you can store out of reach of children and to easily take on vacation with you.

Don't be overwhelmed by this information on mood setting. Pick out one or two ideas in each section, and start building your ambiance skills. Don't neglect the mental, emotional, or environmental atmosphere. Learning to be uninhibited, creative, and playful will help keep long-term sexuality from becoming a routine—and it's fun!

Time Out: 1. What is your best-used sense: sight, smell, taste, hearing, or touch? Select the one least developed and try something in that area tonight.

2. If you were going to spend two hundred dollars to make your bedroom more sexy, what would you buy?

CHAPTER SEVEN

The Joy of Fantasy

OUR MIND AND THE ABILITY to think and imagine are a crucial part of being created in God's image and make us distinct from the animal kingdom. This ability to enjoy mental imagery can be used to expand and enjoy all aspects of our lives, including lovemaking. An active fantasy life can be wonderful for building a great sex life with our mate and companion.

I wonder why it is that often when I mention fantasy people think I am encouraging something very kinky or lustful. Granted, our fantasies can distort and damage our marriages if we take them outside the lines and bring other people or the unrealistic into our lovemaking. But, our minds and imaginations are erotic vehicles that take us into powerful adventures and excitement. In fact, our mind is the most erotic organ in our body.

DEFINING *FANTASY*

You use mental imagery and your imagination to enhance many areas of your life. You pray and build a meaningful concept of God by utilizing your mind and imagination and by letting the Holy Spirit direct your mind. God promises to do "immeasurably more than all we ask or imagine, according to his power that is at work within us" (Eph. 3:20 NIV). You become a wise steward of your time and relationships by building on positive experiences and mistakes, and you use the mind's repository of information to achieve this. The only way you are able to create intimate companionship is to renew your mind as you heal from negative experiences and learn to anticipate pleasure with your mate. All of this is accomplished by employing mental imagery, fantasy, and the imagination.

Sex is not excluded from these other processes. All of them use fantasy and occur in the mind and imagination. Your mind, with the ability to create and store information, is the central part of imagining and experiencing erotic pleasure. That is what sexual fantasy is all about:

your mind, images that are paired with the sexual excitement, and your imagination to give them wings.

First Peter states, "Therefore, prepare your minds for action; be self-controlled . . . Do not conform to the evil desires you had when you lived in ignorance" (1:13–14 NIV). In James we read, "Each one is tempted when he is drawn away by his own desires and enticed. Then, when desire has conceived, it gives birth to sin" (1:14–15 NKJV). Romans 12:2 talks about being "transformed by the renewing of your mind" (NKJV), and Ephesians 4:23 advises to "be renewed in the spirit of your mind" (NKJV).

In applying these passages to fantasy and lovemaking, you need to recognize that sexual desire is never wrong—it is how you choose to use the desire. You can renew your mind and prepare your imagination for the action the Lord wants you to have sexually. You can banish ignorance and sinful lusting or coveting (see Chapter 28).

These passages are encouraging for a great sex life. You can rid yourself of old messages that you must maintain control and never be passionate. You can unleash the playful and sexy parts of yourself as you romp with your mate with a renewed attitude. You can also purge your mind of any thoughts that might get in the way of uninhibited lovemaking with your mate—lustful thoughts of another person, a preoccupation with job or children, even the idea that sex is dirty. You can enjoy mental imagery and not let it become evil. You need to renew your mind so that sex is permissible, fun and, at the appropriate moment, a true priority. You can prepare for action and have a creative sexual mind-set that will result in enticing, dynamic lovemaking.

It's 80 Percent Mental

Sex is perhaps 80 percent fantasy (imagination and mind) and about 20 percent friction. Granted, pleasuring erogenous zones (friction) is fun, but what truly creates the excitement is your mind. With your mind, you can creatively set the mood and build a mental repertoire of erotically arousing experiences and images, as well as utilize your ability to imaginatively play in the joy of the moment.

For simplicity, let's divide fantasy into two areas: (1) the stored sexual information in your mind, which was given its erotic excitement by associating it with hormonal and genital arousal; and (2) your imagination's use of your erotic repertoire to create sexual attitudes and imaginary scenes and stimulate activity and excitement.

An example of the stored part of fantasy is a warm kiss, which is often an important part of making love. Over time, the brain pairs the behavior of kissing with hormonal, emotional, and relational response to stimulate sexual arousal. Kissing your spouse is a turn-on. Though your heterosexual responses were learned and stored from former experiences, making love over a long period of time with your spouse takes those cues and pairs them with your covenant partner. You continually add to that memory bank of erotic thoughts and behaviors and utilize it for enhancing lovemaking.

When you get married, your spouse's mind and your own contain all the sexual data you have read, seen, and experienced. Certain images and ideas are especially erotically charged because you have paired sexual arousal (a sexual relationship, masturbating, hormonal desires) with them. If a spouse continues to build up the nonmarital sexual pairings and collects new data from *other* visual experiences, his or her mate will feel excluded and sexual fantasies will become distorted.

It is important that you erase or refuse to "go there" mentally with some of the sexual learning and experiences from your past. They will detract from your one-flesh lovemaking. I like Proverbs 5:15, which compares a marital sex life to a cistern of water. When we marry, some of us need to drain off a few inches of sludge and distorted sexual images and memories. Carefully choose the fantasies and experiences you wish to store after you are married. The images should be about your mate and should make lovemaking more exciting. Especially guard how you use your stored repository and imagination.

A common plight of many men is that they build in their fantasy worlds ideal women with specific physical attributes, such as big breasted, tall, blonde, and blue-eyed. Yet often the wives they choose are the exact opposite. Men—and women, as well—need to keep storing new sexual information, especially about their mates, as they imagine sexy aspects of their anatomies, and sexy scenes. This is true as we grow older and bodies sag and muscle tone is fading. We must look through the eyes of love with our imaginations and allow our mate to be sexy in new ways.

Fantasy Is NOT Reality

Christ in His teaching stated, "You have heard that it was said to those of old, 'You shall not commit adultery.' But I say to you that whoever looks at a woman to lust for her has already committed adultery with her in his heart" (Matt. 5:27–28 NKJV). The Greek verb for *look* is in the imperfect tense, which is an action that starts in the past and continues into the present. It could be translated "continually look." Christ emphasized the importance of guarding the mental fantasy life. Fantasy is different from sexual actions and at times more complex to manage. He stressed that continual thinking is more likely to lead to an unfaithful heart attitude as well as to sinful behaviors.

This passage offers essential lessons about fantasy becoming sin. The sinful destructiveness of fantasy is relative to the situation and the individual person's inner attitudes. To notice a woman in a bikini or a man's strong hands is one thing. To continually fantasize about your next-door neighbor or a person at work is dangerous. That could much more easily lead to adultery. Christ also encouraged us to be careful how we build mental fantasies. Even though fantasy is not reality or as destructive as actual behavior, Christ warned that your thought life can develop in such a way as to betray your mate in your heart. The specialness of your love and commitment can be diluted—all fantasy is not innocent or productive.

In the letter to the Colossians, Paul encouraged Christians to clean up their thought lives and make wise choices in mentally pursuing sexual cues. Christians should avoid "sexual immorality, impurity, lust, evil desires" (3:5 NIV). Everyone has sexual reactions triggered by cues in the environment. That is not wrong desire but is often reflexive. You can choose what you do with that desire to keep it from evolving into sin. You can control whether you objectify a person or "continually look" to the detriment of your thought life and partnership.

It is not wrong for a man to praise the Lord for heterosexuality and the female form. Fantasies are not behaviors, and visual cues can unintentionally stimulate arousal. But, a male can tune in so much to external environmental cues that he forgets to notice his wife's feminine appeal and have a proper focus on his own special woman.

Similarly, a woman's sexual fantasies are stimulated by sensory data (for example, a romantic movie, a good-looking guy, or an affirming comment on her femininity) that go through the pipeline of her nerves to her genitals and body. A woman's response might be more general and not so genitally focused as a man's, but can also lead to counterproductive fantasy.

Remember that fantasy is not reality but does require discipline so the deeper heart issues of love are protected. Let God be in your bedroom, and He will help you keep imagination pure and growth-producing—to help you keep your desires centered on your lovemaking.

Men and women alike will experience sexual arousal as a part of the sleep cycle, with erections, lubrications, and dreams. This arousal is not unfaithfulness, and if you think about your dreams, they are probably based on your mental story of erotically arousing events or perhaps your emotional struggles at the time. You cannot control dreams, and again, fantasy is *not* reality. A great way to understand your dreams is to deal with the feelings behind them. By not being afraid of your dreams, but through exploring them and praying, you can learn from them and make necessary changes in your life.

Gender Differences

The fantasy lives of men and women are different. Stored erotic data can vary, as well as the manner in which imaginations are employed concerning these images. Saying fantasies are different says nothing about male or female capacities for enjoying fantasy. Distortions also have nothing to do with gender differences. Double standards that are not based in Scripture allow and encourage boys to be more in touch with their sexuality and to notice sexual cues in the environment more, and these same double standards encourage girls to be seductive, fearful, and repressed.

Overall, men seem to be more focused on genitals and explicit sexual activity, and women tend to be more holistic, with an enjoyment of the sensuality and personality behind the body. But men and women should not be stereotyped. Some men appreciate gentle, romantic ambiance more than their wives do. Some women may be very visually stimulated by genitals and enjoy immediate, direct sexual stimulation. There seem to be some general differences, though, that can help you understand the effective use of fantasy in your lovemaking.

Women and men may enjoy different memories of the same sexual encounter. If a couple were given the use of a private house right on the beach, for instance, the woman might remember that one night by moonlight they had made love on a blanket among the dunes between the house and beach. There was the gentle roar of the waves, and her husband had left some soft music playing on the CD player on the deck. They were warm from the day's sun and sensuously rubbed lotion on each other and passionately built up to some great sex. He rubbed her stomach and legs, taking time to enjoy her body. Afterward, they lay together on their backs and talked as they looked at the stars. It was a very bonding and romantic experience for her.

A man, however, might state how exciting it had been to set up the romantic props of the music and blanket. He had gotten an erection just thinking of the coming activity and how great his wife had looked in her bathing suit that day. He might reminisce about how that evening he slowly removed her shorts and T-shirt and the way her body glowed in the light with the highlights of tan lines and nipples and genital area. The lotion was so very sensual, and he remembered the manner in which she had undressed and caressed him. He might also be aroused by the "illicitness" of having sex under the stars as if they were sneaking in a special way to enjoy each other. (Of course, she also might have been aroused by that—husbands and wives are not always that different in their erotic arousal.)

In the above example, there are some differences. The man's attention was directed toward visual stimulation by specific physical attributes and touching of the genital area. The woman reveled in the relational and overall sensual atmosphere and her husband's "slow hands." But she does not want to be stereotyped because she, too, enjoys visual aspects of her husband's body. Fantasy makes for great sex but can be varied from husband to wife and from individual to individual.

Time Out: 1. Think of a sexual experience that you enjoyed with your mate, and each of you describe it fully. How do you two differ? How are you similar?

2. Brainstorm with your partner about how you could increase the use of your imaginations. What three things could you do to stimulate creativity?

Mental Variety

An important question is whether it is wrong to have fantasies of other people and events. When does this become destructive or dangerous? Christians need to come to grips with this issue.

The answer is important to us. Human beings are created with a need for stimulation, adventure, and variety, and sexual fantasy can help provide both. God has shown, though, that any thought or behavior that detracts from enjoying your mate sexually is wrong and outside His blueprint for building intimate companionship and a great sex life.

As it happens so often in applying God's principles to our lives, "All things are lawful for me, but all things are not helpful. All things are lawful for me, but I will not be brought under the power of any" (1 Cor. 6:12 NKJV). Is it destructive to see and be excited by environmental sexual cues? There are few times we can be in public—whether at the beach or shopping malls—without getting sexually stimulated. This is not wrong. But not controlling our eyes, thoughts, and impulses can become sinful and destructive to our relationships.

You may want to become more selective in what movies and television shows you watch. Some movies may stimulate your enjoyment of your spouse; others create sexual imagery that does not help you enhance your sex life. Certain types of romantic novels may be too detracting from your lovemaking and get your mind into potentially dangerous patterns of thinking sexually. So many plots are built on adultery and casual sexual encounters.

Is it wrong to fantasize having sexual activity with an imaginary person or an actor or actress on the screen? Is it okay to think back on past situations that were arousing? We as Christians have been reluctant to talk about these subjects. Everyone has fantasies about other people, and they can be destructive to your commitment to building sexual intimacy. Fantasy is important, but it should be centered on your mate and the fantastic sex life you are creating together.

Fantasy gives your imagination the opportunity to add variety within your marriage without the destructiveness of sampling greener grass. You can go to Hawaii or the Riviera; you can make love on a secluded beach; you can enjoy all over again favorite times with your mate.

One woman was curious about what it would be like to make love to a different man. What she needed, however, was mental variety and a better sex life rather than an entirely different man. She needed to remember that one body is pretty much the same as another. Her more basic curiosity was a special mood, some novel experiences, someone to touch her sexuality in deeper and more exciting ways. An affair may very well not meet these needs and would certainly destroy the honesty and trust of her marriage. If she was willing to work at it with her husband, she could meet her needs wonderfully with him.

A questionable part of fantasy is that, like masturbation, it is at times an individual sexual activity. Christians don't have too much trouble with the mutual part of sexuality, but the individual part is harder to sort out. In fact, the personal fantasies that accompany masturbation or even lovemaking often raise objections. We need to be comfortable with our personal sexuality and revel in our orgasms and feelings, as we create the mood for adventurous intimacy. But fantastic sex is designed to be a mutual experience, and individual fantasy should always enhance, rather than detract from, mutual lovemaking.

Enhancing Lovemaking

Sexual imagery and imagination should be used toward the goal of increasing the enjoyment and intimacy of lovemaking. Here are some rules of thumb that can help you maximize your mental fantasy life. They can help you, whether individually or mutually, to keep your fantasy skills and usage within God's sexual economy as it enhances lovemaking.

Keep environmental cues disciplined. It is great to be heterosexual and enjoy the opposite sex. But you can make choices about how this enjoyment can be controlled. Guys, it helps to employ the one-second rule and keep your gaze moving rather than lingering. You can enjoy and be enriched by variety and romance without detracting from your commitment to enhancing your sex life as you eroticize your mate. If this doesn't happen, and you are fantasizing about something else during lovemaking, you are diminishing your relationship and sexual partnership.

Keep intentional fantasies centered on your mate. One man who went to many conferences built a fantasy in which he met a sexy woman who seduced him in his hotel room. Unfortunately, he never took his wife to the conferences. You know the sad outcome of this story and what happened at a conference. You should keep all fantasies that you willfully (intentionally) create focused on your partner. Sinful diluting of intimacy and acting out sexually are encouraged by continual, intentional fantasies about a person or situation outside your marriage.

Keep the enhancement of your lovemaking the primary focus. Continued fantasies about women with big breasts or men with muscular shoulders are stupid if your spouse is small. The same can be said about not taking the energy to allow your mate to be erotically attractive to you and fantasizing that you are making love to someone else. This can be very demeaning and destructive to your lover and your lovemaking. Create fantasies about you and your mate that are romantic, fun, and realistic.

During and after making love, notice and fantasize about aspects of your spouse that you find erotically attractive. Don't just stop with the physical attributes; go into the soul of your attraction. Look into his or her eyes and feel your love and why his masculinity or her femininity is so deeply attractive. So much is being paired up intimately. Let these feeling-laden images become a part of your increasing store of sexual memories. Turn your imagination loose on ideas that could make you a better lover and your sex life more exciting and intimate.

Keep creative variety. Fantasies can become as routine as your sex life. You need to continually add to your store of sexually arousing imagery and keep creatively utilizing it with your mate. Don't be guilty of a limited repertoire. Men, even more than women, can allow fantasies to be repetitive and boring. Some of them probably date back to high school. Allow your mate and dynamic lovemaking to stimulate your imagination and spice up your fantasy life.

Keep between the lines. Some people and ideas should have tight boundaries placed around them so they are never allowed to create erotic arousal. You may inadvertently get sexual feelings, but you can choose to stop the feelings as completely inappropriate. This can be called for in regards to a neighbor, all the way through to that person in the church choir.

A sense of the unusual, of newness and adventure, enhances sexual excitement and variety. The human mind is naturally curious and loves mystery or new experiences. Your imaginative capacity and fantasy can help fulfill this in many ways. Keep an adventure component in your personality. Fantasy with mystery and novelty can give your love life wings. Mentally making love with your spouse on your office desk may lead to your setting it up and seducing your mate there. Wives and husbands can imagine themselves wild and uninhibited and then practice some of these fantasy behaviors. These lovemaking sessions usually end up with much laughter and a bonding closeness. A great fantasy life and a dynamic sex life are indeed a state of mind. Unleash your childlike wonderment and curiosity as you discover new dimensions of play through fantasy.

ENJOYING FANTASIES

You can take pleasure from your imagination and use it in a healthy and exciting way to increase your sexual intimacy. You can also experience greater joy and variety by increasing your repertoire of stored sexual images and using them more creatively. All this is to say, you should learn to romantically enjoy fantasy with your spouse.

Fantasy Lovemaking

Each mate should get a piece of paper and pencil and take the time to unleash your imagination as you write how you would program your lovemaking for maximum pleasure. How would you start? How would you create atmosphere? What props would you use? What things have you always wanted to include? This is fantasy and not reality, so let your imagination loose.

I laugh as I think of the wonderfully developed fantasies of wives over the years when I have done this exercise. One wife might say, "He met me at the door and had been thoughtful enough to arrange for the kids. We made a leisurely dinner together and talked. We then kissed on the couch and slowly lost our clothes on the way to the bedroom, which had new satin sheets and my favorite gardenia-scented candles." And her husband's fantasy? "She met me at the door nude and we did it in the hallway."

Block out at least an hour for discussion, creative brainstorming, and enjoying this process. One at a time, take your fantasy lovemaking sessions and describe them to your mate. Detach from your own feelings as your mate shares his or her ideal lovemaking. Don't interrupt, but let your mate develop the whole scenario. Sit back and just be an empathetic listener. Abandon your defenses and do nothing but acknowledge your mate's ideas, needs, and feelings. Ask feedback questions to make sure you understand, and then try paraphrasing what you are hearing. Don't assume or mind-read, and above all, don't make any judgments.

After each of you has shared your fantasy sessions, have fun with the following challenges:

1. Share three items from your mate's sexual fantasies that sound particularly exciting to you. Embellish these three ideas with elements from your own fantasy life and have fun laughing, sharing, and fantasizing.

2. Describe three aspects of your lover's fantasies that you don't relate to or might have some problems enjoying. Be a good communicator and don't get stuck on semantics or content, but reveal your needs and feelings on a deeper level. Why would you struggle with those parts of the fantasy? Talk about it as you take risks and disclose more about yourself.

3. Be creative and compile a composite of your fantasies, but don't create just one big scene. Pull your lovemaking apart and make three different scenarios. Laugh and let your imagination get on a roll. Increase your repository of sexual information and ability to fantasize new and different situations.

4. Use your ingenuity. Plan when you will implement one of the above composite lovemaking sessions in the next week. (How might each of you sabotage accomplishing this task this week? This is probably a hindrance to your fantasy and sex life that you need to resolve.) Which session would be good to save for your next getaway?

Acting Out Fantasies

One overburdened wife found vacationing especially romantic. The second honeymoon to Hawaii was a favorite source of her fantasies. She loved the moonlight walks, the sensuous dinner talks, the exciting hike to one lagoon, and having no demands from children. About twice a year, her husband would surprise her with baby-sitting already arranged and meet her at the door in his Hawaiian shirt. They would have loads of fun re-creating her fantasies about their honeymoon in their own home.

Husbands and wives enjoy their mates initiating exciting and different lovemaking. One wife was aware of her husband's fantasy of being surprised sexually as she sweeps him off and enjoys his "irresistible masculine charm." She made reservations at an elegant hotel and made up a plausible story that got him to the hotel lounge at 6:00 P.M. that Friday. Unbeknownst to him, she got off work early and checked in to their room, where she took a leisurely bath and got some props ready. You can imagine the rest when she met her man in the hotel lounge. They didn't leave their room until the 11:00 A.M. checkout time the next morning.

Should you share all of your fantasies with your mate? That probably wouldn't be wise. You may need to make some aspects of your fantasy life more mature as you conform to God's economy for a fulfilling sex life. But discussing fantasies can be arousing and enrich your love

Time Out: 1. Think of your most common sexual fantasies (scenes, settings, objects, ambiances, styles) that could help your mate understand your sexual needs better and be a real turn-on. Strategically share appropriate ones with your partner as you discuss and perhaps incorporate some of them.

2. What three things do you need to do that would better unleash your fantasy life and help you be a better lover? (For example, take the courage to tell your mate some of your fantasies, become more childlike, and tune in to cues in your lovemaking.)

life, and not letting your partner into your fantasies may diminish your love life. It can be great fun to act out some of them as you increase variety and playfulness.

DANGERS TO GUARD AGAINST

Distorting Fantasy

Fantasy can be distorted. As you allow yourself to enjoy fantasy, you must be wisely mature. What exactly gets you thinking outside God's guidelines for great sex and into sinful, destructive lust? The Bible warns that the Lord hates "a heart that devises wicked plans" (Prov. 6:18 NKJV), and it urges that "you put off . . . the old man which grows corrupt according to the deceitful lusts" (Eph. 4:22 NKJV). How can you as a Christian utilize your visual perceptions and the sexual thought processes that follow to sabotage healthy sexuality and intimate companionship? When are you guilty of "wicked plans"?

Destructive lust forgets that every person is special and three-dimensional with a body, soul, and spirit. Lust objectifies (makes a sexual object of) a person and views the person as a detached body with only genitals and erotic appeal but no personality (or soul). Lust can harm other people for personal sexual gratification because it has detached sex from a person and an intimate relationship.

Harmful sexual thinking is immature and practices poor impulse control. You constantly focus on sexual stimuli in the environment; sex becomes a mental preoccupation. Sex invades your total life, assuming too great an importance as you notice every little sexual cue. Sex can take on addictive proportions and sabotage a balanced life and caring relationships.

Damaging sexual fantasy keeps looking at and obsessing about a person or sexual situations outside marriage. This "lusting after" sets up a person until the thinking begins to encourage the likelihood of sinful behaviors and infidelity. Lust is often a detrimental pattern that comes out of and perpetuates a series of poor choices.

Lust diminishes your attraction to your mate and can be insulting to your mate, who comes to feel inferior, embarrassed, or neglected. It detracts from your commitment to building a more exciting sex life with your partner. Sinful fantasy adulterates your enjoyment of your partner rather than enhancing your sexual intimacy together.

Poor Thought Control

The Roman Christians were exhorted, "Do not be conformed to this world, but be transformed by the renewing of your mind"; and "To be spiritually minded is life and peace" (Rom. 12:2; 8:6 NKJV). Paul also encouraged, "Whatever things are true, whatever things are noble, whatever things are just, whatever things are pure, whatever things are lovely, whatever things are of good report . . . meditate on these things" (Phil. 4:8 NKJV). God has given us as human beings the marvelous capacity to choose what we wish to think and fantasize about.

Men don't always have greater sex drives than women. Men more often than women have poor thought control, though both are afflicted with this disease. Seeing an attractive woman at a restaurant and following her across the room as you mentally undress her is wrongly accelerating your sex drive—not a result of your higher sex drive. There's a difference between being highly sexed and allowing one's thought life to run along unchecked (see Chapter 28).

Lust is a fascinating and often poorly understood word. We have already established that we are not talking about enjoying sexual stimuli or creating a fantasy life. Lust is distorted fantasy and especially unchecked sexual thoughts—objectifying and using sexuality in a way that does not produce intimacy or a more fulfilling sex life. We are warned as Christians that "each of you should know how to possess his own vessel [body, especially the mind] in sanctification and honor, not in passion of lust" (1 Thess. 4:4–5 NKJV).

Diminishing Your Mate

The sexual verbs are *relate* and *connect*, and great sex is based on a fun and loving relationship. Your fantasy life—both old and newly input erotic data and the imaginative use of this information—should enhance your intimate companionship. Pining over the lack of breast size or focusing on the muscles of other men is diminishing your spouse and can lead to ineffective fantasies. If you choose to focus on supposed flaws, you will never build the kind of erotic enjoyment of your mate's body that you need for a great sex life.

When you fantasize, fantasize about your mate in exciting situations. Any time your fantasies exclude your mate, you diminish your mate's importance to your emotional and physical fulfillment.

Many mates at times think of something else when they are making love. Is this destructive? One wife confessed that she often planned her week's agenda during the Sunday night sexual session with her husband. Is this always wrong? Yes. Anything that diminishes your mate and your focus on making love is counterproductive.

Is it always damaging to bring erotic fantasies of someone else into married sex? It will not instantly sabotage your love life, but it will not maximize your lovemaking; and it can drain off sexual energy that you could be using to eroticize and focus on your partner. You may be creating a private world in your head to the exclusion of your partner as you simply use his or her body. It diminishes your mate and could come to destroy your mate's erotic attractiveness. If you are feeling bored or turned off, you need to face that and deal with it, not create destructive fantasies.

Immature Patterns

Men often are less holistic in their sexuality than women as they fixate on some narrow focus, neglecting a broad range of fantasies and feelings. Men unfortunately are not alone in creating patterns that restrict God's plan of exciting sexual bonding in marriage.

One woman enjoyed dating, loved to kiss, and all her life had romanticized sex. In her mind, sex was gentle wooing and sexy flirting. After she married, sex became difficult for her. It suddenly involved physical aspects of making love, and she felt she lost all control. As she sought answers, she realized that she had an immature, limiting sexual mind-set that desperately needed an overhaul. Her repertoire of erotically stimulating images, settings, ambiances, and styles required expansion. Not using your imagination and fantasy can be as immature as employing distorted fantasies.

Spectating

Another variety of immaturity and ineffective use of fantasy involves spectating. Mentally, great lovers focus on and revel in the present experience. However, all of us at times mentally leave the scene and watch the lovemaking as if from afar. The wife, who thinks she is taking too long to climax and her husband is growing tired, all of a sudden becomes anxious, spectates, and loses all capacity for arousal. The husband who doubts his ability to get an erection or excite his wife mentally leaves the immediate lovemaking, anxious about his performance. Both are mentally up on the bedpost observing the process, rather than being mentally present and involved. This can obviously be very sabotaging.

You can use your imagination in negative ways as you spectate and borrow trouble or create agendas in your mind rather than enjoy the sexual celebration. Effective fantasy utilizes imaginative capacity to enjoy the party and create new levels of excitement. Keep your mind on your lovemaking, and don't spectate!

Destructive Fantasies

"It all depends" does not apply to all of fantasy. Some types of fantasy are wrong—period. Any fantasy that involves children is wrong. We are responsible for protecting God's little ones, especially those He has entrusted to our care, and ensuring they are not sexualized destructively.

Time Out: 1. Each of us distorts fantasy in some way. Which examples and areas apply to you? What reward do you receive from that distortion that keeps you from changing it? The first step in changing this distortion can be sharing this secret with your mate or a friend.

2. What makes you detach and spectate? Discuss this with your mate, and both of you figure out how to do some prevention, as well as ways to get back into the lovemaking (for example: criticism causes anxiety and detachment; your mate's being more active would get you back into the activity).

Allowing your neighbors' or friends' mates or associates or clients to be sexually arousing and the objects of fantasies is courting disaster. You are in constant contact with these people, and you need to avoid any complicating sexual overtones. Noticing an attractive person on the beach is different from checking out a friend's mate.

Fantasies that involve hurting another person, pain, or domination do not promote loving, growth-producing sexual relating. It is easy to confuse pain and pleasure, but they are obviously very different in their effects on a relationship.

Any fantasy that would lead to adultery is sinful and contrary to the goal of intimate sexuality. Fantasies that dilute your erotic attachment to your mate, even if they don't lead to affairs, are ineffective. The word *adulterate* means "to water down," and your personal fantasy should make your mutual sexual pleasure more exciting—not less.

This is a tough area of sexuality to sort through. There are no easy answers. Talk with a wise friend or your mate about some of the areas and specific behaviors that still have you perplexed. Talk through some of the ideas of this chapter. Please bring your faith into the equation and humbly ask God to shine truth into your life and thinking. God has a way of honoring that request through many meaningful and sometimes surprising avenues.

Do not be afraid of fantasy. It comprises too important a part of intimate lovemaking. Acknowledge the fact that all of us notice and think about a variety of sexual cues in the environment. These cues and sexual desires are not wrong. It is how you choose to discipline your thought life and bring your fantasies into enhancing your sexual partnership that separates sin from appropriate and great lovemaking. Enjoy!

CHAPTER EIGHT

Sexual Communication

MANY LOVING COUPLES never talk about sex together. This is sad, because effective communication is at the heart of falling deeper in love and creating a truly passionate marriage. It isn't easy to create a comfortable sexual vocabulary or develop the ability to dialogue about lovemaking. Perhaps sex was never talked about in your growing-up experiences. Sexual discussions are indeed difficult as they can get into unmet needs and constructive criticism, problem solving with no easy answers, and very private feelings. This is messy to deal with—especially for those who want to be perfect lovers or thought sex would automatically fall into place—and is easier to just avoid.

Lack of sexual communication can be disabling, though. It prevents couples from making needed adjustment for greater pleasure, it robs them of a great aphrodisiac because talking is very sexy, and it blocks them from sharing fantasies and creating erotic, romantic evenings. For many marriages, it is not just sexual talk but communication in general that suffers. Mates often have acute skill deficits in resolving conflict and negotiating tentative solutions.

This chapter tackles three basic skills for effective communication and dialogue and for managing conflict in the partnership. We will then explore the language of lovemaking, from vocabulary to slang to love talk. The sections on coaching with initiating and refusing and maximizing should also help resolve and avoid conflict.

You will also discover that effective communication brings many fun spillovers into your sex life. The more you talk and feel close, the more you will want to make love. The more you talk about sex and your love life, the more satisfying your lovemaking will become. Dialogue is also basic in resolving sexual conflicts.

EMPATHY: THE KEY TO GREAT COMMUNICATION

The essence of effective communication is a dialogue that ends in empathy. One partner has assertively stated his or her reality, and the other partner has been able to walk in his or her shoes to understand and acknowledge that reality. This is what empathy is all about—understanding. It is not *agreeing*, but rather hearing and acknowledging another reality that often differs from our own.

Three Skills for Great Communication

A crucial part of effective communication and avoiding defensiveness is coming into this process with an attitude. Not a bad attitude but a deeply loving one that conveys to your mate, "I like you—you're safe with me. I want you happy and fulfilled." Mature communicators in this dialogue process abandon the need to *win, debate, convince,* or *make a point.* You are creating a dialogue with the goal of exchanging information. Each partner communicates his or her reality while the other truly listens and works through to empathy.

1. Assertively state *your personal reality.* Start with "I" statements that take responsibility without blaming (not "you" turn me off but "I" feel my desire shut down when you grab at me). Assertive communication is direct and respectful without being aggressive or passive. Risk conflict and express your core feelings and needs. Don't get hung up on one point, but express the greater reality and what's going on at gut-level. You are communicating information that your mate really needs in order to have a contented spouse. Share that!

Practice Exercise: In a self-aware, straightforward manner, communicate to your mate what you would like sexually on the coming weekend—what you desire and how you would appreciate your desires being met. Take the courage to assertively express what arouses you and some of your feelings associated with those behaviors. Maybe complete the following sentence: "I wish sexually that you would . . ." Then dialogue about your answers. Remember that you are nondefensively collecting information. Now try this: "I enjoy it when you . . ."

2. Objectively empathize *with your partner's reality.* Express understanding of your partner's message with short, empathetic summaries. Go beyond the surface content to acknowledge the deeper needs and feelings. Remember that empathy is not agreeing that your mate's reality is free of distortions or accepting that the other's feelings are correct and true. It is containing your judgments and feelings while you try to understand his or her reality. You may speak German and have to learn some French to really empathize correctly. Be aware that you mate *will not feel truly heard* until he or she has felt empathy and understanding.

A note for husbands: wives especially need to have their feelings empathized with and acknowledged. My wife is like a broken record and keeps repeating herself until I have empathized with her feelings. Cathy says, "When you jump up to check your e-mails in the mornings, we don't get to cuddle and be close." So of course I respond, "I don't think you understand how busy I am" (male defensiveness at its best), or "If we made love every morning, cuddling would be so much better" (male fix-it and personal agenda mode). She will keep repeating until I acknowledge, "I'm sorry, you love the closeness of mornings and lying on my chest for a few minutes. I know you feel special, and this is connecting for both of us. I can do better. I'll try to call you and hug you more during the day too."

Practice Exercise: Ask your partner to describe a lovemaking session that was very special. Put yourself in your mate's sexual reality, and some deeper needs: variety, tenderness, competence, challenge, affirmation, fun, comfort. Use remarks such as: "What I'm hearing is . . ." or "You must feel . . ." or "You're needing me to . . ." Switch roles after the partner who is conveying his or her reality agrees that the other has understood and the empathy statements are accurate. Empathy skills are crucial to resolving sexual conflicts too.

3. Tenderly negotiate *a partnership reality.* Create tentative solutions. Bargain with the collected information of each reality, as both lovingly compromise. The purpose of dialogue is to mutually meet needs and resolve differences, not to win or make your point. This may mean to agree to disagree while you work on thinking an issue through more and temporarily put it on hold. It could be a behavioral solution negotiated around each mate's needs and feelings, a solution both are willing to try to implement even though it may not be balanced evenly. Few compromises are 50/50, but with dialogue and empathy with each other's souls, it still feels like a compromise even if only 20 percent of your needs are met this time.

In your solutions, neither of you must lose your soul as you lovingly compromise. What I mean by losing your soul is that there are some things, if compromised, that will cause you or your mate to lose an important part of who you are and your deeper values. Love is patient, kind, and protective. Paraphrasing Matthew 16:26: "What does it profit a mate to gain his or her own way if the partner loses his or her soul?" The husband who gave up his request after realizing his wife would lose some of her modesty and self-respect if she gave in to his desire to videotape their lovemaking was indeed wise.

Practice Exercise: Each of you take the information you have collected and propose a tentative solution around a difficulty in your sex life. Make sure neither of you loses his or her soul, but also realize that what goes around comes around in good relationships. The 20/80 compromises even out over time in loving, giving partnerships.

CONFLICT MANAGEMENT IN THE PARTNERSHIP

Both you and your partner are intelligent people with a lot of spunk and opinions. That strength naturally creates conflict. Sexual disagreements can stem from very different needs and expectations. *Learn to manage emotionally loaded topics in the partnership.* There are skills that great communicators utilize to keep negotiation and conflict resolution clean and productive.

Guidelines for Conflict Resolution

Perhaps you and your spouse grew up arguing and enjoy the challenge, or are afraid of conflict and avoid it or distance yourselves when you feel attacked. Or your arguments often end with nothing resolved and anger on both sides. Agree to practice these "fight-management" skills as you institute some rules. The guidelines apply to managing all of your communication more effectively, but they especially apply to conflict resolution.

Stick to the topic. Perhaps you have the habit of switching topics when you're losing. Sometimes one topic suggests another, but it is extremely confusing to get two or three going at once.

Pick your battles and develop your timing. Some things are not worth fighting about. If you have seven points of contention, pick your top two. Otherwise, in your nit-picking you will not be heard when you really need to make a point. Choose carefully the things you cannot live with and accept—make a stand only on those items. Some hills are not worth dying on. Be strategic in timing your conversations and conflict. Don't sit on your feelings, but avoid times when you are extremely hungry, angry, or tired.

Remain courteous. Increased volume, power struggles, scorekeeping, and blaming "you" language are extremely ineffective. Passive withdrawal or aggressive attacking is discourteous and can create a negative atmosphere. Sexual topics can become personally loaded but keep it clean.

Set limits. Know when to stop, even if it means to agree to disagree for now. From midnight to 3:00 A.M. is seldom a productive time. You and your mate know when conflict has become counterproductive or is escalating out of control—stop right then! Remember to include humor and to include a short bathroom or snack break now and then. These help both of you to keep your perspective and limit angry intensity.

Reconcile the relationship (forgive, apologize, emphasize your love). Reconciling is different from agreeing or compromising on the issues of your fight; it is not letting "the sun go down on your wrath" (Eph. 4:26 NKJV). (The sun may go down on your disagreement but hopefully not on your anger.) It is amazing what you can accomplish by saying, "I'm sorry you're upset," "I really do love you," or "Forgive me." Somehow, in the midst of conflict, phrases like this stick in your throat, but if you can apologize and affirm your love, these words have a soothing and healing effect. Humility and gentleness go a long way in managing conflict. Remember, your relationship is much more than this one fight.

Practice Exercise: Start working through, one at a time, the emotionally loaded topics in the sexual area of your relationship—those that have produced ineffective fights in the past. Both of you keep a list of the communication-management "skills" in front of you. Practice sticking to the topic and remaining courteous as you work through the three skills of great communication. Stop at forty-five minutes per session. Be courageous and wise as you look at tough areas (for example, sex during the wife's period, managing the children, language you don't like, more spontaneity, birth control, and so on). Practice your empathy skills and give understanding summaries of the content, feelings, and needs that your partner has expressed.

I cannot stress enough the importance of communication skills in working through sexuality—in engagement, on the honeymoon, and in the years to come. Continue to improve your nonsexual communication so you are even better at your sexual communication. Read a book (a great one is *A Lasting Promise: A Christian Guide to Fighting for Your Marriage* by Stanley, Trathen, McCain, and Bryan [San Francisco: Jossey-Bass, 1998]), watch a video, or listen to an audiotape together on improving communication in your marriage. Talk about what tips and techniques you would like to try and implement.

THE LANGUAGE OF LOVEMAKING

Sex is a difficult, private topic. Couples can often make love more easily than they can talk about it. Assertively asking for what they need does not come easily for many people, especially in the sexual arena. Sexual problems and sexual ignorance, with unresolved anger and hurt, can also impede sexual communication. Each partnership needs erotic verbal and nonverbal skills in this area.

Vocabulary and Slang

Before getting into sexual vocabulary in general, let me comment about male and female slang. If the male genital slang is not funny, it is aggressive and harsh. The female slang, if not demeaning, is silly and suggestive. This is a sad and destructive distortion of God's gift of sexuality. Christians need to reclaim sex from the world and bring back to making love the beauty and joy that God intended. Slang is certainly an area where we can practice not buying in to sinful, destructive values.

In developing a sexual vocabulary, you may be wondering if slang is ever appropriate. Of course, slang is permissible and fun and erotic. Your pet names for body parts and secret vocabulary shared by only the two of you contain a lot of slang. And as a couple you will find other words expressive and arousing. As Christians, however, we must be careful to avoid the very negative attitudes and ideas about sex that society over the centuries has incorporated into slang. We never want to be funny at someone's expense, aggressive, demeaning, a silly kind of seductive, or suggestive.

The renowned semanticist S. I. Hayakawa said that all language and words are symbols and we give them their meanings and impact. That is especially true of slang. Remember two points as you keep your language within God's guidelines:

1. You have the necessity of building an erotic vocabulary so you can enjoy the gift of making love with the comfort and flair God desires.

2. The vocabulary must enhance the loving, exciting process of making love. Each partner should be able to associate the same symbolic meaning with the vocabulary as it becomes playful and arousing. If any language is demeaning, offensive, harmfully aggressive, or cheap to either mate, it should be avoided.

You should know the correct biological terms for parts of the human body. That is a good starting point. One woman grew up in a home where sex was never discussed. She and her husband had some very frustrating times in the early part of their marriage. She did not have

Time Out: 1. Turn to Chapter 3 and read to each other some of the information on sexual parts as you repeat the correct biological terms to each other.

2. Have fun the next time you are making love by creating some pet names for activities and body parts. (I often laugh in counseling sessions when clients talk about "Big John" or "Shamu" and wanting to "dive into your pool, but you fell asleep.") Tell your mate of two slang words you find exciting and two that you feel would decrease your sexual enjoyment and arousal.

an adequate vocabulary, and neither did he. He had picked up some slang from the locker room and peers, but that didn't help. She was not orgasmic when they married and was given to yeast infections, but they couldn't comfortably discuss these problems.

The wife bought a book on becoming orgasmic and began becoming more comfortable with her body and sex in general. She learned exactly where her clitoris was and how it functioned. They both laughed as they practiced vocabulary together because they had never said many of the words aloud before.

Learn to converse openly about making love without shame or embarrassment, and talk during sex. Expand your vocabulary, and adapt slang that both of you enjoy. Sex is your playground and great communication translates into having more fun.

Nonverbal Signals

Build up a fun and useful repertoire of nonverbal language. Experts speculate that anywhere from 65 to 95 percent of communication is nonverbal, so it is no wonder that great lovers master this aspect of connecting. Try not to mind-read or assume; check out or establish some of the nonverbal signals verbally. Perhaps gentle pressure with a hand signals the desire to shift into another position. Groans, sighs, and exclamations may signal degrees of arousal and when to proceed to another phase of lovemaking. Nonverbal communication helps orchestrate a sex life that will grow ever more comfortable and meaningful.

Develop a nonverbal signal that indicates your desire for sexual activity. Without allowing it to completely lose its subtlety, make sure the nonverbal vocabulary is accurate and obvious enough. It may be a passionate hug or kiss. Sometimes an amorous look or a soft kiss on the back of the neck is all it takes. A husband related that his wife usually initiated her desire for sex with a certain nightgown. He thought the nonverbal signal was okay but wished, after eight years, she would buy another gown.

Nonverbal communication evolves with most lovers. Don't just use it as a signal to orchestrate—get excited and involved as you express and increase your arousal. It is difficult for most people to relax control and truly get excited, not only in sex but even on a roller coaster or at a ball game. Give yourself permission to be uninhibited and make noises during sex. Groan, breathe loudly, exclaim in excitement, purr with pleasure, squeal with delight, and allow your nonverbal communication to be truly expressive.

A wife complained that her husband never made noises during lovemaking, which made it difficult to read his level of excitement. I suggested that making noises could be his homework for the coming two weeks. I asked in his next session if he had been able to groan. He said he had. I then asked if his wife had picked up on his groaning, and he said that he had pointed it out. I laughed and thought to myself, *How erotic!* "Honey, that was a groan, and I think I am getting somewhat excited and wanted you to know."

Remember not to get lazy or assume or completely rely on your nonverbal communication. Some messages need to be verbally communicated and feedback exchanged. Lack of communication can become amusing. A wife finally disclosed to her husband, "I wish you wouldn't stick your tongue in my ear during lovemaking." The husband quickly retorted, "I thought that turned you on. Why didn't you say something two years ago?" She replied, "I liked it two years ago." People change, and a continuing verbal dialogue is irreplaceable for true sexiness to flourish in intimate companionships and love lives.

Time Out: 1. What are some of the nonverbal signals you currently enjoy in making love? Think of one area you would like to signal your partner better nonverbally, and add it to your bag of techniques.

2. Make love this week, but agree ahead of time that you will make more noise than is usual for the two of you—exaggerate and enjoy it.

Love Talk

How much do you talk before sex? During sex? After sex? Talking really is a great way to enhance your sex life. One couple stumbled on to the importance of talk one night as they were making plans for their summer vacation. It was after the wife had become more adept with her sexual vocabulary, and both felt less inhibited about sex in general. They were working through plans to go to the Caribbean and spend a long-anticipated week in the islands. She had bought a cute bathing suit and, after modeling it for her husband, asked how he would like to take it off on some deserted beach. They then digressed into how much they were looking forward to time alone and some fun sex.

The husband related how seeing the hotel room and Jacuzzi in the travel brochure had made him excited as he fantasized being with her on that king-sized bed after some time in the Jacuzzi together. She remarked how wonderful it felt after sunbathing to lie on cool sheets, bodies entwined. She even found it erotic the way their bodies perspired while making love during the summertime. As they sat there talking about sex, they could see that both were becoming very aroused. The evening concluded with his slowly taking off her bathing suit in the bedroom and their having a very enjoyable sexual encounter.

Each of three areas of erotic communication—before, during, and after making love—has its unique excitement and sexual stimulation.

1. Love talk before. This couple discovered that just engaging in sexual talk made them feel closer, more comfortable with sex, and aroused. They made a special effort to include the topic of sex at least once a week in their discussions. They tuned in to conversation triggers (a television show, a new bathing suit, a joke) more readily and just talked about sex more.

They discussed why they, like many couples, had seemed in the past to unconsciously avoid communicating about sex. Some of it was a lack of vocabulary, and some of it might have been an unwillingness to take the risk to be that intimate with each other. They realized that they did not trust each other or feel comfortable enough to discuss a variety of relational and sexual topics. Their closeness grew as they discussed her insecure perfectionism and his feeling he could never make enough money to satisfy her. One weekend they jumped into the topic of his getting a vasectomy, with many raw nerves being exposed, but they came to a much better understanding of the needs and feelings of both.

In fantasizing about the Caribbean getaway, they got into another great type of before-sex talk: sharing fantasies! It is fun to enjoy, before the fact, some of the things you would like to do. Often it is crucial to creating the ambiance. They also took the time, as suggested elsewhere in this book, to relate to each other their ideal sexual encounters and to incorporate some of these ideas into their lovemaking. The less inhibited they became in their sexual talk, the more fun they had. It did not have to lead anywhere, either. It was enjoyable to get somewhat aroused and then go on to another topic.

She started to tease more and make sexually suggestive comments like the one about the bathing suit and a deserted beach. He would tease her in turn. He would phone her at her job and say things or express them in confidential e-mails, and she would laugh in delight but be a little embarrassed, as if somehow her office mates could read her mind. They might be at a friend's house waiting for them to answer the door, and she would surprise him with a suggestive sexual comment. Certain parts of his anatomy would respond in embarrassing ways and she would laugh, delighting in her feminine power.

2. Love talk during. During sex, the idea is to relax and let the talk be free-flowing from what you are feeling and sensing. Sometimes you and your mate will be on a common theme, and at other times each will pursue personal images—both can be connecting and stimulating sexually. The wife might say, "You sure are hitting the right spot inside me." And the husband might reply, "You feel so good, I wish I could do this all night." Or the husband might go off on his own tangent: "I'm glad you're feeling excited. That dance you did to seduce me tonight was unbelievable."

During making love, you can also tease and talk about fantasies. This talk can be very erotic

Time Out: The next time you make love, try practicing a stream-of-consciousness flow of conversation—both of you keep up a running commentary on what you are feeling and sensing. It will be tremendously exciting.

as both get into creating the mood. Tell your partner what you want and need sexually in a given session. If something pops into your mind that you haven't tried in a while, bring it up, and both may enter into the activity with gusto. Erotic communication has so much potential.

3. *Love talk after.* In Chapter 4 we discussed the afterglow phase of sexual activity: the time after each partner has been satisfied and bodies and emotions are returning to their normal state. It is a time that is important for couples to connect and enjoy the connection, but this resolution phase is fraught with pitfalls. Wives often need to empty the bladder and clean up, while husbands feel so relaxed that they might roll over and go to sleep. Both can end up feeling frustrated and ruin the warm connecting that just occurred.

It should be a time of talking and warm reminiscing and reaffirming your love for each other—appreciating how truly close you two have become. You are perhaps closest to the Garden of Eden at this time in your intimate connection—like Adam and Eve, during your lovemaking, you have become naked without any shame.

Time Out: Discuss with your partner what kind of affirmation and talking and holding would be special and affirming for you in the love talk after sex. It's a different kind of love talk, but it's so bonding. Even a simple "Wow, anticipating another forty years is awesome" takes on special significance during this vulnerable, united time. Wives especially feel vulnerable and need this affirmation because they have both physically and emotionally opened themselves up to their husbands.

COACHING

A wife may think her husband is supposed to know all about sex. Or a couple may wonder why they are the only couple in the world whose sex life has not automatically fallen into place. After all, if making love is supposed to be such a natural thing, why are they struggling? The truth is that, like marriage in general, two unique male and female persons getting together will have differences. No matter how technically skilled they are, their sexual relationship will be a blending of two unique bodies and varying attitudes and needs—which will continue to vary over many years and different life tasks.

Coaching is all about assertively expressing your sexual needs and feelings, learning to problem-solve in difficult areas, and helping your mate understand you. All couples have to gain skills in coaching, whether it is initiating and refusing sex or encouraging what you enjoy. Like other aspects of communication, these skills don't come naturally. You can't immediately know exactly all the things that pleasure your partner. Throughout the years together, the stresses of life, the aging process, children, and many other issues will give you new reasons for readjusting your sex life.

This section considers three areas of making love that will need some coaching. First, how do you initiate and refuse sexual activity graciously, without feeling pressured or resorting to pouting? Second, how can you maximize your sex life by coaching what you need, what turns you on, and what turns you off? Finally, what are some pointers on problem solving so stressors and difficulties can be worked through with no lasting roadblocks to a great sex life?

Initiating and Refusing

Consider these comments:

"My husband is so uncreative in the way he approaches me for sex."
"Why is it that every time I turn him down, and it isn't that often, he pouts?"
"I would love for my mate to be more aggressive in initiating sex."
"I love my wife, but I'm not always instantly ready to make love like she expects."

All successful lovers have to polish initiating and refusing. No couple is immune from some misunderstandings in this area of sexual communication and attitudes.

Think for a moment about what is at stake that makes initiating and refusing become so symbolic and filled with disappointments and hurt feelings. First, initiating and refusing make one vulnerable to rejection and feelings of abandonment. Second, ineffective initiating attempts can make a person feel pushed, controlled, and treated like a sexual object. Third, much of initiating is nonverbal and therefore open to misinterpretation. Fourth, initiating, or the lack thereof, becomes synonymous with sexual desire and sexual attractiveness. Fifth, initiating or refusing sex means coordinating two unique people with different needs and priorities on any given day or hour.

No wonder this is a loaded topic that must be discussed with both partners open to coaching! Great lovers take the time and energy to understand their mates and make changes.

Time Out: Switch roles. Role-play being your mate and demonstrate how you would like him or her to initiate and refuse lovemaking. Remember you are not yourself but living in your mate's reality. Keep your partner's needs and attitudes in mind as you model initiating and refusing. In this positive way coach your mate on the things you appreciate and the things you would like to be eliminated. Practice both nonverbal and verbal techniques as you smooth the process and make it honest and loving.

Maximizing Coaching

In your sex life there are some things your mate does that really turn you on and others that really turn you off. You have to tell your partner what you want and what you dislike, including specific behaviors and attitudes that are appreciated or get in the way. You want to maximize your sex life? Talk! Emphasize and practice the positive!

Here are some important guidelines for giving helpful suggestions as you coach your mate and maximize your sex life:

1. Major coaching should be done fully clothed as you dialogue about your sex life. Subjects could be poor hygiene, inhibitions, boredom, pushiness, and/or technique deficits.

2. Minor adjusting needs comfortable nonverbal and verbal language that can be done non-threateningly. For example, you might say, "That hurts." "Slow down." "You're on my arm." "More." "Shift."

3. Keep your coaching adult-to-adult as you teach without becoming parental or condescending. Stay humble and self-confident as you listen to criticism. Allow yourself to be in a nondefensive learning mode, and create dialogue. This is a partnership.

4. Focus on the positive! The primary goal of coaching is not to correct what's wrong. It is to maximize the strengths, bring the best out in players—not simply to correct imperfection.

5. Great coaching employs many methods. Demonstrate by doing it on yourself or guiding your mate's hand, dialogue and exchange information, buy books and use them as your assistant coaches, go to a sex therapist, and start with small changes.

6. Know thyself! Acquire wisdom! It is tough coaching if you are not sure what you need or want. Read; experiment; give yourself permission to be uninhibitedly sexual as you become truly self-aware. Great coaches know and utilize each player's strengths and abilities.

Overcoming Roadblocks

Quite often couples feel that they are the only ones whose sex life isn't easy and effortless. However, it wouldn't surprise me if over 50 percent of normal, loving couples have had some kind of sexual difficulty in the past year. All marriages encounter roadblocks to making love. It may be a lack of desire, finding time and energy, temporary impotence, an inability to let go of control, problems reaching a climax, or an unresolved affair.

All the things you have already read about sexual communication especially apply to roadblocks. You can't sweep them under the rug because they won't go away. They can be embarrassing to discuss, and they are emotionally loaded.

Communication skills really count now. Choose a setting where there is plenty of time and privacy. Keep clarifying the message as you focus and really try to understand your mate's needs and feelings. Detach from your anger and fear as you listen and acknowledge your partner's assertive sharing of what is happening. Get a dialogue going.

Time Out: Practice this assignment frequently. Fully clothed, sit with your lover and discuss what modifications you would like to make in your sex life. Be specific, and explain what you wish your mate would do more and less of. Arrange a time for a lovemaking session in which you institute and practice one mate's suggestions and a separate time for the other's suggestions. Be sure to use the six ideas for maximizing coaching of your sex life.

You may need some professional help, but first read an appropriate chapter in this book or another that deals with your problem, and start talking. Sexual communication has some marvelous healing capacities. A central part of most sexual difficulties is anxiety (fears, worry, guilt) or anger (irritation, disappointment, disrespect, hostility). Talking about the difficulty and acknowledging its impact keep lovers from being so anxious and avoiding sex. The anxiety and guilt of impotence or climaxing too slowly can cause partners to wonder if it will happen again with each lovemaking session. Talking it through encourages enjoyment of the moment instead of panic.

Anger and disappointment can quickly distance lovers as hurt and disrespect grow. It is painful and tough at times, but there is no substitute for talking through the problem. Talking defuses the tension, creates understanding and acceptance, and promotes changes. Yes, it may take professional assistance from a sex or marital therapist, but start your own honest, open dialogue.

Time Out: Pick a roadblock in your sexual relationship, and do some reading and research on the problem. Rehearse in your mind what you would like to say, and choose a strategic time for this discussion. Talk!

Great lovers have to be able to communicate. Husbands and wives, especially husbands, need to take responsibility to learn effective communication skills. Develop a great sexual vocabulary, and enjoy erotic communication. Talk before, during, and after you make love as you enhance the entire experience. God has given you a wonderful aphrodisiac in your ability to communicate. Make use of it!

CHAPTER NINE

Sensuous Massage

THIS CHAPTER WAS ENCOURAGED by missionary friends who are a pretty unique couple. During every furlough they choose one class or educational experience to enrich their marriage. This past furlough their choice was massage, and they swore it helped revolutionize their relationship and lovemaking. This book stresses the importance of building a loving, nurturing relationship for lovemaking to flourish. Massage indeed is a marvelous way to accomplish the goal of feeling connected and deepening your intimate companionship.

Massage has been shown to have profound effects on the one giving the massage as well as the person receiving it. A massage reduces stress, blood pressure goes down, and a relaxed, comfortable, nurturing atmosphere is encouraged within the companionship.

In this chapter you will first learn an exercise called *sensate focus,* which is sensual touching for your personal pleasure. The following three sections explain and demonstrate sensuous massage (with helpful illustrations): how to set the stage for massage; basic techniques to get you started; and massage on various parts of the body from face to feet, with ways to increase the sensuous pleasure as you apply these techniques. The last section details ways to utilize massage as you incorporate it into more intimate stroking.

SENSATE FOCUS

In Chapter 3 we talked about sensate focus as a means of exploring erogenous zones. Remember what a marvelous gift God has given you with your skin and its sensory nerve endings? If you can learn to relax, get comfortable with touching and being touched, and focus on your sensual feelings, you can embark on a wonderful journey of pleasure and bonding. Your ability to enjoy touching can be the foundation for enriching your marriage and creating some fantastic lovemaking.

Sensate focus develops the art of sensual touching. It is often a prescribed part of sex therapy because it takes the focus off performing and places it on mutual sharing and sensuality. Sensate focus and massage will enhance your ability as a lover to be sensual and to give and receive nurturing touch. It also is very bonding and increases a shared sense of partnership and intimacy.

In this exercise, both partners are nude, and the temperature is set at a comfortable level. The active partner is in charge of setting the ambiance (music, lighting) and choosing the place. The bed is excellent for enjoying this experience of sensuality and touch. Do not touch the genitals or breasts as you learn to enjoy the whole body—this is a sensual as well as an erotic activity. To make this easy and comfortable to include in your repertoire or intimate activities, block out two fifteen-minute sessions in a week, and each of you be the active partner once. Sometimes you may wish to block out thirty minutes and each take the role of giver and receiver.

Mates will have to be able to assume two different roles as they enjoy the experience of sensate focus. To relax and revel in sensuality, do not have intercourse or manual stimulation of the genitals for the remainder of the day after sensate focus. The focus is on touch and its sensual, erogenous nature, even though the exercise is done with both partners nude.

The Active Toucher

In sensate focus, the active mate touches the passive partner in ways that feel good to the toucher. This touching is oriented toward individual pleasure and sensuality, not attending to the partner's desires. The toucher focuses only on personal feelings and enjoyment of the mate's body. There are no performance needs.

Experiment with a variety of touches and strokes on any area other than genitals and breasts. It is often helpful to start with the touchee lying on his or her stomach. Begin at the top of the head and slowly work your way down to the feet. Have the passive partner roll over, and work from the feet to the head. It is best not to have any communication at this point but to revel in individual sensations. If you are aware of areas of the body that your partner does not like to have touched, in love and respect stay away from these areas.

The Passive Touchee

The other half of sensate focus involves the touchee, who lies passively and allows the active partner to touch the body. Often the touches that pleasure the active toucher give stimulation and pleasure to the passive mate, too. The passive partner can increase self-awareness by noticing which areas and types of touching give the greatest pleasure. You can ask for these to be repeated while making love at a different time. The touchee is also learning about the lover—what kind of touching and strokes the toucher usually enjoys to give and receive.

Don't confine your touching when you're the active partner by this information. Do your active touching for yourself.

You will find this a very bonding and warmly connecting exercise. In previous chapters, you have explored the need to get beyond performance and to selfishly delight in sensuality for yourself. Sensate focus will do this in marvelous ways.

Note: Sensate focus can also be done with feedback from the touchee in a more active manner. This feedback can help the toucher give strokes, rhythms, and pressure that feel best to the touchee. This makes it a learning experience and more for the touchee's pleasure.

SETTING THE STAGE FOR MASSAGE

Tools

There really are few preparations or necessary items other than some oil and a quiet, warm place to lie during the massage.

Oils. Natural oils like coconut, sesame, safflower, almond, soy, or avocado work well. Some natural oils like olive, peanut, or corn oil can be too thick and don't spread or absorb as easily. Adding some scent to these oils or burning already scented oil can add to this sensuous experience. Be sure to warm both the oil and your hands before applying, and use only enough oil so the hands move smoothly over the skin—don't saturate to a greasy feel.

Two types of containers work well for storing the oil during the massage. You can put it in a shallow bowl and dip your hand in it. Perhaps even better is a plastic squeeze bottle that allows you to control the amount and won't spill if it turns over. This also allows you to place the oil on the skin and massage it in, or you can squeeze some on the back of your hand and massage it in while maintaining your rhythm.

Table or mat. A bed does not work well because it is too soft and will prevent firm, even pressure. If you have a table that comes to your upper thigh, find a mat or a piece of foam rubber or use blankets and towels to put over it.

You may not have a table of about thirty inches in height, but don't let that be a roadblock. Put a mat or blankets and towels on the floor. You can get a mat or a piece of foam at a sporting goods store and create a comfortable pallet. Place a pillow under your knees to soften the floor as you give the massage.

Movements

Be sure to remove your jewelry and warm your hands. Massage is lovingly nurturing your mate's body, and these are common courtesies to enhance the experience. You may want to buy a flannel sheet to drape the parts of the body you are not massaging. Keep towels handy to roll up under the neck or other areas that need support.

Rhythms. A soothing and sensuous massage should maintain a smooth and even rhythm with strokes that flow into one another. It should have a relaxing, almost hypnotic effect. One technique for accomplishing this is trying to always have at least one hand on the body at all times. You will become more adept as you practice. Don't worry, it will feel great regardless. As you practice, a natural rhythm will come more easily.

Pressure. A common mistake is thinking that massage, to be effective, must always be firm. Sometimes a light stroke or a hand lying on a body part will start nerves and skin to tingling and will feel very sensuous. The reason the table should come to the upper thigh is that the pressure in massage should be given by leaning your body weight into the person—not straining your back or shoulder muscles. It is helpful to face the way you are stroking and be able to move around the person as you go from legs to back to abdomen.

Breathing and relaxation. Massage should be a stress reliever, both physically and mentally. Put on some relaxing music and dim the lights. It helps to practice diaphragmatic breathing for stress management: draw deep breaths clear into your stomach and gently let them out. You can practice diaphragmatic breathing by resting a hand on your partner's stomach as your partner breathes deeply and slowly, causing your hand to rise and fall. The one giving the massage also needs to breathe deeply and be relaxed; the goal is to avoid communicating stress and tenseness. You will be amazed how relaxed you feel after giving a massage if you allow yourself to calm down and get into the sensuous flow. Slow down your mind and choose to focus on the sensuous massage rather than everything you need to be doing. This is a marvelous gift God has given you: you can mentally choose to relax and tune out the world's worries for a time.

Sequences. You will establish some sequences that will feel good to you and your mate. This chapter starts with the back and shoulders, then moves to feet and legs, then hands, abdomen, chest, and face. Because of time limitations, you may wish to do mini-massages in which you do shoulders and face, or you may wish to focus on the lower and upper back. Sometimes it will be meaningful and relaxing to stick to one part of the anatomy, such as feet or face. Create different sequences that connect and relax you as a couple. A full body massage could take at least an hour, so you will have to adapt your massage to accommodate your time schedule.

If there is a problem with sensitivity or ticklishness, try a firmer touch. If that doesn't work, move on to a less ticklish part; often you can come back later. The person being massaged often finds that the ticklishness is more mental and will go away as relaxation increases. Massage not only helps a person relax and enjoy a very sensuous experience but also is very beneficial health-wise. Massage accelerates the flow of blood in the body without straining the heart. The blood removes the waste from muscles and tissues and can promote healing and physical well-being.

BASIC TECHNIQUES OF MASSAGE

Massage is not complex. This section develops basic movements that you will need to master to pleasure and relax your mate. Many other techniques of massage are simply variations. We will demonstrate on the back and arm so you can practice quite easily as you learn.

Stroking

You will use stroking the most in your massage as you glide your hands over the skin with modified pressure. You will use this technique often (for example, applying oil) in a simple stroking motion as you rub an area with fingertips or entire hands. Remember the importance of a steady rhythm in which you vary the pressure and speed of the movements. Here are seven variations of stroking motions.

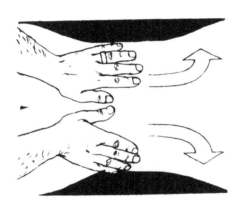

1. Fan stroking. Start with hands together and move them upward, applying pressure with palms and heels of your hands as you lean into the stroke.

Maintain gentle pressure as you mold hands to body and slide them up the abdomen and lower back.

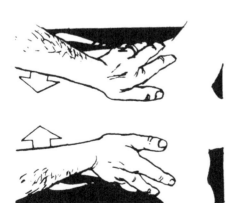

Fan hands out and lessen pressure as you glide them down and around the sides.

With light pressure move hands back into position to begin the stroke again.

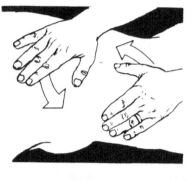

2. Circle stroking. Make a continuous circular motion with hands rotating in a wide curve, with firmer pressure on the upward stroke.

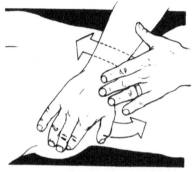

One hand does a complete circle, and the other hand crosses over in a half circle.

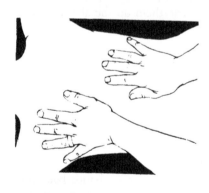

3. Alternate stroking. One hand strokes upward while the other hand glides downward in alternating motions—the upward stroke can be firmer as you vary pressure.

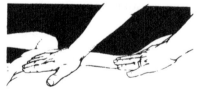

4. Sequential stroking. Stroke one hand soothingly down the area, followed immediately by the other in a rhythmic, pawing sequence as you lift the lower hand and begin again. Try with very light pressure as well as firmer.

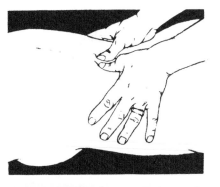

5. *Thumb stroking.* Place your thumbs on the sides of the spine and slowly move them up and back down with firm, even pressure.

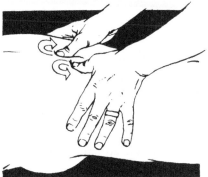

Apply pressure on an area with only the thumbs in small, firm, circular movements.

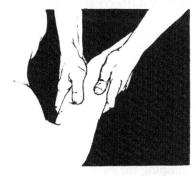

Stroke upward with one thumb and fan outward as you begin stroking upward a little higher with the other thumb and fan outward, repeating the sequence up the limb.

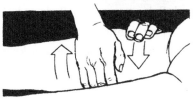

6. *Friction stroking.* Circle leg with hands placed side by side and create friction with firm pressure and alternative hand strokes.

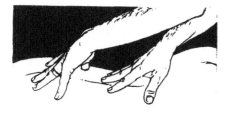

7. Brush stroking. With fingertips or the entire hand, sensitize the skin by *very* lightly brushing an area of the body—often used at the end of massaging a given part of the body.

Kneading

Kneading is a technique that you can use on larger areas (the soft tissue of the lower back) as well as smaller fleshy areas (shoulders, thighs, and calves). It is much like kneading dough and relaxes muscles as it stimulates blood circulation. You can vary the pressure and rate of kneading as you wish, harder to get to deeper muscles or lighter to just sensuously stimulate the skin.

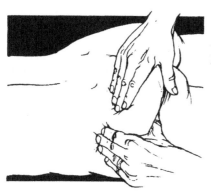

To knead, place hands on the area and squeeze and roll the flesh between the thumb and fingers of one hand as the other hand and fingers apply pressure.

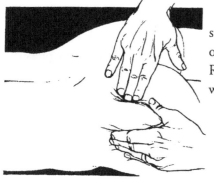

Glide the hand grasping the flesh toward the pressure of the other hand. Release; grasp the flesh with the other hand as you repeat motion with that hand. Rhythmically squeeze, push, and release as you knead with alternating hands.

Knuckling

In this technique the knuckles apply small circular strokes and create a pleasant rippling effect. This stroke is effective on back, shoulders, and chest. It can also be enjoyed on the palms of the hands or soles of the feet.

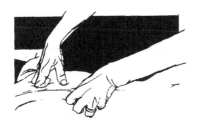

Curl your fingers into loose fists, keeping the middle joints of the fingers against the skin. Now ripple your fingers around in small, circular motions.

Pummeling

The important part of this technique, whether you are using a loose fist or relaxed hand, is to use bouncy motions and not strike the flesh. Pull your hand away as soon as it touches the skin so there is no bruising pressure. It helps to keep the wrists loose and hands and fingers relaxed so you can hear them slapping together, and the motion should be brisk as you rapidly stimulate. Sometimes pummeling might be better reserved for the end of the massage, though it can be relaxing if done more gently. It is great for fleshy areas like the back or thighs, where there are heavier muscles.

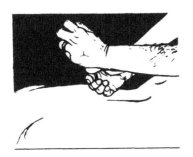

Relax your wrists and hands and apply brisk, alternating movements with your hands in a light, bouncy motion.

Passive Touching

You don't always have to be actively stroking or massaging a body area. Simply placing a hand on a spot as the partner's body feels the warmth or pressure (if applied) really feels good as tissue is stimulated by the passive touch. Passive touch also includes pulling or rotating a part of the body to loosen up and exercise joints without actively stroking.

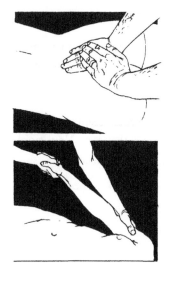

1. Pressure. Place your hands over the tailbone area and leave them there lightly for thirty seconds—now lean your hands in with pressure but no movement.

2. Lifting, pulling, and rotating. Lift your partner's arm up and down several times and gently pull up on it; now slowly rotate it in a circular motion several times, hold it a few seconds, and then lay it down.

SENSUOUS MASSAGE

Let's now look at areas of the body where you can bring tension release and sensuous pleasure to your mate with massage. The illustrations include a variety of techniques, but use your creativity as you improvise and create your own sequences. You won't believe what this sensuous nurturing will do for your friendship and love life. As you conclude the massage on each area, gently caress that area and hold your hands there a few seconds to seal the nurturing of that part.

Back Massage

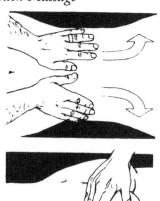

1. Fan stroking. Begin with hands on lower back with thumbs on each side of the spinal cord. Apply firm pressure as you move upward and fan out to shoulders. Squeeze firmly and stroke down over your partner's sides and back to the spinal column.

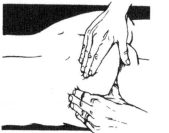

2. Kneading. Begin with the fleshy area of the lower right side and knead up and include the shoulder. Move over to the left shoulder and knead down the left side and work across the buttocks area and back to the right lower back.

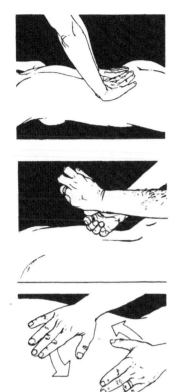

3. Passive touching. Place hands over the kidneys as your partner feels warmth and tingling. Put one hand on the tailbone and the other on the spinal column under the shoulder blades and gently press. Position heels of hands next to spinal column and press. Work your way up to the neck—gently applying pressure every few inches. Leave hands over kidney area for a few seconds.

4. Pummeling. Lightly begin pummeling with loose fists the fleshy area of the back on either side of the spinal column and the entire shoulder area.

5. Circle stroking. Start with broad circle strokes on the upper back and work your way down. Do smaller circles as you thoroughly massage both left and right sides. Remember to lightly caress the entire area and leave your hands on the middle of your mate's back for a moment to gently seal the nurturing.

Foot Massage

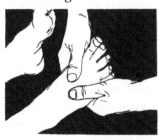

1. Stroking. Do one foot at a time. Grasp it firmly as you stroke it from ankle to heel and down the arch to the toes. Hold foot with both hands and do thumb strokes on back of the foot; stroke between the tendons and up over the arch and around the base of the ankle.

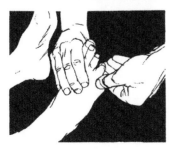

2. Toe massage. Grasp toes with your hand and wiggle and bend them. Massage each toe separately; gently squeeze and pull each toe. Hold the toes between hands and rub rapidly.

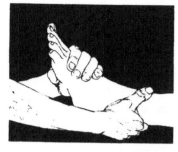

3. Passive touching. Grasp the ankle, and with the other hand, manipulate the foot; hold and apply pressure with thumbs at various points of the arch.

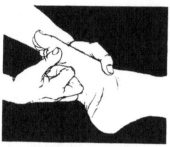

4. Knuckling. Place one hand over the top of the foot and knuckle the arch from heel to toes. Gently caress and hold the foot a minute. Go to the other foot.

Leg Massage

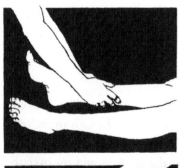

1. Stroking. Begin at the ankle, and using an alternating stroke, go up the sides of the left leg. Then repeat on the right leg. Now with one hand's fingertips on the shin and the other grasping the calf, apply alternating friction stokes as you encircle and work up the calf and thigh.

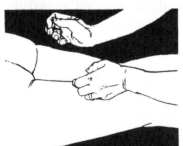

2. Pummeling. With partner on stomach, begin pummeling the calf and work your way up to the thigh. Carefully work on the upper thighs and buttocks areas in a rapid motion.

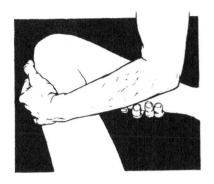

3. Passive touching. Have partner lie on back and place one of your hands under the calf and the other palm on the thigh as you softly apply pressure on both. Lift the leg and manipulate the knee and the hip joint with lifting and rotating.

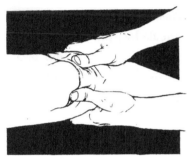

4. Thumb stroking. Grasp the knee with both hands and carefully massage with thumbs, using thumbs in small circle strokes to deeply massage. Try the same stroke on the upper thigh as you squeeze with hands, lightly caress the entire leg, and gently hold the calf and then the thigh for a moment.

Hand Massage

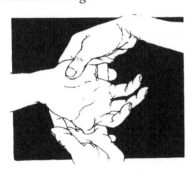

1. Thumb stroking. Lock your little fingers under the thumb and little finger of your partner's hand and massage the palm from fingers to wrist thoroughly with your thumbs.

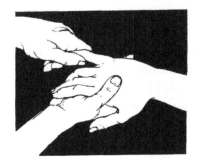

2. Finger massage. Grasp and stroke each finger as you also rotate and lightly pull. Take your index finger and thumb and rub at the base of each finger.

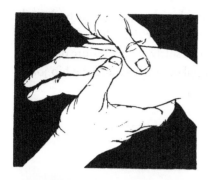

3. Passive touching. Holding your partner's arm just above the wrist, manipulate and bend each finger and the wrist. Then grasp the hand between your hands and press and release several times.

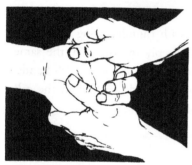

4. Thumb kneading. Focus on your partner's thumbs as you grasp and knead the fleshy palm and work your way up to the joints. Gently tug the thumb back. Conclude by caressing and holding your partner's hand between yours.

Abdomen Massage

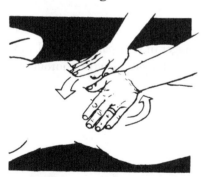

1. Circle stroking. Start with circular stroking using the navel as the center point and gently sweep in larger clockwise circles around the entire abdomen area, lapping over the sides.

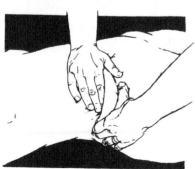

2. Kneading. Place yourself beside your partner. Start with the hip away from you and knead up the side to ribs, then work across the upper abdomen and down (the side closest to you) to the hip and knead across the lower abdomen. On areas with less flesh use fingers and thumb to knead in a lighter fashion.

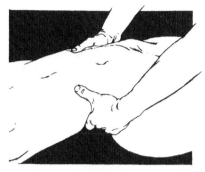

3. Passive touching. Maneuver so you can place the heels of your hands on the hipbones with fingertips touching, and gently press on the abdomen. Reach under your partner's back with your fingers meeting on the spine and gently press upward. Go back to the abdomen, then press gently and relax and press again.

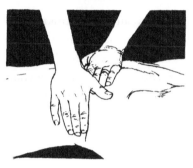

4. Sequential stroking. One hand follows the other as you start stroking on the sides with long movements up over the navel to the other side. Change sides and repeat with a smooth rhythm. Conclude with caressing the abdominal area, placing hands softly on your mate's stomach for a few seconds.

Chest and Neck Massage

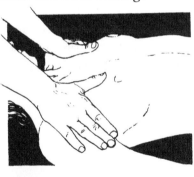

1. Fan stroking. Position yourself behind your partner's head and place hands below the collarbone. Press downward to the chest, then fan across the pectoral muscles to the shoulders and bring your fingers, with pressure, up the back of the shoulders and neck, then back to original position. Repeat.

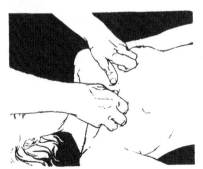

2. Knuckling. Using a knuckling stroke, ripple the muscles of the chest and shoulders and the back of the shoulders and around the back of the neck.

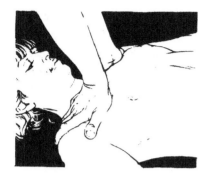

3. *Passive touching.* Place the palms of your hands on the shoulders with your fingers under the shoulder blades, then press down. Release and press again. Gently hold the head by placing your hands at the base of the skull, and slowly, without jerking, apply traction by pulling away from the head/shoulders, then rotate while the neck is loose.

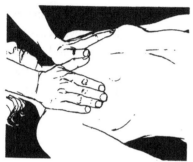

4. *Alternate stroking.* Begin alternate stroking on your partner's chest and work around to the shoulders and then to the back of the neck and shoulders. Conclude by caressing the entire area and resting your hands on your mate's upper chest for a few seconds.

Face Massage

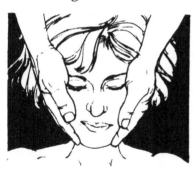

1. *Stroking.* Take your hands and softly stroke and cup the entire face—reaching under the jaw, over the cheeks, down the nose, and across the forehead and eyes.

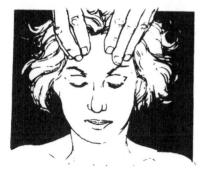

2. *Stroking with fingertips.* Do small circles with both hands, using your fingertips on the temples, jaw, base of skull, and carefully around the eyes and forehead.

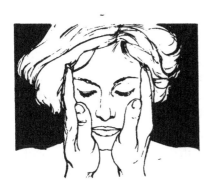

3. *Passive touching.* With your hands cupping the face, gently press on temple areas. Rest fingertips on the eyes. Press on the forehead with one hand over the other.

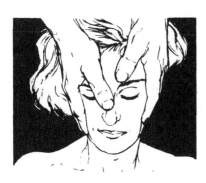

4. *Alternate stroking.* Place hands on the cheeks and do alternate stroking as you loosen the mouth and stoke up into the hairline and down to the tip of the jaw. Conclude by caressing your mate's face and gently cupping it between your hands for a few seconds.

MASSAGE TO ENHANCE LOVEMAKING

Massage will help you as a couple feel more sensuous and close. By its very relaxing and nurturing nature, it will be an aphrodisiac to your sex life. Massage can't help but teach you to be a more gentle and sensitive lover and bring you as one-flesh companions into a more bonded, caring, and stress-free relationship.

Here are some suggestions for applying the massage techniques you are mastering to more erogenous loveplay. Please keep in mind that you can destroy the soothing, sensuous experience of massage if you keep it too erotically charged. Overall, let the occasional surges of sexual feelings that come with such an intimate activity be enjoyed but not acted upon. That is why it may be wise to strategically drape your partner's body as you focus on relaxing and nurturing. Designate the times when the massage will be a prelude or part of making love and when it will be a separate event.

In the following activities, use plenty of warmed oil because the massage will be on tender areas of the body. All focus on nongenital erogenous zones and may be activities you choose to do in beginning loveplay as you increase arousal. Making love to your mate's body is such an exciting and varied process. Massage emphasizes this fact in fun and sensual ways.

Circular Sensuality

Begin a gentle, circular stroking of the chest area, starting at the collarbone and shoulder area. Use both hands in a wide, circular motion. Slowly, an inch at a time, lower the circle and massage down over the abdomen, over the pubic area, until the movements are circling the genital area with the top end of the circle on the pubic bone and the lower end over the thighs. Now start the circle moving back up to the upper chest again. This can be very arousing visually and sensually as you allow your hands to follow the contours of the body with fingers and palms lightly caressing. Don't linger on nipples or the genital area—just keep rhythmic, sensual motions.

Kneading

Have your partner lie on his or her stomach, and begin with a kneading motion on the left thigh, starting at the knee and working up over the buttocks area to the lower back. Now sensuously knead the right thigh in the same fashion. Have your partner roll over, and knead from knee to pelvic bone. Do this softly, but squeeze the flesh in a full way that manipulates the thigh and genital area as you knead.

Intimate Fan Stroking

Have your partner lie on his or her stomach, and stand (if your partner is on a table) or kneel between your partner's legs, facing the buttocks. Begin with the palms of your hands on the calf of the back of one leg (placed slightly toward the inner part of the leg) and fingers pointing upward toward the buttocks. Slowly push up with the heel of the palm in a firm stroke and do a fan motion with your fingers up over the leg to the outer side and back down. Slowly work your way up the thighs toward the buttocks an inch or two at a time as you repeat the fan motion until the top of the stroke is fanning gently down over the outer back/abdomen and hip area. Then do the other leg.

Sensual Stroking

Sit or stand beside your partner, who is lying facedown, and do a sequential stroke beginning at the left knee and working your way up almost in a wavelike motion—gently stroking at the inner thigh in a hand-over-hand sensuous rhythm that is relaxing and erotically arousing. You can continue this sequential stroking in a sideways fashion up over the buttocks area and the back. Switch to the right side and come back down to the knee. Have your partner roll over. Begin at the top of the chest and work down the side of the body over the abdomen, pubic area, and inner thighs. Switch sides and repeat from thighs up to the chest. (Try this with knuckling for a different sensation.)

Skin Tingles

Have your partner lie on his or her stomach. Start at the base of the skull with one hand and slowly move it, hardly touching the skin, in one continuous brush stroke down the body to the ankles and very softly back up, conforming to the contours of the body. Repeat several times, going down the right and left sides of the body. Now with your fingertips, lightly stroke all over the body as the skin tingles.

Have your mate roll over and face up. Do small, circular motions lightly with both hands over the whole body from face to feet for several minutes. Hardly touch the skin with very light strokes on the chest, breasts, abdomen, shoulders, thighs, legs, hands—the whole front of the body. This exercise is very sensually arousing and can awaken and stimulate the skin. Finish by lightly stroking with the fingertips.

Let massage be another way of enjoying your one-flesh companionship. Don't get too technical, but practice enough to become comfortable. You may wish to buy a whole book on massage and learn more specific ways to relax and stimulate various parts of the body. Go to a bookstore, look over what is available, and pick one that meets your needs. You also may want to invest in a massage table, or make one, as my missionary friends did. Great lovers have mastered the art of sensuous touching. Massage is a marvelous way to develop that skill as you relieve stress and grow more intimately connected to your mate in the process.

CHAPTER TEN

Making Love with Clothes On

MANY COUPLES EARNESTLY SEARCH for a deeper intimacy in their marriages. They wish longingly to feel more in love and recapture some of the passion of their dating days. If only they could be playful soul mates and enjoy a fun companionship. Making love, of all marital activities, should be a powerful agent in creating this type of intimate bonding.

What happens to sabotage lovemaking so it doesn't create this loving closeness? I think the biggest culprit is that married partners forget the important concept of making love with their clothes on. In an exciting, intertwining way, sex should permeate the whole marital relationship. Perhaps the word *foreplay* should be banned. *Loveplay* more aptly describes what God intended for couples who are sexually bonding. It does not depend on having your clothes off and reaching a climax. Making love is so much more than intercourse.

In the Song of Solomon the wife speaks about her mate and making love in a beautifully poetic fashion:

> His mouth is most sweet,
> Yes, he is altogether lovely.
> This is my beloved,
> And this is my friend . . .
> My beloved has gone to his garden,
> To the beds of spices,
> To feed his flock in the gardens,
> And to gather lilies.
> I am my beloved's,
> And my beloved is mine. (5:16; 6:2–3 NKJV)

Kissing, cuddling, and giving long, romantic looks with some "lily gathering" should be daily or even hourly activities as you keep your mate present in your thoughts and life.

Time Out: Close your eyes and get comfortable. Allow your imagination to take you back in time to when you first met and were getting to know and love your mate. Remember some of your first dates and times alone together. Recall your feelings and the many things that initially attracted you to each other. Fantasize about some of those early sexual feelings. Recollect and re-create those times when you intimately bonded with your clothes on and it had nothing to do with genital sexuality.

The goal of this chapter is to help you feel a deeper sense of intimate companionship as you learn to make love as a total part of your relationship. It reviews the important concept of pair bonding and the need to be sexually complex and balanced, because genital focus alone can be impoverishing to a fun love life. It then describes and encourages a sexual celebration for two that is not centered on the goal of intercourse. Creative techniques for erotic fun with clothes on close out the chapter.

When you were dating and putting your best foot forward, you abandoned your defenses and allowed yourself to be intimate and uninhibited. You may feel uncomfortable with the deep kind of intimacy encouraged in this chapter. In order to really feel in love and sexually alive, you will have to let down your walls and defenses and need for control all over again. This type of intimacy requires trusting and being vulnerable and living joyfully in the present moment.

PAIR BONDING

Loveplay and intimate bonding are a great prescription for your sex life. Forget about intercourse and some of your other favorite sexual focuses for a little while. Create some alone time with your partner. Then fix some popcorn, put on some music, sit on the couch with your sweetheart, and let yourself be transported back in time to your courting days. Recapture some of the magic of those days when just looking into each other's eyes and holding hands was a spiritual experience with a physical rush of feelings. Remember when you made love for hours with little or no physical touch and your souls communed.

Sociologist Desmond Morris addressed this important concept and process in his book *Intimate Behaviour* and called it "pair formation" or "pair bonding." He observed humans in their courting behaviors and saw a process that often included all or most of twelve separate steps. Each step is progressively different and important. The needs of an initial step cannot be met by skipping ahead to another. Lovers often hope that genital-to-genital involvement will instantly create intimacy. They fail to realize, to their great detriment, that intimate bonding is indeed a process.

I have taken the concept of pair bonding and applied it to the sexual enrichment of a marriage and the importance of making love with clothes on. Even though intercourse is an important part of married love, mates need to continually incorporate each of the twelve steps. Here is a simple summary (from Desmond Morris's work) of these important steps that can help you build or recapture a deeper romance and intimacy.[1]

12 Steps of Pair Bonding

1. Eye to body. Our senses feed our mind information about another person. This includes sexual information, but it is a more total observation. We sort and assess this information as we define attractiveness. We sum up and ponder in our mind the personal and physical qualities that are appealing to us.

2. Eye to eye. People usually watch one another privately and do not directly look into each other's eyes. Strangers will often break eye contact because this is an invasion of privacy. A friendly smile or an inviting look is often the beginning of more intimate contact. The old song "Drink to Me Only with Thine Eyes" emphasizes a crucial bonding behavior.

3. Voice to voice. Often initial verbal contact is quite casual but furthers the bonding process. The connecting conversation allows more information to be exchanged. Accents, tones of voice, vocabularies, and styles of communication and thinking all give valuable knowledge to the pair becoming intimately involved.

4. Hand to hand. Hand to hand or arm may be more of a supportive behavior at first, as one person assists the other out of a car or lightly supplies directional guidance. It may be a disguised intimacy and lead to more hand-holding if there is a mutual inclination and desire for closeness. Both partners are aware that this is symbolic of a bonding sequence that may in time involve richer intimacies.

5. Arm to shoulder. The previous steps can be more casual in nature, but this step intentionally brings the partner into closer body contact. An arm around the shoulder communicates a message of close friendship and perhaps love. It draws the partners together and indicates a deeper desire for intimate companionship.

6. Arm to waist. This is a more direct statement of sexual and romantic interest. The arm is around the waist and closer to the private areas of the body. Arm to waist is indicative of a growing intimacy and amorous bonding. Like the preceding step, it brings the trunks of the bodies into contact in an increasing intimacy.

7. Mouth to mouth. Kissing on the mouth with the accompanying behavior of a close, frontal embrace is a big step forward in pair bonding. This is the initial step that can create erotic and genital arousal, especially with prolonged and intimate kissing. The man and woman are becoming lovers and are enjoying sexual arousal, with an intimate closeness developing.

8. Hand to head. Perhaps as an accompanying behavior to the intimate kissing, the hands touch and caress the partner's head. The defensive walls are let down and bonding occurs as fingers tenderly stoke the face, hair, ears, and neck. Sometimes the hand will lovingly clasp the head in a communication of caring and intimate possessiveness.

9. Hand to body. Intimacy deepens as the hands explore the partner's body with touching, rubbing, squeezing, and gentle fondling. The trust and bonding is deepening with caressing of the more intimate areas and further sexual arousal. Often couples who do not wish to proceed to completion in making love will stop at this step.

10. Mouth to breast. With this step the bonding behaviors have become private and a new level of intimacy has been reached. The first nine steps, with the exception of caressing a more intimate part of the body, might be expressed in public and the pair bonding developed without a need for privacy. The female breast is covered in most societies, and its exposure is symbolic of advanced intimacy. The mouth caressing and suckling the breast is the last of the pregenital bonding behaviors. This step is usually the prelude of stimulation to an orgasm, rather than a more general step in loveplay.

11. Hand to genital. This is an advanced step in pair bonding. Touching the lover's genitals implies a sufficient level of trust and bond of attachment for deeper intimacies. This touching often begins in a teasing, caressing manner. As arousal increases, the partner proceeds to a tender, rhythmic rubbing that stimulates arousal. This step can include the intimate behaviors of stroking the penis, fondling the labia and clitoris, and inserting fingers into the vagina. Manual stimulation can also lead to the partners trusting each other in the sharing of a climax.

12. Genital to genital. The final stage of pair formation includes intercourse and the potential for creating a life. Each preceding step will have deepened the bond of attachment and intimate connection. The intimacy of intercourse is built on the earlier bonding behaviors that have created a partnership to provide for the possibility of pregnancy. The design is that the couple remain bonded beyond the satisfaction of the sex drive in orgasm. The couple will have created an intimacy deeper and more long lasting than sexual arousal and consummation.

If you want to feel more deeply in love and expand into a full-time lover, devote some time to each of these steps. Let's take them one at a time and explore how each can enrich your sex life. Ralph Waldo Emerson stated that "foolish consistency is the hobgoblin of little minds." No one wants to be categorized as having a little mind and neglecting effective ways to enrich sexuality. Everyone at times gets into a destructive "consistency." That is why this chapter de-emphasizes orgasm and intercourse in making love. You need to expand your sexual realities. Certainly you want to be a wise lover characterized by emotional depth and an enriching complexity.

A holistic view of making love is an attitude from which exciting behaviors flow. There are great returns in practicing better body and mind control—in not being ruled by the heat of the moment. God intended His one-flesh concept to include a lot more than intercourse.

In the first three steps couples learn and share information that builds companionship and sets the stage for sexual connectedness. In these steps there is no erotic touching. Steps four through nine encourage a fun sexuality that is not genitally focused. They are less erotic in nature than the last three steps. As you practice these steps, you will find it exciting to make love with your clothes on.

1. Eye to body. This step includes much more than observing or staring at select parts of your mate's nude body. Become a student of your spouse's body as you fall more deeply in love. No one perfectly meets Hollywood standards, but everyone has many endearing qualities. Examples are dimples, hairy legs, expressive hands, the face lit up with a smile, startling blue eyes, the shape of the nose, the calves, and the body intensity when sharing a story or working in the yard.

Practice Exercise: Let the word *bedroom* trigger in your mind an opportunity to carefully observe. So often *bedroom* triggers the idea of sleep or a place for active sex play. The bedroom is actually a marvelous place to study your mate and notice some things that you passed over. Focus on noticing, accepting, and enjoying as you tune in to your mate's masculinity or femininity when putting on clothes, reading a book, or simply bustling about. Observe your mate peacefully sleeping at night and feel happy for this companion God has given you.

2. Eye to eye. Do you two look into each other's souls anymore? Eye-to-eye contact connects two individuals in this special way. Romantic dinners are integral for staying in love. They are sensual feasts, and they create a context for much eye-to-eye bonding. In the busyness of life, lovers forget to make eye contact when they are talking—or for that matter, when they are making love. The eyes express so much: acceptance, excitement, a longing to understand, and sexual desire.

Practice Exercise: Look into your mate's eyes whenever possible. See if you don't feel more connected and in love after a couple of days of doing this. Communicate warmth, acceptance, and appreciation with this eye contact.

3. Voice to voice. Isn't it amusing how much time adolescents can spend on the phone? Perhaps you remember when you and your mate first met and started dating—an hour-long phone conversation was not that unusual. Your voice and speech patterns are unique and can trigger warmth and enjoyment in your partner. The chapter on sexual communication noted how erotic talking about sex can be, whether in bed or with all of your clothes on. Learn to love your mate's voice as you connect through intimate conversations. Husbands may have to work harder on just engaging in connecting chitchat and meeting their wives' greater need for conversation, which is a crucial part of intimate companionship.

Practice Exercise: Stop reading right now and say to your mate, "I love you!" It may necessitate a phone call. Make contact voice to voice!

4. Hand to hand. Holding hands has special meaning. This behavior symbolizes trust, protection, and caring. An excellent example is a child who holds an adult's hand almost instinctively. When lovers hold hands, they convey this idea of trust and togetherness as well as acknowledge sexual bondedness. Holding your mate's hand in public demonstrates the one-flesh companionship you two have created and are continually creating. Gently squeezing your partner's hand when you are in the car says you think of and value this love relationship. It's a fun way to make love without taking your clothes off.

Practice Exercise: Unless you are different from most couples (if so, I congratulate you), you have pretty much quit holding hands. Make a mental note to hold hands the next time you are leaving church, driving to Mom's, or sitting on the couch.

5. Arm to shoulder. Commitment is a vital component of fun sex. On the one hand, it is saying, "We can count on each other, and together we will build one great sex life." On the other hand, it is saying, "Forget about the sexual transmission of HIV or other STDs, sweetheart; we're clean, and our fidelity will keep us that way." A partnership is comforting, and two can be better than one. It is great to feel an arm around your shoulder and have a lover to help you achieve your personal goals as well as your sexual potential.

Practice Exercise: Commitment involves a series of daily choices that protect your marriage and your sex life. Have you made any poor choices recently? How about serving on that extra committee, working late, or not exercising? How could you rectify these destructive choices this week and get that arm more firmly back around his or her shoulder?

6. Arm to waist. So many pop songs emphasize getting closer. This deepening of intimacy is a complex task. Intercourse and genital intimacy won't eliminate the need for preliminary buildup and loveplay. Remember a key concept of pair bonding: you can't meet the needs of one step by skipping ahead to another! Arm to waist provides a different closeness from genital to genital. This closeness can be exemplified by a full body hug where you pull your mate tight and revel in the warmth of each other's closeness. Sexually, this would be more like being on first base: sharing fantasies, caressing and holding, talking, and drawing close. These activities can be enhanced by keeping your clothes on as you reach out and pull your mate close.

Practice Exercise: At least four times this week, embrace your mate in a bear hug for ten seconds (you'll be amazed how long that is), kiss the neck, and express your love. You will be surprised what this arm-to-waist activity will do for helping you feel in love and increasing sexual desire.

7. Mouth to mouth. Mouth to mouth creates a sensuous, experiential bonding. Emotions and minds and bodies connect in a special manner, and there is fusion in a romantic and erotic rush of feelings. You allow your partner deeper into your private spaces as you actually kiss and exchange body fluids; you experience a scary but exciting lowering of your ego boundaries and a melding with another person. There is almost no need for talking in this step. The action speaks for itself: *Let me gaze into your eyes and passionately kiss your lips. You are mine and I am yours.*

Practice Exercise: Married couples can forget the importance of kissing. Put on some soft music, wrap your arms around each other, and get body to body as you gaze into each other's eyes. Close your eyes and focus your whole mind and senses on slow, sensual kissing as you bond.

8. Hand to head. This is trust! You may not like people to muss your hair up, caress your face, or touch your head. My mom, my daughter, and my granddaughter are the only ones apart from my wife who touch my head. But we can feel safe with our spouse. Hand to head is so tender and intimate.

Practice Exercise: Place your head in your mate's lap so that you can be caressed and nurtured. It may feel uncomfortable at first, but try to relax. Try some facial massage (explained in the last chapter). You may discover you also don't know how to relax and let your mate nurture you during lovemaking.

9. Hand to body. Start on the outside of the clothes and keep away from the erogenous zones. The husband can unbutton the wife's blouse or the wife can pull down the husband's zipper later. This is sensual exploring and relaxing caressing. Giving and receiving sensual pleasure are possible for every lover. Read the chapter on sensuous massage and get creative in this hand-to-body bonding. Learn to enjoy level-two erogenous zones. You are nurturing and accepting this person you love. You are saying, "Your body is unique and I enjoy it. You are one sensuous person!" Your clothes will be a signal to go slow and build this hand-to-body experience. Pretend you are making love with your clothes on.

Practice Exercise: Get in your car and find a safe parking place (it may be in your garage). Have some fun hand-to-body contact or get steamy without taking clothes off or following through.

10. Mouth to breast. Now the husband can unfasten his wife's bra and allow another level of pair bonding. What might the male be experiencing? Dependency and closeness, acknowledgment of his sexual needs, appreciation of her need to nurture, sexual arousal in enjoyment of this special symbol of femininity, and a desire to stimulate his mate. What might the female be experiencing? Intimacy and vulnerability in sharing a special part of her body, pleasure in nurturing her man, sexual arousal, and realization of the sexy power of her feminine self. This is fusion on a deeper level than simply nibbling on erotic tissue. Mouth to breast is symbolic! You are acknowledging the fact that you depend on each other to create this great sexual magnetic field of excitement. God's magnificent design of complementary differences is being celebrated with male and female needing each other. The female can also enjoy the male body by nibbling on his nipples, neck, and stomach as she sensuously bonds by placing her mouth on his erogenous zones. He may feel reluctant at first, but he, too, can enjoy the mouth-to-breast foreplay.

Practice Exercise: When the mood is right, the wife can invite her husband to make love to her breasts. He can pull her blouse up, but the rest of the clothes stay on. Allow yourself to enjoy the pleasure and the symbolic nature of this love-play. Salute your mutual ability to meet needs and merge into warm closeness. Then reverse roles.

11. Hand to genital. This level of intimacy expresses that each is completely the other's to enjoy. To hold your husband's testicles in your hand, with their sensual softness, truly symbolizes his trust and sexual surrender. To tenderly and voluptuously slip your finger into your wife's vagina demonstrates her confidence in and love for you. Be sensuous and go slowly as you become a total lover.

Practice Exercise: Undo zippers and belts but again keep clothes on, and preferably do this in the dark. This is a tactile adventure and experience in sexual bonding. Loosen clothes and underwear as needed as you slowly touch and explore genitals in a renewed way. No orgasms—you are making love with clothes on. Your mind and emotions are tracing and memorizing favorite sensations through your fingers. You are strengthening attachment and trust.

12. Genital to genital. We are to remember that "the two shall become one flesh" (Matt. 19:5 NKJV). Somehow we were created with an intense enjoyment of and need for this genital union. Never forget the emotional and spiritual closeness of this final step of pair bonding. Never forfeit the sheer sexual excitement of this lover's embrace. This step involves intercourse, even though this chapter is trying to de-emphasize this aspect of making love. Allow this to be playful and focused as you keep as many of your clothes on as possible. Don't climax—this is genital-to-genital bonding. Isn't it exciting to think that you will repeat this act countless times over the coming years? The sexual potential and promise of an intimate marriage are amazing.

Practice Exercise: Get each other excited with some face-to-face and hand-to-body connecting, then very slowly let vagina contain penis. Hold each other in this embrace for a few minutes. Stop for now and do something else companionable. This step obviously takes mutual resolve and willpower but will teach some important lessons on making love all the time.

ROMANTIC FUN WITH CLOTHES ON

This section offers more suggestions for making love without the urgency to head for the bedroom and get nude. These activities further underscore the spirit of erotic fun with clothes on—subtle, pervasive, spontaneous, tantalizing, and sensuous loveplay.

Sensual Exploring

How do you think Marco Polo felt enjoying marvelous new experiences daily? Great lovers have the qualities of a famous explorer: curiosity, adventure, and a desire for more knowledge and new discoveries. Your mate's body can be your undiscovered territory if you are willing to enjoy eye-to-body and hand-to-body bonding in innovative ways. This exploring can be done nude, but doing it clothed has special excitement. It allows you to concentrate on exposed parts like face, hands, and feet without genital distraction.

It is easy to build the attitudes of a sensual explorer, letting your fingers do the walking. Gently explore curves and crannies; feel the beauty of the human body and the softness of a cheek or firmness of a shoulder. Drink up your lover's uniqueness as you touch and memorize some of your favorite sensations. Close your eyes and focus on hand-to-body contact as you lightly run fingertips over your partner.

Part of the fun of making love with clothes on is the sensuous texture of fabric and the way it alters the feel of the body under it. Gently stroke your mate's back with a T-shirt on, and feel the soft warmth of the flesh underneath. Wife, stroke your husband's genitals with his underwear on. Now repeat, caressing the body with a more silky fabric—the experience is entirely different. Stand up facing your mate and massage his upper arms with his suit coat on. Husband, lightly touch your wife's hips and buttocks with a slip or pantyhose over them. Expand beyond erogenous zones and become a sensual explorer!

Physical Affection Versus Grabbing or Controlling

"I wish we could hug without him grabbing me." One wife related how she and her female friends at work were laughing in frustrated amusement about how their husbands' hands were "homing devices." This irritating male habit is certainly not consistent with the idea of making love with clothes on. Couples, wives especially, need physical affection and warm nurturing gestures that are not always focused on the breasts or buttocks or genitals. Maybe you did not grow up in a home in which physical affection was demonstrated freely. You may need to learn physical nurture that is not overtly sexual.

Perhaps it is not fair to pick on men. Some women also have trouble allowing easy physical affection without its heading in a sexual direction. More often, however, the female counterpart to grabbing is needing control. Making love with clothes on can be hampered by always wanting exactly the right time and place. Yes, it can be a nuisance to stop and get romantic when you are intensely involved in a project. And yes, when you are busy, sex may be the furthest thing from your mind. But part of making love all the time involves relaxing control and enjoying your mate.

After your mate has had a shower, take a towel and dry off his or her body. Who cares if you have an hour before you head for church. This will take five minutes. Massage the scalp, rub the back, pat the face, and nurture your mate. Like other making-love-with-clothes-on gestures, the emphasis is not on visual or even physical stimulation but on touching and enjoying with a cloth boundary. Let it be a subtle sexual experience.

Dressing Up

Clothes are fun erotically. They stimulate the imagination and increase anticipation. Imagine what is under a robe or a strategically draped towel. Use your creativity and dress up for your mate. Flatter your strengths, and flaunt your masculinity or femininity. Build a private wardrobe designed for making love and increasing sexual attractiveness.

Clothing doesn't have to stimulate erotic thought to enhance your ability to make love to your mate all the time. Maybe you enjoy dressing up for a wedding or a night on the town. Making love with clothes on is getting excited by your mate's appearance in evening clothes, admiring that new tennis outfit or colorful top, appreciating a particular piece of jewelry, and delighting in the love and joy of eye-to-body pair bonding. Dress up for your mate, and watch your intimacy grow deeper.

Unexpected Treats

Variety and the unexpected do indeed create spice in life. Part of the fun of making love with clothes on is spontaneously enjoying hand-to-body, hand-to-genital, and genital-to-genital encounters while clothed. Unzipping pants in the privacy of a car or home in order to share some quick contact is tremendously exciting. Stay loose, and don't get goal oriented—just enjoy the short encounter.

So much of your time is spent clothed, so plan treats for your mate. Buy an outfit with convenient buttons or zippers. Let the erotic and romantic pervade your relationship. Encourage that occasional foray beneath the clothing as you keep the unexpected alive.

A Striptease for One

Be intimate and trusting and allow yourself to be totally naked and unashamed with your mate. Falling deeper in love is a marvelous process. In the context of this safe relationship of marriage it is bonding to do some stripteasing and self-disclosing. Baring your soul is usually more difficult than taking your clothes off, but both are important. Orchestrating your private striptease for your mate can be another playful aspect of making love with your clothes on.

I am talking to both husband and wife, and I am not encouraging you to get completely nude. Wife, put on your husband's shirt over a funny T-shirt and wear some sexy lingerie under that. Take your time in slowly pulling off various garments as you eat supper or do some other activity together. Right now in your closet and drawers you have all the garments for a fantastic show. Maybe include a fancy dress, your bathing suit, and the lavender bra and panties. Get creative and have some fun being silly together.

Husband, find out what garments are sexy to your wife and what aspects of your body trigger erotic thoughts. If it is your hairy legs or muscled shoulders, start off with them covered and show them off as the striptease proceeds. Buy a muscle shirt or brightly colored gym shorts. Be subtle, and arouse your mate with innuendo and hidden secrets. Maybe do the unexpected by buying a crazy for-you-only item of apparel and setting the stage so you can slowly strip. This is pair bonding and loveplay. You are building that deeper intimacy you have been searching for. Throw caution to the wind, and let the clown and entertainer in you take over.

CHAPTER ELEVEN

Mutual Pleasuring

GOD GAVE US SUCH A PRICELESS and unique gift in demonstrating and creating love through sexual intimacy. Making love encourages mates to focus on fun, be lighthearted, indulge curiosity and playfulness, and experience some awesome feelings. In sex, lovers are supposed to get out of their controlled, everyday adult routine and create a bonding, erotic, and adventurous experience together. What glue and recreation and nurturing and three-dimensional fun this sexual connecting is. True sexual lovers will never be simply roommates.

This chapter focuses on the sensual pleasuring of your mate's level-one and level-two erogenous zones, without a demand for intercourse or orgasms. Nondemanding genital pleasuring does not mean you must exclude intercourse and orgasms. It simply means that bonding, affectionate sex can be hampered if it is always goal-oriented, rushing into intercourse or producing a climax. The chapter starts off with describing the concept of pleasuring and distinguishes isolating masturbation from personal pleasure. It develops two comfortable positions for you and your mate to pleasure each other and enjoy genital sensuality. It concludes with some suggestions for including nondemanding genital pleasuring in your repertoire as another way to make love.

PLEASURING: MUTUAL AND PERSONAL

Pleasure is an interesting word. Somehow it almost does not seem to fit within Christian values. It feels self-centered and selfish. The truth of the matter is that God gave us our erotic sensuality to enjoy. The sin is not in experiencing pleasure but in calling pleasure sinful when it isn't.

Enjoying Pleasuring

Many Christians think they don't deserve pleasure, sexual or otherwise. Perhaps it does seem very self-centered and contrary to our hardworking, self-sacrificing American Christian ethic. The truth is, however, that God created humans with the ability to experience and enjoy pleasurable feelings. And marriage enables mates to help each other overcome inhibitions and enhance the ability to become aroused and both relax and revel in sexual joy.

Enjoying genital pleasuring that is slow and bonding without pressure and demands is critical to a truly intimate, nurturing, and exciting sex life. You need to be able to make love for half an hour to a couple of hours at a time. You have already explored the enjoyment of sensual massage. Pleasuring is a more focused sensual massage. It requires that you notice and give yourself permission to enjoy your sexual feelings, and find relaxed and comfortable positions that enhance the process and help you luxuriate and focus in on your sensuality and sexual pleasure.

Experiencing Personal and Mutual Pleasure

In working through and understanding experiencing personal pleasure, we need to discuss the concept of masturbation. The word *masturbation* conjures up all kinds of taboos and guilt. Myths existed even in medical textbooks into the 1930s about masturbation causing psychoses, "lunacy," blindness, and many other mental and physical problems. Supposedly, people could identify such self-abusers by the way they walked and their stunted physical development. Obviously, this is not true, psychologically or medically.

In terms of morality, the Bible is silent on the topic of masturbation. It does not say the behavior is right or wrong to do. Like some other sexual behaviors, we keep it in accord with God's sexual economy by applying other scriptural principles.

Christianity has been reluctant to deal with masturbation and has even fostered some of the myths about it. One such myth is denouncing masturbation by calling it onanism and saying that Scripture is clear on this point. This is a gross misinterpretation of the Genesis account. In the story, Onan's brother died, and the custom was for Onan to impregnate his sister-in-law so she could have children to carry on his brother's name. Onan apparently wanted the inheritance for himself and his own children, so he selfishly practiced the withdrawal method of birth control: "But Onan knew that the offspring would not be his; so whenever he lay with his brother's wife, he spilled his semen on the ground to keep from producing offspring for his brother" (Gen. 38:9 NIV).

Some of the prohibition against masturbation seems to have evolved from the early church doctrine on birth control. Within marriage, masturbation was viewed as a form of preventing conception. It also was seen as promoting uncontrolled lust and self-centered sex.

In looking at the scriptural guidelines on masturbation, four ideas seem important in defining our theology and practice within God's sexual guidelines:

1. God created sexuality to reveal Himself and His love of intimate relationships. His sexual verbs are *relate* and *connect*. Masturbation at best is incomplete and may take the edge off of hormonal desire but is a solitary activity. It becomes a detour to intimacy in marriage because our hormonal desire should drive us to each other—not to nonintimate masturbating. Genital pleasuring as a solitary activity can create a secret world that diminishes your mate and excludes you from a more exciting sex life. Masturbation can signal laziness or a fear of intimacy.

2. Any sexual behavior that becomes a habit can be detrimental to and narrow your sex life. This is true of simply getting locked into a routine that excludes spontaneity or focuses only on intercourse. It is also true of masturbating, which can create a habitual kind of sex that detracts from making love and locks in a type of erotic arousal that your mate cannot duplicate. The apostle Paul wisely wrote, "All things are lawful for me, but all things are not helpful. All things are lawful for me, but I will not be brought under the power of any" (1 Cor. 6:12 NKJV).

3. In any type of sexual pleasuring, you must guard your fantasy and thought life. In Chapter 7, we explored the importance of keeping sexual desire and fantasy within God's guidelines. The bottom line was allowing sexual thinking to promote intimacy with your mate and not have your partnership adulterated by fantasizing about other people. If you use masturbation as a solitary activity to release sexual tension while separated from your mate, you run the risks with your thought life as well as not allowing your mate to create intimate connecting, which is the deeper need—not just need for release.

4. Sexually compulsive or addictive persons should never masturbate. Chapter 28 discusses sex addiction. A simple definition would be someone who exclusively uses sex to destructively control and alter feelings, much as others use alcohol or food. Masturbation becomes an isolating activity and builds a secret world, separate from the mate, in which sex becomes a drug to combat boredom or relieve stress or alleviate guilt. As with any drug or surge of adrenaline, sex outside the concept of a loving relationship takes bigger doses and can lead to destructive behaviors like exhibitionism, voyeurism, and hours spent watching pornography.

Married couples need to establish the difference between isolating masturbation and personal and mutual pleasuring. Most couples are fine as long as they are stimulating each other to an orgasm, manually or orally. They enjoy this as loveplay and pleasuring, with no question of masturbation. It becomes more questionable if pleasuring includes touching yourself, even if your mate is present and participating. It can somehow feel wrong even if done in the context of lovemaking.

Because of the excessive baggage the word *masturbation* carries with it, it is preferable to use the descriptive words *genital pleasuring* in the context of making love. This is a behavior that can be done to yourself (personal) and to your mate (mutual). We have already established that great sex is built on enjoying your own feelings uninhibitedly, which also arouses your mate. Sometimes in the excitement of making love or the nature of some lovemaking positions, it will be natural and arousing to increase the stimulation of your genitals by stroking yourself. This is true of the husband as he grows older and needs more direct stimulation of the penis to gain and maintain an erection.

I think, especially as a wife is working to become more easily orgasmic, personal pleasuring can be a gift to the marriage in self-discovery. Mates can learn about their arousal patterns and what type of stroking feels best on which areas of their bodies. Husbands and wives can also demonstrate to their partner what feels most arousing. If we aren't careful, we can become legalistic in never touching ourselves. I remember the female client who stated she liked the husband-on-top position of intercourse but that she also enjoyed continued stimulation of the clitoris during his thrusting. I suggested that the most effective way to do that during this position was for her to reach down and stimulate her own clitoris. She exclaimed, "I couldn't do that! That would be touching myself."

Lovemaking is a mutual celebration, whether we are stimulating our own body or our mate's body. We are sharing pleasure and arousal. Work beyond the fear of self-stimulation or being selfish and learn to play together.

I include three different aspects of genital pleasuring from which I have banned the word *masturbation*—and thus the idea "Yuck, I'm touching myself": (1) pleasuring each other's and our own genitals indiscriminately as a part of making love and enjoying arousal that can create pleasure and lead to a climax; (2) stimulating yourself during sexual interaction to maintain or increase arousal; and (3) arousing yourself apart from your mate as a learning experience to increase personal awareness of pleasuring and how to more easily be aroused, which will be incorporated later into lovemaking. (If genital pleasuring is utilized for releasing sexual tension in the unavailability of your mate, this area will have to be thought through more carefully in the context of your marriage and masturbation.)

Positions for Genital Pleasuring

Here are two relaxing positions that lend themselves to nondemanding genital pleasuring of various kinds. In each position, you may wish to lie on pillows or use the back of the bed to prop up and get comfortable.

1. Sitting or lying with legs overlapped. You can experiment with whose legs are better on top in the overlapping process. Size and whether you are the pleasurer or the pleasuree can make a difference. The pleasuree may wish to lie down with knees bent and focus on personal pleasure, while the pleasurer props against the back of the bed with pillows in a sitting position. Both may wish to face each other, sitting and look deeply into each other's eyes. This position lends itself to communicating and exchanging nonverbal signs of pleasure.

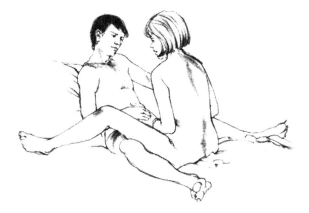

Fig. 11.1. Sitting with legs overlapped

2. Sitting with back to chest. This position has the pleasuree sitting comfortably between the legs of the pleasurer, leaning back against his or her chest to be cuddled and pleasured. The hands of the pleasurer have access to the chest and genitals of the partner. The pleasurer can be propped up against the back of the bed for comfort. An important part of nondemanding genital pleasuring is feeling close and connected as you give your mate pleasure and in turn sensuously enjoy your mate's body. This position allows special closeness as you cuddle up close to your partner and enjoy the delight of the hands. Another important aspect of mutual pleasuring is feeling supported and comfortable physically. This position helps prevent aching backs and sore knees.

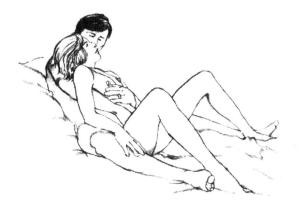

Fig. 11.2. Sitting with back to chest

Making Love with Genital Pleasuring

Helen and George valued the sexual part of their relationship. But the longer they were married, the more neglected and routine it became. Their biggest disagreement sexually was about George's greater need for sexual frequency and release and Helen's feeling pressured to perform. Both wished they could put more of the sparkle of earlier years back into their love-making. (With some other couples, the roles of George and Helen are reversed, with the wife feeling a lack of frequency and sexual attention.)

Practicing genital pleasuring became a key source of making changes as intercourse was de-emphasized. Helen did not want to have an orgasm every time they made love. George felt that he wasn't a very good lover or did not have as much fun unless she wholeheartedly entered the process and he brought her to a climax. Learning the pleasuring positions and starting off with genital exploration and slow, sensual massage of the genital areas got them back into the habit of taking more time to play and build excitement. It was done in a non-demanding fashion so that Helen could relax but not climax unless she so desired.

Genital Exploration and Massage

They began by sitting with legs overlapped, and through sensual touching, they explored each other's genital area from top to bottom. With Helen lying back, George started with her outer vulval lips and moved to the inner lips and the clitoral area and finally into her vagina. He did this gently, with plenty of lubrication. He found his index finger to be most sensitive to the nerve endings. During this entire process, they communicated with each other about what felt most sensitive to her and what was particularly sensual to him as he experienced her body. Part of the time he closed his eyes so he could focus on his sense of touch and revel in her softness.

Helen then explored George, beginning with the base of his penis between the scrotal sac and the perineum at the external point of the prostate. With her fingers and her whole hand she then caressed his testicles and proceeded up to his penis, where she explored the shaft, top to bottom. Extra care was taken for the head of the penis, with its ridges and sensitive nerve endings.

They took their time doing this exercise, stretching it out over most of an hour. They repeated it within the week, and later discussed that it was an entirely different experience to explore each other's body the second time. They were becoming more aware of each other's skin and softness, and this kind of touching seemed more sensual and exciting.

In the coming weeks they progressed to genital massage. He enjoyed having her sit with her back to his chest as she propped her knees up and leaned comfortably back. He had easy access to her genitals while he held her warmly to him. It also allowed nongenital caressing of face, neck, tummy, and thighs. She liked to kneel between his legs facing his genitals. She could easily use both hands and seemed to get less tired as they adapted their own fun routine and variants of the pleasuring positions.

At first, George's ego was a little offended when she offered to show him what felt good to her, and he kept his hand too rigid for Helen to place his hand over hers and guide. As he relaxed it, she was able to demonstrate some of the touches that she found most arousing. She took his relaxed index finger and placed her index finger over it as she caressed her clitoris. He showed her places on his penis that were especially sensitive and placed his hand around hers as she massaged his penis, to help her learn the firmness and rhythms he appreciated the most.

They liked to use coconut oil as a lubricant even though it was not water soluble. (You as a couple can experiment with what feels and smells and tastes best to you—depending perhaps on the type of genital massage you wish to engage in on a particular occasion.) Both were pleased that the genital exploration and massage increased the wife's pleasure and desire for sex. She felt more attended to and loved the closeness. The husband developed greater sensuality. Both welcomed it as they expanded their repertoire for erotic arousal to include some very stimulating touching.

Nurturing Through Orgasms

George had a higher desire for sexual activity than Helen did. She explained that it wasn't that she didn't like sex or didn't have a desire to make love. She just did not want to become actively involved on some evenings when she was fatigued. The following technique revolutionized their sex life. At least once a week, she pleasured him to an orgasm without her active participation.

She would slip off her nightgown and gently hold his testicles while he stroked himself to a climax. She did not mind his fondling her breasts, and she appreciated the pleasure she brought him even with the minimal involvement. Sometimes she would place her hand over his and in other small ways would be supportive. She snuggled close to him and afterward used a warm washcloth to help him clean up. Often that type of sexual activity would not take more than ten minutes, but he found it nurturing and fulfilling, and they still felt like they were making love.

They grew closer as they eliminated one of their nagging problems, and George felt sexually satisfied. His wife promised him that once a week she would wholeheartedly engage herself in making love and it would not always be a quickie. But in between, she would focus on meeting his needs. Both were able to work through the difference between "duty sex" that felt unfulfilling to both and nurturing sex that was participative, but in varying degrees.

Helen was happy to be able to nurture without thinking about birth control (they used a diaphragm) and cleaning herself up afterward. At times she was just distracted and tired from the kids and did not feel up to active lovemaking. Sometimes as he began getting aroused, she would decide she was in the mood and would insert the diaphragm. At those times she might not be as active, but some of the fatigue would melt away as they made love.

For other couples, the husband may pleasure his wife when he is not in the mood or feels tired. Nurturing through orgasm can be a loving compromise in a sexual partnership and not have to involve duty or pity sex.

Overcoming Anatomical Difference with Genital Pleasuring

The greatest source of male sexual arousal is the head of the penis, while female arousal is centered in the clitoris. During intercourse the penis is being constantly stimulated—but the clitoris isn't. The pleasuring position of sitting with legs overlapped allows a better match-up of the most sensitive parts of the male and female anatomy. It is an exciting, connecting, and very accessible position for pleasuring both partners. The hands are free to caress and massage both genital and nongenital parts of the body; and you are eye to eye and mouth to mouth, so verbal and nonverbal communication is facilitated with long, sexy looks and interchanges of how you are feeling. Again, be sure sensitive tissue is lubricated as you enjoy these husband-and-wife variants of this pleasuring position.

In the first scenario, you, the wife, are the pleasurer as you sit with legs overlapping. Start with caressing his face and chest and connecting with him physically. As you continue to do this with one hand, take your other hand and play with his testicles and penis. Now direct your full attention to the penis. Have him close his eyes and revel in the sensations as you run fingers up and down and stroke the shaft and head. Build the excitement as you use the stimulation that can create a climax. As he approaches an orgasm, stop your active stroking of the penis.

Now direct your attention to yourself as you use his penis as a wand to stimulate your genital area. Lovers find the penis is a marvelous tool for stimulating the clitoral region. He may lose some of his arousal, but that is good as you prolong this pleasuring session. He will enjoy your continued penile touching as well as your participation in experiencing your own pleasure. Go slow at first, and stimulate your whole vulval area as you keep coming back to the clitoris. Bring yourself to a climax first if you so desire. When you have enjoyed your genital stimulation enough, focus back on his sensations and build him to an orgasm.

In the second exercise, you, the husband, are the pleasurer. Start with a hug, and caress her back and face, sucking her fingers and lightly kissing her arms, running fingers teasingly over her breasts and stomach as you approach and back off from the nipples. You are arousing and connecting with your lover before approaching direct genital stimulation. As she becomes aroused and desires more genital excitement, have her lie back with her legs continuing to overlap yours. Arouse your penis to a full erection, and use it to slowly stimulate the whole vulval area as you spread her lips apart and lightly caress.

As she becomes more aroused, use your penis to increase the stimulation of the clitoris. Let her guide you in what area feels best and what motions are more arousing. As you use your wrist and arm to create vibrating sensations, you can also stroke the shaft of the penis as a part of these motions, continuing to also increase your sexual buildup. Be creative as you vibrate faster, then slow down some; apply lighter pressure and more direct pressure; turn your penis down to the vagina and back up to the clitoris. Entice and tease as you take plenty of time to enjoy each other and slowly build to a climax. After she has had an orgasm, you can bring yourself to one, also.

Coaching the Pleasure

Teaching your mate what feels sensual and arousing to you can include guiding hands and fingers to create the touch you desire. Utilize several of the pleasuring positions as you alternate blocks of pleasuring time. This will challenge you as a couple in many growth-producing ways. It will require you to tune in to your own pleasure as you instruct your mate about what you desire and find stimulating. It will perfect your coaching techniques: verbally, in talking about what you desire, and nonverbally, in hand-guiding and illustrating motions. You will become more comfortable in asking for what you want and demonstrating your desires. These are vital skills for a great sex life over the next fifty years or more.

The Pleasure of Oral Stimulation

In the same way that kissing and intimately sharing mouths bring erotic arousal and intimate bonding, oral stimulation of the genitals can build trust and be exciting for mates. A quick bath and good hygiene are crucial for this genital pleasuring. If seepage bothers you, keep a warm washcloth handy and gently wipe as needed. Don't worry about his climaxing in your mouth—you as wife are assertive and can ask for what you do and don't want. Actively share your needs and sensibilities.

Remember that Scripture is silent on the topic of oral sex. This does not make it right or wrong. You as mates will have to sort and pray through various behaviors as you choose what to include in your repertoire of lovemaking. Never make your mate feel guilty or inhibited because he or she does not feel comfortable with a given behavior. The object is to be playful, lovingly connected, and creatively varied. This can obviously be accomplished without focusing on one type of genital pleasuring.

Trusting your genitals to your mate's mouth is warmly intimate. The genitals are called the "privates" for a reason. Husbands are very protective of the penis and testicles. To allow the partner complete access is an important commitment, as they feel very vulnerable and in turn arousingly close. Wives have sometimes bought in to the notion that somehow they are dirty down there, or they have left their genitals to remain as an unknown area. To have the husband intimately scrutinizing and enjoying this part of the body takes special trust and openness.

Here are a few suggestions for wife and husband to enhance this variety of genital pleasuring:

Wife, use your lips as buffers for your teeth in order to prevent damage to sensitive tissue. Use tongue and mouth to tease the head of the penis, as you manually stroke the shaft of the penis and create firmer stimulation. Allow your mouth to create a vacuum effect—the stronger the sucking action, the more pleasurable the feelings produced. The head of the penis is the most sensitive part—don't worry about trying to take more of the penis in your mouth.

Husband, tease with your tongue as you flick it lightly over the vulval area. Kiss and gently suck the entirety of it. If your tongue gets tired, hold it firm and create rubbing sensations by moving your entire head side to side. You can also create sucking motions with your mouth over the clitoris to produce a climax. Keep teeth covered and employ variety until she actively approaches an orgasm.

Oral sex can be interspersed with other types of genital pleasuring in a nondemanding, emotionally connecting manner. It can be more exciting at times if combined with simultaneous manual stimulation. While enjoying oral sex, you can keep your hands active, too: as clitoris is sucked or penis and testicles are stroked, fingers are inserted in vagina or back and chest is caressed, buttocks are massaged, and skin is teased. Inhibition vanishes and control is relaxed as partners revel in each other's sensuality and sexuality.

Genital pleasuring may not come easily to you or feel comfortable. You may need practice tuning in to the pleasurable sensations of your body and allowing excitement to build.

Listen to your body and enjoy the natural sexual feelings. God meant covenant lovers to be aroused by pleasuring the genital area. Respond to rhythmic stimulation, breathe more rapidly, and allow your automatic responses to flow without inhibitions. Let go of your embarrassment and need for control as you feast and relax in the excitement of mutual pleasuring. You are creating a special intimacy.

Keep balanced in your lovemaking, and don't just focus on intercourse and orgasm. This may seem odd advice when the next chapter is completely focused on intercourse, but you need variety. Always keep in mind that sex is not the only facet of your companionship. Enjoy your wonderful marital partnership as you play together in a variety of ways.

CHAPTER TWELVE

Creative Intercourse

A NEW CLIENT OPENED UP a session by saying there were over four hundred positions of intercourse and he wanted to learn them all. This was probably a comment on his obsessive-compulsiveness rather than his desire to be a playful lover. I quickly replied that there were actually only about eight basic types of positions because we are limited by anatomy and flexibility. After these eight basics, then there are variants like husband on top with toes crossed, or wife on top with eyes closed.

In reality, unleashing a childlike curiosity, becoming delightfully uninhibited, trying new things, and being playmates are the vital components of exciting intercourse. Your minds and relationship can take these uninspired techniques and bring them alive. The imagination, with some practice and experimenting, can create great variety and immense romantic pleasure.

PLAYFUL, CREATIVE SENSUALITY + KNOWLEDGE + PRACTICE = CREATIVE INTERCOURSE

You as a lover provide the fusion, sensuality, and excitement to intercourse. You as a couple become adept and then can choose when and where you want to enjoy these positions, whether on a soft mattress, under the stars, or in the shower. You control the candlelight, music, lotions, lubrication, and ambiance.

PLAYFUL, CREATIVE SENSUALITY

Enjoy the total array of your senses and lovingly enhance touch as you employ the suggestions and encouragement of earlier chapters. Go slow and build tension as you sensuously progress through the lovemaking process.

You can enjoy intercourse in different ways during the arousal and plateau phases of the sexual cycle. Let intercourse and various positions be interspersed throughout the arousal activities as you warmly connect as well as build tension. Each position will offer a new variety of ways to stimulate, touch, and take pleasure from each other's body. Also, allow your hands and mouth to keep actively caressing and stroking throughout intercourse. Focus in on yourself and your partner as you experience this inimitable, soulful, body-to-body connection.

Knowledge

Stimulating intercourse is developed through a knowledge of male and female anatomy. Figure 12.1 shows the physiology of intercourse with the penis in the vagina and the man on top. Notice where the penis touches in the vagina: six o'clock, twelve o'clock, and the outer third of the vagina are the most sensitive. The head of the penis and the coronal ridge create the greatest arousal in the male. The vagina or the penis is angled differently for every individual, and each couple needs to find those positions that feel best for them. Never put up with physical discomfort, but make necessary adjustments to receive the most pleasure.

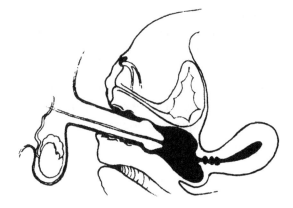

Fig. 12.1. Penis in vagina with man on top

Becoming a great technical lover in intercourse is more than just knowing physiology and the various positions. The actual entry of the penis into the vagina can be new and exciting every time. Intercourse and the bonding one-flesh experience of lovers joining bodies should be an emotional and mental rush as well. Slow your mind and focus on the actual physical feelings of entry; don't take it routinely. As one partner separates the outer vulval lips and guides the penis in, each can delight again in the other's body. Over the many years together, this scintillating connection you enjoy can have a delightful electricity every time you experience it anew.

Make sure the lubrication (artificial, or the seepage at the tip of the penis) has been gently spread over the head of the penis and the vaginal lubrication has wet the mouth of the vagina. (Dry skin chafes and hurts; be sure the vagina is lubricated.) The husband should take care not to simply shove in and start vigorously thrusting. Part the outer lips with their pubic hair, and position the penis at the mouth of the vagina or allow the penis to sensually slide down the inner labial channel to the vagina. Slowly and gently push the penis in, reveling in the sensations. Thrust partway in a time or two with tender care as lubrication is spread, and enjoy the feeling of it. Perhaps lightly shove the penis all the way in and start to thrust, the husband wiggling his penis by using his PC muscle and the wife tightening hers; feel warm and close in this one-flesh embrace. Allow the vagina to lovingly contain its partner.

Practice different rhythms of coital thrusting with pelvic muscles as both partners push to meet each other or one controls a given movement. The outer third of the vagina is particularly sensitive—the husband can practice quick, shallow thrusting at the mouth of the vagina, flicking the penis in and out. It is a myth that deep, strong thrusting is the greatest turn-on, though it can be very exciting for both partners, especially as excitement builds. Intermittently varying rates and depth of thrusting is a crucial skill of the mature lover. Intercourse thrusting might be charted like this: slow-deep, rapid-shallow, stop, rapid-deep, stop, rapid-deep, slow-shallow, slow-deeper, stop, rapid-shallow, and so on.

Luxuriate in developing a variety of rhythms. When the wife is on top and in other positions, she can control penetration and pace the movement, bouncing and moving in ways that produce great feelings for her and her mate. Take care of muscles and ligaments; most of us are not gymnasts.

As excitement builds and orgasm approaches, the movements and rhythms of both partners will probably increase in intensity and rapidity. Again, movements do not have to be rough or painful. Muscle contractions, facial grimaces, exclamations of excitement, and rapid breathing will be a part of intercourse. Throughout the activity and especially toward orgasm, the wife can enjoy contracting the PC muscle. Remember, it is not abnormal for a male to climax in two to three minutes if actively thrusting. Throughout the process, practice stopping and starting, occasionally slowing down, and squeezing the male PC muscles (see Chapter 21) to prevent premature ejaculation. (It may also be helpful to read the last section in Chapter 17 on increasing arousal and becoming orgasmic during intercourse.)

The stimulation and arousal caused by the angle and depth of the penis penetrating the vagina will vary from woman to woman. Talk and experiment. Varying the position will create different angles or allow deeper penetration—enjoy what is exciting to you. Some find a lateral or scissors position, with the side of the vagina being stimulated, very arousing. The twelve o'clock (toward the belly button) and six o'clock (toward the anal area) parts of the vagina have many nerve endings, as does the the G spot. Positions that stroke these areas (man-on-top; rear-entry spoons) are often physically exciting to the woman.

With intercourse, as with all of sexual activity, enjoyment and passion will be enhanced by your imaginations and stored erotic stimuli. Certain positions can excite the visual sense of the husband, and others the romantic, connecting needs of the wife. Invent a fun repertoire together. Celebrate the bonding, nurturing, and excitement of intercourse. It is indeed a fun playground activity for the loving, creative couple. At times forgo any movement and just lie in each other's arms—basking in the warmth of a one-flesh, intercourse, "I'm-so-glad-to-have-you" bear hug.

You as a couple should consider seven items in finding positions of intercourse that provide variety, meet different needs, and enhance your lovemaking.

1. Are you comfortably supported so muscles don't grow weary and neither partner feels squashed or smothered?

2. Does the position allow for good penetration—not too deep or too shallow—and is the penis hitting the right spots in the vagina?

3. Is there visual contact and is it sexy—with the husband and wife enjoying a view of each other's genitals and body with penis and vagina thrusting, and both appreciating eye-to-eye connection? Remember your eyes and souls are connecting along with your bodies.

4. Does the position allow manual or oral contact with the body, breasts, or genitals? Can you kiss, cuddle, and caress—stroke scrotum or clitoris while thrusting?

5. Are you positioned with enough leverage to create easy, thrusting movements so that husband or wife or both can produce exciting friction?

6. Does it encourage creative lovemaking? Can you enjoy it in the shower? Can you accomplish it partially clothed? Does it allow either partner to take a more dominant role as desired?

7. Are there special needs? Can it work in pregnancy, can it work with a partial erection, can it lessen pressure on hips or knees, or can it help control the depth of thrusting?

PRACTICE

You know the old saying that "practice makes perfect." Any new position will be awkward at first and perhaps not as fun, warmly connecting, or erotically arousing as ones you are used to. Practice is important so that you as a couple can quickly begin to enjoy different positions in an adept and relaxed manner. They say that if you use new vocabulary words three times in your conversation, they are yours for life. Do this with positions of intercourse, too.

Practice the following positions in two different ways. First, do some preliminary learning with the book beside you as you learn the position and try it out. Second, incorporate the new position into your lovemaking over the next week or two as you truly make it yours.

Be playful and creative as you make up some of your own variations to try. Also practice shifting into a new position from an existing position without removing the penis. This creates fun moves and erotic loveplay.

EIGHT TYPES OF INTERCOURSE POSITIONS

The rest of this chapter develops eight basic types of intercourse positions. Under some types, two or three alternate positions are described. Relax and play at acquiring this knowledge. Learn what fits you both, but be creative and try some new positions. Consider when a given position would most enhance your lovemaking. Men and women have different physical and psychological makeups and will have differing preferences about what is exciting to them. Remember that you as unique lovers take this knowledge and give it playful, creative sensuality.

1. *Wife on Top*

The wife-on-top positions are favorites for several reasons. For the husband who has a bad back or knees, this position takes the pressure off and allows his wife to be the active participant. It is also the needed position for a couple with disabilities who want to press into the vagina the flaccid penis of the husband. The positions are visually very arousing to the male, and the female is more in control of her own stimulation. Many women find being on top positions the vagina and clitoris to achieve orgasm more readily during intercourse. The husband's hands are also nicely placed to stimulate the clitoris as needed.

Kneeling. The wife kneels while she straddles her husband. She can use a number of angles: a backward tilt as she supports herself with arms straight and hands on his legs or the bed, a 90-degree upright stance with bouncing motions or a 45-degree forward tilt with weight on arms or forearms propped on pillows. This position allows the woman to control the depth of penile penetration and orchestrate the movement of the penis in the vagina with the clitoris against the pelvic bone. It may be easier for her to guide the penis into the vagina. It is also pleasurable to simply let the erect penis lie on his stomach and, with proper lubrication, rub the clitoral area back and forth with a rocking motion across the hard penis, without vaginal penetration.

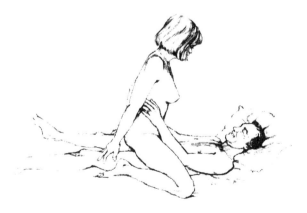

Fig. 12.2. Wife on top, kneeling

The husband can also thrust with pelvic motions. This position is fun for the husband because his wife's breasts are near his face and mouth, and the pubic area is very visible. The wife can enjoy the easy access her husband has to massage the clitoris with his thumbs. For variation and different sensations, the wife can kneel facing away from the husband. Remember, the penis only has so much flexibility. You won't snap it off, but sudden movements to sit straight up may scare him and cause some discomfort.

Prone. The wife lies comfortably on top with her legs straddling his body or between his legs, finding leverage with her feet and knees. She may also wish to prop her shins and feet insteps on top of her husband's lower legs and hold her feet against his feet to gain leverage for giving thrusting motions. In this prone position, as well as others, it is easier to insert the penis in a corollary position (wife kneeling) and then ease into the position desired. Or, when the husband is on top, simply roll over so that the wife is prone on top. The woman-on-top position allows the wife to take the lead in a fun, selfish way, using her husband's body for her pleasure.

2. Side by Side

Couples enjoy side-by-side positions because bodies are comfortably close and facing each other for cuddling and kissing. Bodies are well supported, and both partners can control and contribute to coital thrusting while they caress and stroke.

Relax and enjoy the total experience of intercourse. Look at each other and delight in your mate's arousal and in the beauty of the body. Gently caress skin and revel in the texture. Talk and give verbal and nonverbal exchanges of love and excitement. Close your eyes and focus on the specific pleasure of the penis in the vagina—go slow, with light, feathery motions; rapidly thrust with penis touching only the outer inch of the vagina; try deeper penetration—then stop and lie in each other's arms for a minute. Creative intercourse is making love, not just building to an orgasm.

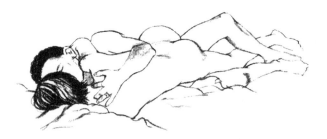

Fig. 12.3. Side by side, wife straddling husband's leg

Wife straddling husband's leg. The husband lies comfortably on his side, with his bottom leg extended straight, his other leg bent at the knee, and his foot on the bed. The wife lies on her side and straddles the top, bent leg, with her lower leg between his legs and her top leg thrown over his torso. This positions the penis at the vagina (with proper shifting) for easy access with either partner guiding it in. Again, pillows under heads or sides increase comfort.

Couple embracing chest to chest. The wife lies on her side with the husband facing her in a mutual embrace. This may be most easily achieved by rolling over onto the sides from the wife-on-top or husband-on-top position. The husband's top arm and hand are free to caress his wife's buttocks and back. This can be a fun, bonding embrace as you adjust the underneath arms for greatest comfort, and both supply movement.

3. Husband on Top

This has often been called the missionary position because, according to legend, the Hawaiians did not employ this position. They were surprised to discover that the missionaries to their land used it exclusively. It may be an apocryphal story, but this standard position is often thought of as uncreative or elementary. Actually, it is pleasurable in various ways. It allows deep penetration, active thrusting by the husband, and a total body hug with much eye-to-eye lovemaking.

Legs between. The husband lies on top of his wife and supports his weight with his knees and elbows or arms. His legs are together between her legs and give leverage for easy pelvic thrusting. Variations of this position are the wife's raising her legs and scissoring them around the husband's torso or raising her legs to rest on his shoulders. Be gentle. This position offers perhaps the deepest penetration of any position.

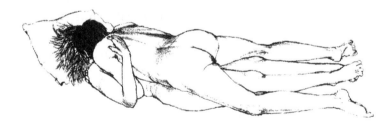

Fig. 12.4. Husband on top, legs straddling

Legs straddling. It is easier for the husband to start with legs together and the penis inserted in the vagina. Now, with the penis remaining inserted, he can gently shift one of his legs outside one of his wife's legs as he straddles that leg. For different sensations, he can shift his other leg from between to outside as he straddles with both legs outside his wife's legs. This allows his wife to clamp or scissor her legs together and produce greater friction on the penis in her vagina. The husband has an easy, swinging motion of the pelvis and can raise up on his knees and elbows to relieve any excess pressure on his wife.

The husband-on-top position gives an ability to be body to body in a special one-flesh hug. At times, just lie there and enjoy this intercourse embrace, remembering your commitment and love for each other as you savor the skin-to-skin contact.

4. Crosswise

Both crosswise positions are great for freeing hands to stimulate the clitoris and caress bodies. While the husband is thrusting, the wife can caress his testicles or scissor two of her fingers around his thrusting penis to increase stimulation. She can also stimulate herself or hold his hand as he stimulates her clitoral area. The husband can maneuver his body (collapsing the straight + into a collapsed cross X), while keeping the penis in the vagina so that he is able to nibble at her breasts and enjoy kissing, too, in these positions.

Wife's legs over. The husband lies on his side facing the wife, crosswise on the bed. His wife lies on her back and creates a cross of their bodies by resting her legs over his thighs with one leg toward his waist and the other leg toward his knees, allowing easy penetration by the penis. The husband creates the thrusting motion with pelvic movement.

Scissors. The husband lies crosswise on the bed with his head to the wife's right, and she lies on her back. This time the wife's right leg is propped over her husband's thighs, and her left leg is scissored between her husband's legs. If the husband is left-handed, he scissors her right leg, placing his head on her left side. This leaves manipulation and penetration of the penis to be controlled easily by the husband.

Scissors is an ideal position for using the penis as a wand to stimulate the vulva and clitoris. The husband can hold his erect penis and, with the wife's instructions, learn the right rhythms and pressure and placement to help her achieve an orgasm. If the wrist grows tired, he can use more of the entire arm, like painting, to vibrate and massage the clitoris. This can

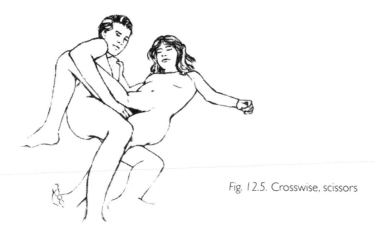

Fig. 12.5. Crosswise, scissors

be interspersed with vaginal thrusting to keep the whole area lubricated. As she approaches a climax, the wife may want the husband to switch to vaginal stimulation alone.

Either crosswise position works well during pregnancy. From the scissor position, the couple can maneuver into the rear-entry spoons position without withdrawing the penis. The wife rolls on her side with her back toward the husband. The husband gently unscissors her leg, then slides his legs so they are behind hers in a spoon position as he thrusts against her buttocks.

5. Rear Entry

The rear-entry positions, especially the lying-down spoons or both kneeling on or by the bed, are great during pregnancy. The wife should be comfortably supported with pillows as needed, and thrusting should be as gentle as desired.

Spoons. The husband faces his wife's back, like two spoons cradling. The penis can be inserted with the husband separating legs and outer vulval lips while the wife guides the penis into the vagina. Male pelvic thrusting bumps softly against her buttocks as the penis stimulates the front of the vagina and the G spot.

The husband can enjoy caressing his wife's stomach and breasts and stimulating her clitoris with his free hand. The wife often likes this angle of the penis with slow or vigorous thrusting that is exciting but not too deep. Both are comfortable with less demand on muscles and joints—a great position for aging bodies or for a break from more active loveplay.

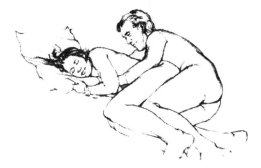

Fig. 12.6. Rear-entry, spoons

Kneeling in husband's lap. The husband kneels with knees together and back propped upright. The wife kneels with her back to him, straddling his legs and propping herself in his lap—carefully inserting the penis as a mutual effort. He can place his hands on her hips to help control movement as she moves up and down, and he can create some pelvic thrusting. She may wish to bend forward and brace herself with her arms. This position leaves the husband's hands free to caress, while the wife can control depth and positioning of the penis with pelvic and leg movement.

Both kneeling. The husband kneels behind his wife, who is kneeling, bent at the waist with forearms and head resting comfortably on a pillow or the edge of the bed. The husband sep-arates the outer lips from the rear and gently inserts his penis into the vagina. This position may seem awkward to the wife, but it is very visually stimulating to the husband. He has an exciting view of waist and hips and his penis penetrating the vulval area. It also allows easy thrusting motions from slow to vigorous and stimulation of the sensitive twelve-o'-clock part of the vagina.

Another variant of this position is for the wife to slide down into a prone position on the bed, with a pillow under her stomach propping her buttocks and genital area up. The hus-band lies down on her back with his legs between her legs and inserts his penis. He can get leverage for thrusting with his feet and knees as he hugs her from the back.

6. Standing

The standing positions encourage creative intercourse without the need for a bed. They are fun for rooms of the house other than the bedroom.

From the back. This is similar to both kneeling, only both partners are standing. The wife bends at the waist and supports her weight with her hands on a bed, a table, or shower fixtures. The husband stands or crouches behind her and, separating outer labia with one hand, inserts the penis. This can be a fun position for a quickie in the kitchen or a romp in the shower.

Facing, with wife on one leg. The wife faces the husband and raises her left leg, which he cradles with his right hand, and they mutually insert the penis. If the husband is much taller than the wife, she may need to stand on a small stool or pillow. This position permits eye-to-eye contact and a chance to mutually hug and caress.

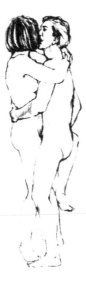

Fig. 12.7. Standing, facing with wife on one leg

7. Face to Face

These face-to-face positions will remind you of the wife-on-top and the rear-entry kneeling (only reversed) positions of intercourse. The fun comes in as you stay creatively sensual and are willing to experiment. As playfulness and curiosity take over, you can create many hybrids on your own.

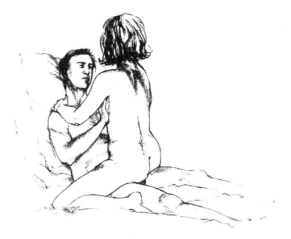

Fig. 12.8. Husband sitting, wife kneeling

Husband sitting and wife kneeling. The husband sits upright with his back propped against pillows, while his wife kneels astride his lap, facing him with her legs around his thighs. This position allows for fun hugging and kissing and provides close body contact but not much leverage for thrusting. Movement can be assisted by the husband's hands placed under his wife's buttocks and by her legs creating bouncing motions with her hands on his shoulders. The penis can be mutually inserted, and because this position allows for deep penetration, care must be taken for comfort. This is a good position if the husband has back problems, because he can be comfortable with his back propped with pillows.

Wife lying down and husband kneeling. The husband kneels and his wife, lying on her back, places her legs over his thighs with knees bent and feet flat on the bed. It may help to prop a pillow under her head and shoulders or position a pillow under her buttocks to position the penis better. This is a good position for using the penis to stimulate the clitoris. If the angle is too much to allow easy penetration, the husband may wish to bend forward and cradle his wife's legs with his hands under her buttocks or waist so access is more comfortable. This allows pelvic thrusting as well as adjustments and movement with his arms. This position can be gentle if the wife has arthritic or damaged knees. Again, husband and wife are face-to-face so they can enjoy each other visually. (For variety, have the wife flip over onto her stomach with the insteps of her feet on the husband's shoulders—use imagination and creativity.)

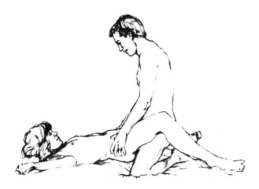

Fig. 12.9. Face-to-face, wife supine and husband kneeling

8. Partner and Props

In the chapter on setting moods, we explored the utilization of props, from candles to showers to pillows. These positions use the furniture around your house as props as you increase your erotic playing together.

Sitting on a chair. The husband sits up straight on a chair that allows the wife to sit in his lap facing and straddling him. The penis is inserted with mutual effort. It is helpful if the wife's feet touch the floor or are propped up on pillows to ease insertion and to help create movement. This position, like other face-to-face positions, allows visual contact and kissing and holding and whispering or breathing in ears. The hands are free so the husband can caress back and buttocks. He may try cradling her buttocks in his hands to help produce movement with his arms. A variant of this position is to have the wife turn around and face away. Again, it is helpful if her feet can touch the floor. The husband can stroke breasts and clitoris while she reaches down and stimulates his penis with her fingers.

This position, like some of the other sitting positions, does not allow a great deal of thrusting motion. It can be quietly erotic; the connecting of intercourse does not always have to lead to rapid movement or produce a climax. Sitting positions can be playful, and they add variety.

Wife on the edge. This position is important for men with bad backs or women during pregnancy. The bed is a comfortable object for the wife to be on the edge of, but don't limit creativity. Dining room tables, kitchen counters, couches, and easy chairs work well, too. Many beds are too low and pillows will be needed or the man will have to lower his body.

The wife is positioned at the edge of the bed, sofa, or table. Her legs are around her husband's torso, resting comfortably on his thighs, with his arms supporting and clamping them to his body. The husband kneels or stands, depending on the height of the object the wife is on, so his penis is accessible to her vagina. He has an easy thrusting motion, and the wife may not be fully reclined but propped up on the pillows of an easy chair and can have access to stroking and caressing herself and her husband.

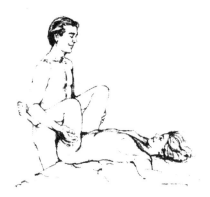

Fig. 12.10. Wife on the edge

This position is very visually stimulating to the husband: he can observe the vulval area and the penis thrusting in and out. It is exciting to the wife as well: she can observe her partner's arousal by her body while experiencing her own visual excitement, and her vagina and clitoris receive excellent friction in this position. The wife-on-the-edge position works well during later stages of pregnancy or when the fatigued wife wants her husband to take the active role. It lends itself to all rooms of the house and provides some fun variation because it can be enjoyed without removing or wrinkling clothing.

You now have a good working knowledge of the basic positions and many variations. It is now up to you to bring them alive in your lovemaking. Be curious and experimental as you take the risks to try new position and learn them well enough that they become comfortable. Truly frolic and laugh and love as you enjoy making intercourse a fun part of your sex life. Create your own variations and become lovingly at ease with a wide variety of moves and rhythms.

May God always be in your bedroom as you grow increasingly comfortable with His gift of erotic play, and may you enjoy the specialness of one-flesh union as symbolized in intercourse. Use your God-given imagination and sensuality as you seek out positions especially suited to your bodies and those that can be very arousing to you as a couple. You have been given a rich and exciting treasure in the complexity and simplicity of sexual intercourse. Celebrate!

CHAPTER THIRTEEN

Making Love to Your Wife

MEN DESPERATELY WANT to be competent at all that they do. Making love can seem a real setup, because your wife will often be a deep mystery to you. Women are so beautifully complex. You think you know a lot and you're trying to be a great lover, but then you hit another bump in the road. Let's try to understand some of this mystery so that making love to your wife can become more exciting and less frustrating for both of you.

UNIQUELY FEMALE

Begin this journey by trying to walk in your wife's shoes as you grow in understanding and skills. There is a uniqueness to her that is helpful to know. It is fascinating that both of these statements are true in God's design: "Men and women are more similar than they are different." "Men and women are really wired differently." This chapter can help you empathize with some of the common differences in her reality.

Warmly Connected Soul Mates

In the wise, biblical way of "becoming one flesh," women don't divorce sex as easily from the relational and emotional aspects as men can. A woman wants to feel cared about and emotionally connected before sexual activity can have appeal. For her, fun sex flows out of an intimate companionship that is emotionally close, with plenty of physical affection and quality time together. Conveying this attitude and these feelings is *not something you can do quickly in the hour before you want sex*. Intimate connecting involves daily and hourly choices. Pay attention to her: give her two compliments every day, tell her things you notice and appreciate about her, and come out of your cave and talk more.

Your tenderness and attentiveness may be more erotic to your wife than great techniques. Doing the dishes, calling her during the day, or tenderly listening can be a sexual turn-on, if she knows you are doing this from the heart and not for the purpose of getting sex. Time spent in loveplay draws her closer than time spent producing orgasms. The different paths to the souls of men and women could be charted as follows:

- *Men:* Physical activity → connects the soul → leads to emotional closeness
- *Women:* Emotional closeness → connects the soul → opens the door to physical activity

Vive la Romance

People are not born romantic. Romance is a combination of skills and attitudes that are learned. What is this romance that women yearn for and need to have included in their sex lives and relationships? The words *special sweetheart* describe the attitude your wife desires from you. Your passionate focus on her, as if she is the only woman in the world, makes her feel special.

Women are certainly on target in demanding romance as a necessary component of making love. *Vive la romance!* Great sex does indeed originate from your imaginative creativity and those mushy cards, erotic, candlelit bedrooms, sexy dates, and holding hands.

Consistently Inconsistent

You may wonder why your wife is physically inconsistent. On one evening she may like oral arousal or enjoy her breasts and nipples being caressed, and at another time she may not want that particular stimulation at all. Her body and reactions do not stay consistent, and you get confused. The fact is, she does change in what is arousing to her. Sometimes her clitoris is more sensitive than at other times, and a particular stroke is more irritating than exciting. A firm, rapid stroke might feel good later on in a lovemaking session but is annoying for her initially. Your penis is very consistent, and most times it responds to firm stimulation. But your wife's body does not function in this way.

Develop a series of strategies for making love. Become adept at smoothly switching gears, from strategy A to strategy B to strategy E, depending on where your wife is in a given lovemaking session. Encourage her to say what she wants. Sometimes she may just want to nurture you, and you may climax as quickly as you want to. At other times she may desire gentle massage of nonerogenous zones or her breasts. Expect inconsistency and revel in your fast footwork and improvisational skills. Become a skilled lover as you vary approaches and rhythms and types of stimulation. She will love your spontaneous variety and your lack of irritability or pouting.

Your wife may also not have the same consistent type of desire that you do. This may be hormonal, and you can enjoy certain times in her menstrual cycle. The inconsistency may also be relational and environmental, and you can help make changes to alleviate stress and create romance. Your desires are just different in what you find stimulating and arousing—in what turns you on and turns you off. Her desire is probably more receptive than assertive, as she thinks about sex less consistently than you, but can often find interest when approached. Talk about it and negotiate.

Vulnerable to Distraction

Husbands can falsely assume that their wives don't like sex as much as they do. They don't understand that their wives are more easily distracted by their environment and their inner attitudes and feelings. When she is fatigued, fearful the kids will come pounding on the door any minute, struggling with body image, or feeling hurt, she may be unable to focus on sex and her desire to make love will be on the back burner.

Your wife, more than you, may have to fight distractions during actual lovemaking to be able to focus on her own arousal. The wise husband minimizes distractions (for example, bedroom picked up, phone calls made) and helps his wife begin to make love (romantic suggestion when leaving for work, sexy kissing in living room when he comes home) even before the bedroom. Be sensitive to her concerns. You are less susceptible to distractions and often want to make love without the mood having to be exactly right. As you are more supportive and involved, she may be in the mood more often. Your wife will find making love more appealing and restorative as the distractions are acknowledged and controlled.

Making Love an Emotional Choice with a Warm-Up Time

Your wife is more likely to make a cognitive decision when she wants to make love and appreciates having the opportunity to create the right mental and emotional attitude. It isn't the more immediate, hormonal surge that it can be with you. Wives love surprises and being spontaneous, but they are usually not crazy about quickies or jumping into bed the minute the vacation destination is reached.

Sex is more purposeful, romantic, and intimate with a woman. She will not think of sex as often as you do, but this is not for lack of desire. My colleague Debra Taylor, in the research for her coauthored book, *Secrets of Eve*, found many women actively thought about sex only twice a month. *You can learn a lot from each other* with your wife's emotional decision (sometimes this decision is made when you initiate) to nurture and be with you, and your impulsive readiness to jump right in.

Your wife has to want sex and choose to make love in ways that are consistent with how she is feeling, with emotional and affectionate attachment. The timing must be appropriate, with plenty of loveplay as her body and emotions are "primed" and she is allowed to choose to respond in her own passionate way. Women often take fifteen to twenty minutes to reach an orgasm. This is part physical and part because she needs time to overcome distractions as she mentally and emotionally allows arousal. You were ready when she took her shirt off, but she will take time. When lovemaking occurs and she is willingly involved, she can respond with receptive desire and a passionate enjoyment that will surprise you.

Gentle and Teasing and Slow—Then Vigorous

Wives often complain their husbands are too direct, speedy, or entirely too predictable. Men often have a real skill deficit in the art of touching softly, approaching gently, and keeping a teasing variety in lovemaking. There can be too much pawing and grabbing and going straight for genital arousal.

Especially in initial loveplay, women often prefer gentle, teasing caresses, and may like intercourse to start off with easy, shallow thrusts. She may like to flirt and start making love with clothes still on. She may love it when you tease her body and softly blow in her ear, kiss her neck, and do not immediately head for her breasts or genitals. The pleasure will gradually grow and will be exciting when you take the time to playfully torment her by coming on, then backing off. Teasingly touch nipples and genitals but keep moving to new spots.

Slow is the operative word in fantastic sex. Teasing arousal by its very nature takes time but a gradual, unhurried, leisurely pace will be greatly appreciated by your mate. Often she will take longer to reach arousal, and this will allow her that time to enter into the lovemaking fully.

As you follow her lead, your wife depends on you to create the rhythm of your lovemaking. She will not always want it slow and soft. As she becomes aroused the pace can get vigorous and fast. Then you can think of what feels good to you and duplicate it with her. She will want stronger stimulation of the clitoral area and intercourse can be a wilder experience. Genital pleasuring can become the focus and orgasm more the intent.

Multiorgasmic

Women are multiorgasmic; men are not. A woman can have a series of orgasms, one right after the other. Men have a recuperative time between orgasms that can increase from minutes to hours with age. Some wives may experience two or more separate orgasms in a couple of minutes with a short pause or rest between each, or enjoy an extended orgasm that spasms for some seconds of time.

But don't get hung up on numbers or multiple orgasms! Help your wife enjoy her orgasmic potential, but let go of any need to create more or deeper climaxes. She won't be keeping score as long as you are growing in your lovemaking skills. The intensity and amounts of the orgasm will follow and will vary from session to session of lovemaking.

Erotic Symbolism and Sensuality

What do women find sexy in men? Gentle or sexy or attentive looks are turn-ons. Stomachs and buttocks that are kept in shape are often on the list, along with grooming in general. Talking and being vulnerable are important; the ability to express feelings is very attractive and arouses erotic feelings. Minds are often considered sexy, and men are pleasing who can be passionate about life or a cause. Wives are excited by their husband's ability to take charge but not be controlling. They want a skilled lover who can take them into passion assertively.

Your wife may enjoy smells and sounds and touch in ways you never thought to appreciate. Silk or satin negligees, warm lotion, fragrant flowers, or rollicking jazz enhance the experience. Making love can become more interesting and arousing as you learn from her sensual temperament and incorporate a wider range of erotically stimulating symbols. Don't get hung up on what you think is sexy and sensual but learn from her, with respect. Peach-colored satin draped sexily over a breast may be more sensuous than the black-lace cutout you had in mind.

FOR MEN ONLY

Men can shoot themselves in the foot on their way to becoming the world's greatest lovers. In this section, we will consider how easy it is for men to miss the mark and sacrifice quality sexual bonding. We need to truly love our wives with passion, wisdom, and depth.

3-D Women

Men have a difficult time letting women be three-dimensional, with body, soul, and spirit. The preoccupation with the body aspect of sex actually puts a damper on the true fun God intended. Husbands who learn to notice and make love to the total person create an awesome passion with a deeper sexual connecting. Practice 3-D sex.

Body. Observe her eyes, which are the windows to the soul. Is she happy, sad, tired, excited? Look at less common but very feminine body parts such as earlobes, hands, mouth, and posture.

Soul. Be aware of emotions. What is her style of enjoying life and people? Observe her mind and heart—know that she needs attention and affirmation, not lust.

Spirit. Know she wants someone special in her life to adore and cherish her. Think of her need for intimate connecting: Has she allowed God to meet deep, inner desires too?

Male Mythology

Probably the most prevalent male myth concerns the size of the penis. Do some self-talk and get over any feeling of inferiority. It's not the size that counts but how you enjoy sensuality and use it. Remember the old saying: "It's not the size of the boat, but the motion of the ocean."

Along with the size-of-penis myth is the idea that a woman is turned on by hard, deep thrusting in intercourse. Your wife will enjoy and be more turned on by softer, smoother, and *at times* more rapid motions in intercourse as you make love to her tender genitals. A variant of this myth is that a really sexy wife will want her husband to take her immediately and then will go into fits of ecstasy as his penis fills her vagina.

Another devastating myth is that men know all about sex and are always ready to go sexually. We have our knowledge and desire deficits just like women, but we often feel guilty admitting them. All of us, as lovers, feel very deficient and inhibited at times.

Start letting go of your myths. You probably have heard some story of a woman who wanted sex all the time. I call this the "nympho myth," and yet 68 percent of women (the bell-shaped curve) will fall into the middle or average part of desire. (See Figure 13.1.) Another 14 percent will have lower or higher desire, with only 2 percent being on the extremes. Your wife is probably quite average in desire, and you don't have to be a sexual machine. Don't assume that problems are all hers or yours. Look at ways that you both might be contributing to a lack of sexual frequency, and pay attention to other concerns in your lovemaking.

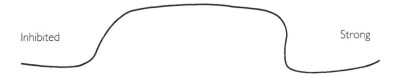

Inhibited   Strong

Fig. 13.1. Women's sex drive

Macho Sensitivity

Your wife will be able to blossom as a woman and as a lover as you are able to sensitively understand and affirm her. You may need to start with affirming yourself and your body image and sexual self-esteem. Accept the size of your penis, trust your ability to acquire whatever skills you need to be an adept lover, and exercise your romantic creativity. Here are some ideas to practice that can help you be a sensitive, focused lover:

Get a Ph.D. in "My Wife." Listen to her, observe her, increase your attention span, ask questions, try different things as you collect information, and be willing to make changes to please her. Husbands, your wives' femininity is precious and unique. Take the time to read a great book called *Secrets of Eve* (Hart, Weber, and Taylor, 1998) and learn more of how she is wired sexually and what it will take to make her truly flourish; she will get turned on that you care enough to read a book about her! Remember that it's not how hard you try but how smart you try. As much as you wish it, she will not respond like you, so you are going to have to learn some new skills.

Gain a working knowledge of feelings. It is especially important sexually that you learn to empathize and express excitement, dissatisfaction, gentleness, joy and happiness, contentment, discomfort, and pleasure.

Cultivate softness, humility, gentleness, and love. Learn to have a light touch and a soft, empathetic approach. Practice gentle responses and the strategy of going slow. Cultivate this feminine side of your masculine personality. It is a vital part of being a sensitive and adept lover.

Forget your obsessions. You have some fantasies and things you find sexy that your wife never will. She may never want to make love on an elevator or have oral sex on an airplane. Men can wreck a great sex life by obsessing on something we think is the ultimate in erotic adventure or the only symbol of real variety.

One of these obsessions I commonly encounter is anal sex. The vaginal tissue, with its lubrication and muscle, was designed for childbirth and intercourse, but the anus was not. The anus was meant to push out waste, not sustain vigorous thrusting. With hemorrhoids and the fragility of the rectal tissue, it is better not to make it an organ of sexual play. Also, the many bacteria in the anus can interfere with the bacterial balance in the vagina and cause infections. Let go of your fetishes and obsessions so they don't destroy your ability to really have fun.

You may also become obsessed with some part of her body that you wish was sexier. *Do not—and I repeat—do not, tell her these things.* You may make a passing statement, "I wish you had less pubic hair/bigger breasts/more of a waist," and then forget you ever said it. She remembers and reminds you eighteen years later. Confess it to a buddy so he can tell you to grow up. Let go of your obsessions so you can enjoy the fullness of a great sex life and the sexiness of your wife without shooting yourself in the foot.

Passionate Leader

Most wives want husbands who are strong and confident and can provide unasked-for nurturing. They would like men who are not always predictable but have spontaneous energy and mystery. Wives at times want to be "taken"—not in a demanding or abusive way, but out of a passionate desire for their femininity from a self-confident husband. They want to be swept off their feet and romantically enjoyed in wild and wonderful ways.

They also desire men who have sexual expertise but are able to implement suggestions without pouting and shutting down. They love men who are secure enough to appreciate and follow their lead at times as well. Men have such a strong need to be competent that it is tough for us not to take personally any coaching or criticism. There may be times you feel embarrassed because your wife has refused something or given alternate suggestions. In the typical fashion of a male with egg on his face, don't continue the behavior and hope your wife will eventually find it okay. "No," "Maybe tomorrow," or "That is bothering me" mean exactly that. Quit selling yourself short by persisting and hoping she will change.

Don't be predictable. Surprises bring a jolt of energy to the relationship as you increase your image of being mysterious, romantic, and passionate. She may think she has you figured out, but keep her off balance with impromptu romantic flourishes. Learn how to "take" her with strong, gentle leadership. Mystery, variety, and strength are very sexy to your wife. Keep humble and secure and nondefensive as you evolve into a passionate leader.

DAVID'S SLING AND HARP

David was a man after God's own heart as he tried to remain within God's guidelines and humbly welcome the revelation of new truth in his life. He made some serious mistakes but repented and made changes. This man was also a strong leader as he protected Israel with a sling against Goliath.

David was a man's man and a part of that was his great sensitivity. The powerful warrior and king played a harp. He was passionate as he built relationships, danced before the ark, and loved deeply. With his harp, he would soothe and entertain with an empathetic touch.

Your wife needs you to be her David with a sling as you provide a protective covering of attentiveness and romantic leadership. She desires you to be sensitive and to gently soothe her, to entertain, and to be playful. This will not always be an easy job.

Having a great sex life and being a strong and sensitive leader are built on some mundane but important things. Prioritize them into your behavior and make your wife feel special. Remember David's sling and harp. Emotional connection and nurturing behaviors precede sexual readiness and arousal. The following activities can make your wife feel tremendously in love and alive.

The Art of Kissing

Women enjoy variety in kissing, and the mouth can be extremely sensuous.

Butterfly kisses. Lightly kiss all over her face and body, keeping lips soft and gentle. Kiss her eyelids, behind her ear, her neck, between her breasts, and all over her stomach and thighs. Be light and teasing, like a butterfly flitting about.

Gently sucking. Practice this kiss by taking your fingertip and placing it between your lips and lightly touch your tongue to the fingertip—now pull your finger out of your mouth with a gentle sucking motion. Try this on your wife's nipple, her fingers or toes, her neck, or her lower lip.

Warm, connecting kisses. Plant a warm, juicy kiss on your wife's cheek or forehead as you walk by. It is almost like the family kiss that communicates greeting, love, and "you're my special person." It lets her know you enjoy her companionship and not just the sexual relationship. Hugging her, rubbing her shoulders or feet, and holding her hand in public convey this idea in warm and emotionally connecting ways, too.

Deep kissing. There is something passionate and intimate about sharing mouths and tongues. Here, as in all of sex, good hygiene applies. Bad breath is out. Brush your teeth before you go to bed. Don't fill her mouth with your tongue or shove it down her throat. Long, exciting kisses where you have to come up for breath should vary between playful tongue contact (don't immediately go beyond her teeth), warm and easy nibbling of her lower lip or earlobe, and deep, passionate sharing of tongues and souls. Breathe heavy and allow yourself to become aroused as you make kissing a drawn-out affair.

Practice long hugs, also. It is amazing, at first, how long a thirty-second hug can seem when compared to an ordinary hug. You will be pleasantly surprised how bonding they will become. The dutiful hug or quick peck on the cheek does not accomplish what a longer hug or kiss will for creating the feelings of being in love.

Making Love to Her Breasts

Breasts and nipples are very symbolic of femininity. They are erotically charged and an important part of the sexual anatomy to both you and your wife. Compliment, appreciate, admire, and enjoy them—don't grab, squeeze, or instantly rub.

Making love to your wife's breasts, like all of making love, should teasingly progress from light touches to more direct stimulation. Lightly brush your hand over the entire breast and her stomach without lingering on the nipples. Take a finger and move lightly in circles around the nipple and move the circle out to include the complete breast, and them move to the other breast. Women love circular, teasing touches rather than direct assaults on their erotic parts. Avoid contact with the nipples at first. Put your fingertips together and place them on the nipple. Open your fingers and slide them over the breast until the palm is resting on the nipple.

Lightly rub the palm of your hand on the erect nipple. Now progress to more direct stimulation with light tongue movement and soft, nibbling kisses. Enjoy the closeness as this moves into warm sucking and intimate arousal. Caress her face and body as you continue making love to her breasts.

Private Intimacy

Part of the beauty and bonding nature of making love is choosing to allow another person, your special mate, into the most private areas of your life and body. Your wife allows you, her husband, to explore and enjoy her vulva, vagina, and clitoris in ways she has probably never even done herself. You need an intimate understanding of her body, especially her clitoris.

The clitoris is the central organ for stimulating sexual arousal in your mate. Expecting your wife to have an orgasm through vaginal stimulation alone (without carefully stimulating the clitoral area) is like her expecting you to climax by rubbing your testicles (without stimulating your penis). The clitoris is another part of the female anatomy that will need an indirect approach. Don't head for it immediately.

Again, the art of teasing comes into play. With a soft, extremely light touch, caress thighs and stomach and outer lips and pubic hair—varying the motion from circles to pats to gentle, long strokes. Don't focus yet. Keep teasing. Try closing your hand and forming a V with your index and middle finger. Gently walk these two fingers over her torso and legs, like a horse slowly and playfully galloping in a teasing manner. Stiffen the same two fingers and run the V softly over her outer lips, starting down at her vagina and up to her navel; then reverse, back down and gently up again, and gallop some more.

As she gets more excited, take thumb and middle finger, and rub the outer lips together over the clitoral area as you stimulate her more directly. Remember that the clitoris needs to be kept lubricated during lovemaking. Vaginal secretions, saliva, seminal fluid, or artificial lubricants can be used. It is very sensitive tissue and can be irritated quickly, which is obviously a turn-off. Unlike in the vagina, the lubrication does not appear naturally.

Women vary in the way they desire clitoral stimulation. Learn what your wife appreciates the most. Let her place her hand over your hand as you relax it, and let her guide your fingers as to the amount of pressure and rhythms she finds most exciting. It may be direct as she gets aroused or may remain quite indirect. You can feel her clitoris get hard as you caress the top of the clitoral hood—it feels like a small electrical cord under the skin. Some women experience a more intense orgasm through external stimulation of the clitoris without the penis in the vagina. You may wish to vary the way you bring her to a climax and sometimes just pleasure her without intercourse until she has climaxed.

The mouth and tongue can stimulate the clitoral area in a very sensual manner. Oral sex, like many other enjoyable techniques, depends on a couple's sensitivities. In fun and loving sexual activity, you are always sensitive to your mate's likes and dislikes. This is especially true of oral sex. There seems to be nothing contrary to Scripture in having oral sex unless you engage in it to the exclusion of all else or force it on your mate.

Power positions. There are three positions of intercourse that your wife will find especially exciting because they enable you to provide direct stimulation to her clitoris: (1) the scissors position, as you also use your penis as a magic wand to stimulate her clitoris; (2) the husband in back in the spoon position, as you massage her back and thighs and bottom; and (3) the wife-on-top position, with her ability to take control in fun ways. (For details, see Chapter 12.)

The G spot. In the early 1950s, German physician Ernst Grafenberg described a place within a woman's vagina that has since been named the Grafenberg, or G, spot. The G spot is located about an inch or two into the vagina at the twelve-o'-clock position toward the navel. It is about the size of a nickel and seems analogous to the prostate in the male. When stimulated, it can become smoother and firmer than other vaginal wall tissue. While books have been written about this phenomenon, many sex therapists think it has been greatly overrated.

The fact of the matter is that the vagina is sensitive and certain parts like the G spot can create more intense physical sensations. That is why different positions of intercourse feel different as the penis rubs various parts of the vagina. An excellent exercise for husband and wife to conduct every now and then is genital exploration. After your wife is relaxed, take a finger and explore her vagina as she tells you what areas are most sensitive. Try to find the G spot. Often six o'clock toward the anus and twelve o'clock toward the clitoris are very sensitive, having many nerve endings.

God has given you a precious gift in creating for you your own special woman and putting you into a one-flesh companionship with her. Together you two can enjoy excitement and intimacy! Maximize His gift as you humbly and wisely become a skilled and passionate leader and lover.

Time Out: Men, pick out two ways you want to become a passionate leader for your wife. Really surprise her and discuss this with her so you can get her input and desires. We sometimes have difficulty setting her needs as our priorities and truly following through—make sure you don't drop the ball with this one as you practice these leadership skills.

CHAPTER FOURTEEN

Making Love to Your Husband

MANY TIMES YOU HAVE PROBABLY been amazed at the way your husband thinks and acts sexually. From the male perspective, there are few situations where sex doesn't add some spice and enhance the relationship. He can seem so one-track and grabby. I remember the wife who told me sex was her husband's solution to much of what he encountered in life. If he got a raise, celebrate with sex; if he got frustrated or disappointed, cheer up with sex.

Making love is perhaps the primary means your husband uses to feel connected to you. He expresses emotional vulnerability and physical closeness in a special way during your lovemaking. He also utilizes his sexual feelings to create variety and excitement in his life, perhaps letting sex have too prominent a place in his thinking and needs. As you read the following pages, you will discover he has a different sexual reality from yours. You may have to make some changes in the way you think, feel, and act to please him and improve your love life. But you will probably discover you are more similar sexually than you are different.

I must also state that some couples reading this book will find their situation reversed, with the wife having the higher urge for lovemaking. In the complexity of today's world, men can be overwhelmed and feel incompetent, sublimate their desire into accomplishing tasks or be extremely stressed by work and parenting, possess a fear of intimacy, or get their feelings hurt. The goal, regardless of which partner is more amorous, is to heal, understand, negotiate, and create a passionate and frequent sex life. Even if your husband doesn't fit the male stereotype, some of these differences will apply.

UNIQUELY MALE

Are men different or simply more immature sexually than women? Some of your husband's actions and attitudes may stem from immaturity, with some needed changes being helpful.

Much of his thinking and behavior, though, is due to the fact that you and he are wired differently. This section explains some of these distinctions.

No Menstrual Cycle, More Apparent Desire

Female hormonal fluctuation is tied in to the menstrual cycle. Obviously, men do not experience this cycle. The primary hormone in the male, testosterone, remains at a steady level within the male body until aging has some effects. Though this is not always true, many women find some of their sexual desire tied to the hormonal cycle while men do not experience this phenomenon. A man's testosterone (which is the hormone that creates desire in both men and women) creates a fairly consistent desire.

That the male desire is apparently stronger may also be a psychological as well as a biological occurrence. Because of the double standard in our society, boys are given a freer rein to their sexual curiosity and experimentation. They are encouraged to tune in to sex more as they, at an earlier age, build a strong visual arousal to sexual cues.

Because men use making love as a primary way of connecting with their mates, their sexual desire can seem greater because the sexual part of the relationship may carry the load of maintaining intimacy. The need for more sexual activity can stem from an inability to connect in other ways, like conversations and nonsexual touching. But men are not sexual machines always switched on. They can be angry or stressed out or have defensive walls up that can sabotage their ability to relate sexually.

Visually Specific and Genitally Focused with Mental Imagery

You can't have helped seeing how your husband is prone to noticing parts of the female anatomy. Research has shown that both men and women are aroused by visual stimulation, but they have different styles. A woman can drive by a cute male jogger, notice his strong physique, and immediately forget the visual stimulus. A man can see a female jogger and almost drive off the road trying to see in the rearview mirror what her breasts are like. He is more specific and obvious in his pursuit of visual sexual cues. If he sees you in panties, he doesn't stop there. He mentally takes one cue and tunes in to other sexual cues almost reflexively in his fantasy life.

It is fun for men and women to help expand each other's mental imagery and use of fantasy. While the husband is tuning in to her bikini bottom and hidden genitals, the wife is noticing his gentle strength, feeling the soft breeze, and dreaming of making love in a secluded spot on the beach.

Men, in general, have to work harder to discipline their thought lives and tune out some of the sexual cues in the environment. They can more easily depersonalize sex as they tune in to erogenous zones more quickly than their wives do. That can lead to objectifying a woman and seeing her as a sexual object rather than as a total person. But there is a positive side to this trait: Focusing visually on sexuality can also be exciting as your husband appreciates and affirms your femininity. His excitement and arousal can be contagious. You may find yourself tuning in to sexual cues more readily and learning from his openness to physical sexuality.

Great sex is built on going from general arousal to stimulating specific locations. You naturally tend to enjoy the general and teasing arousal, while he more enjoys the excitement of specific locations. It is fun to combine these different styles. You will find that a part of you enjoys a focus on erotic zones, and he can appreciate a more general, sensual approach. Each of you may find similarities you didn't know existed.

Immediate and Quicker

Your husband has a tendency towards a more immediate sexual arousal and gratification with his visual specificity, genital focus, and mental imagery. You may enjoy an occasional spontaneous and quick encounter, but not as much as he does. In the sexual cycle, wives will ordinarily take longer to reach an orgasm. He will climax more rapidly. This difference in quickness will require some accommodation.

Wives may sometimes wonder if their husbands have remained sexual adolescents (even though it adds zest to their lovemaking). He thinks about sex a lot; he tends to forget consequences and jump into pleasure, whether it means being late to a party or messing up her lipstick; he touches and grabs at what he likes; he loves the excitement of the moment, even if brief, and then savors these incidents to talk and think about later. He often has a short attention span sexually and will skip to something that seems to offer more fun. These qualities in your mate can be endearing, even though sometimes they drive you crazy.

Predictable

What turns you on physically today might vary tomorrow. Sometimes you want direct clitoral stimulation, and sometimes you don't. But your husband is very predictable. If you appeal to him visually or rub his penis, he gets excited.

In some ways it can be fun that your husband is an easy read. When you take risks and initiate something silly or different, it will seldom flop. Try to remember to include visual stimuli, some immediate gratification, and friction on specific locations. You have a lot of power in a fun, sexual way because he responds so predictably.

TURNING YOURSELF ON

Every wife should be able to tune in to and enjoy the wonderful gift of femininity and the capacity for sexual pleasure that God has given her. You may be wondering, in a chapter devoted to turning your husband on, why a whole section is now being devoted to turning yourself on. The answer is twofold. First, your husband is sexually excited by the sounds and sights of you tuning in to your own sexual pleasure and intensely enjoying the whole process. Do you want to turn him on and be a great lover? Learn to be intensely turned on yourself! Second, you face more hurdles in getting turned on, and it helps to be self-aware as you appropriate God's unique gift of your feminine sexiness.

Permission for Pleasure

God has given us a sexual celebration in marriage. The sad fact is that in Christianity, sex has often been feared and not talked about. Part of the distortion and confusion is created because of the silence as well as negative messages. Anyone becomes suspicious about a topic that is constantly avoided. You may have to erase the mental tapes playing in your head from Mom or Dad, the church, or society to truly enjoy sex and let it be a celebration.

Women often struggle with relaxing control and abandoning themselves to pleasure. Some of this may be due to unfortunate double standards. The brunt of maintaining sexual control in dating relationships is placed on girls. God, in His sexual economy, makes both sexes responsible for healthy boundaries. The unhappy truth is that so often boys try to "score," and girls slap hands and try to keep from getting taken advantage of, hurt, or pregnant. Wives can have a difficult time relaxing control and giving themselves permission to enjoy sexual pleasure, even in a committed and loving marital relationship.

Women also have a natural modesty that needs to be honored. They usually don't prance around naked in the locker room like men do. This is not immaturity and an inability to be "naked and unashamed" but a God-given tendency to treat bodies and sexuality with care and respect. In marriage, there is room to keep this innate modesty but also to open up to the pleasures of romping and squealing and tuning in to your child ego state, which is where great sex occurs.

Tuning In to Cues

From boyhood on, men seem to tune in to sexuality more overtly and, in an unfair way, are regarded as the sexual experts. Girls are taught psychologically to control sexual impulses and do not tune in to sexuality as readily. Even their genitals are more hidden and not grasped every time they urinate as men's are. The environment also takes a toll on sexual desire. In the midst of busyness and children, husbands often fear their wives could go days without sex being that much of a priority.

God gave each woman responsibility for her own body and for learning to experience sexual pleasure. Perhaps you are disappointed that lovemaking hasn't fallen into place as easily as you expected it to or you are not easily orgasmic. Don't be too hard on yourself. You won't think of sex as often as your husband does and your sexual desire will be expressed differently. You usually will have to take longer to become orgasmic, but this can be good as the sexual process is slowed down and enjoyed.

Do take control of your sexuality and tune in to cues more readily, for your own pleasure and your husband's. Here are ten conscious choices that you can make—and women are much more likely to make conscious sexual choices than men—to focus in on sexual cues and keep lovemaking on the front burner of your marriage:

1. Budget and spend a certain amount of money each month on your sex life.

2. Every now and then wear a sexy piece of lingerie underneath your clothing all day and allow its unusual feel to remind you of sex constantly.

3. Don't wear any underwear to a social gathering, and tell your husband on the way out the door. You will drive him crazy while you stay aroused.

4. Plan a sexual surprise at least once a month in which you try to blindside your husband in an arousing sexual way.

5. Keep a mental note, and regardless of fatigue or low interest, initiate sex at least once a week.

6. Have fun with your husband's visual arousal, and flaunt your nude body at unusual times just to enjoy his reactions.

7. Take a bubble bath and indulge in other sensual delights at the end of a tiring day—it is a great aphrodisiac and tunes you in to your body. In the midst of all your demands, you must learn to be self-nurturing. It will keep you sexier.

8. Create romantic sexual fantasies while driving in the car and share them with your mate at the end of your day. You will have to consciously think about sex more.

9. Use a special perfume that you have associated in your mind with making love, and wear it on the evening or the day you anticipate sexual activity.

10. Practice Kegel exercises.

Kegel Exercises

These popular exercises are named after Dr. Arnold Kegel, who developed them in the 1950s to help women with urinary incontinence. The exercises involve the pubococcygeal (PC) muscle, which connects from the pubic bone in front to the coccyx, or end of the tailbone, in back. It is one of the muscles that contracts during orgasm, increases genital awareness, and can tighten the vaginal opening. To locate this muscle, you can practice stopping the flow of urine; it can quite easily, in this fashion, be distinguished from the buttocks muscles. You may feel it by inserting a finger in your vagina and trying to squeeze down on the finger.

Here are three different types of exercises that you can practice to strengthen your PC muscle. They are easy to practice while in the car, while on the telephone, or while watching television. Greater PC muscle control can increase sexual stimulation during intercourse and also help your husband's arousal.

1. Get familiar with your PC muscle as you contract and immediately relax it. Do this rapidly five times as you inhale and then exhale. Repeat five times.

2. Tighten the PC muscle for a three-second count (one thousand one, one thousand two, one thousand three) as you inhale, then exhale, and relax. Repeat ten times and then rest. Try to practice several times a day as the muscle is strengthened.

3. Pretend your husband's penis is at the mouth of your vagina and you are trying to suck it into your vagina by pulling with your PC muscle. Pull for three seconds and relax. Repeat ten times and then rest.

Celebrating Uniqueness

Sex therapist Debra Taylor coauthored an eye-opening book called *Secrets of Eve* that polled two thousand Christian women. In describing what women like most about sex, physical release was fourth behind physical closeness, emotional connection, and time together. Orgasms are not as crucial as emotional closeness and relational intimacy.

We often have defined sexual desire through male eyes. We need to understand that desire is complex and experienced differently, with varying accelerators and styles. Desire can come in two main types: assertive and receptive. Receptive desire responds more than initiates and can be nurturing. You may like sex but at times have a more passive desire. When activated by your husband's initiating, you can enjoy and get involved or even aroused sexually—though you hadn't thought of sexual activity for days. You also can help your husband understand that sometimes your active, assertive desire comes at the wrong times, but he never sees it because he's at work. I laugh because more than one husband has answered, "Give me a call and I'll come home right then."

Frequently a woman does not have a desire problem but she has a fatigue problem. Or, the "problem" is simply that women do not think about sex as often as men do. Learn about yourself and celebrate that unique brand of sexual interacting that you bring to this one-flesh relationship.

Assertive Demands

You, as a woman, may enjoy a slower pace than your husband and need different types of touching. A basic part of turning yourself on is to assertively express your needs. Sometimes you may want to cuddle and be held tight and have it lead nowhere. You may not like to always be the one to go first in having an orgasm. Now and again you may enjoy the intensity of a type of thrusting in a particular position of intercourse. Become very direct in your requests, especially in the excitement of the moment as you become a comfortable coach regarding your own needs.

The more demanding you become about your sexual needs, the more you may turn on your husband or allow yourself to experience more pleasure. Both of you can gain skills in sexual self-awareness and assertive communication. In creating a balance that works, husbands and wives have to acknowledge and accept that their desire, as to type and timing of sexual activity, will not always match.

Sometimes you need to say no to lovemaking. How can you not feel pressured, if you don't give yourself permission to sometimes say you are truly not in the mood? When you are able to assertively say no, you are then able to say yes to varying levels of involvement in lovemaking without acting from obligation. (Note: If you are *never* in the mood, then something is wrong and you need to seek help. See Chapter 18.) Sometimes you will not desire to engage heavily yourself but choose to meet his sexual needs in a nurturing way. If you stay assertive, you will keep from engaging in "duty/pity" sex, which is not fun for either partner.

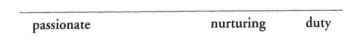

Fig. 14.1. Levels of personal involvement in lovemaking continuum

This may be an issue for the two of you to work out. Duty sex is an obligation out of guilt with neither partner enjoying any real connection. Pity sex is giving the mate sex because he or she seems to be so needy or frustrated. There is a continuum from duty up to passionate involvement. (See Figure 14.1.) Nurturing sex can be a variety of receptive desire and is honoring the higher need of one's partner but done willingly with various levels of participation. This was talked about in Chapter 11 and will be discussed further in Chapter 18, and at times it seems a meaningful compromise.

I laughed when one of my female clients with four children came in and stated assertively, "I've thought this through and discussed it with Mike. Here is what I am willing to do right now. Once a week I will actively get involved and enjoy orgasms and excitement. Once a week I could enjoy a quickie. This can be intercourse without me reaching a climax to give him his time to connect. And maybe once a week, I can manually pleasure him." Bless her heart, and may we all be equally as assertive and compassionately understanding.

PASSIONATE POWER

You have tremendous power to arouse your husband. He desires and needs you. (A crucial note: Sometimes you won't turn him on. Don't assume he's gay, having an affair, or that you're not attractive. Be a detective and explore what is going on in his life. Persist through to healing and change even if it takes professional help.) You may be reluctant to use your feminine power, not wanting it to degenerate into destructive manipulation. But healthy and skillful sexual influencing results in a win-win situation, not the win-lose or lose-lose interaction of harmful sexual games. Your feminine power actually arouses you sexually and plays a part in your assertive sexual desire. This is called alluring desire and is a fun aspect of who you are as a woman.

Correctly using passionate power or alluring desire is *not* meeting him at the door in see-through lingerie so you can manipulate a designer dress out of him when you honestly cannot afford one. Healthy sexual power is *not* cutting off sex so he will straighten up and make needed changes. Actively seducing your husband by playing on his visual nature so he grins all day and you delight in your femininity, or fun flirting and teasing that increase the playfulness and fun in your sexual companionship are examples of a definite win-win and worth cultivating.

Openly Visual

Trying to be more openly visual to turn on your husband will be at first like writing with your left hand when you are right-handed. It will have to be a conscious act of the will. Remember, men are aroused by seeing the female form, and the more obvious sexual parts (breasts, genitals, hips) are more powerful. Views and actions that would do nothing for you will have amazing results on your mate.

Play on his attraction to your femininity. Go upstairs in front of him and put an exaggerated swing in your hips, knowing he is noticing and getting excited. Alone with him in his office or at home, assume a less modest sitting position—flashing him images of things to come. In lovemaking, remember to increase his visual excitement. Certain positions are more stimulating, like when you are on top, and you can encourage his exploration and enjoyment of your genitals and breasts.

Immediate

Your husband wants to quickly touch what he visually enjoys. Work out some appropriate compromises in which you satisfy his need for immediate gratification, but keep balance in your sex life for both your sakes. Enjoy quickies but also teach him to postpone pleasure and not leap right to intercourse for at least five minutes. Let him nibble, but help him understand he may have to wait—you still need to get to church in thirty minutes. Your openness to his reactiveness and quickness will help him back off and go more slowly.

Teasingly Seductive

Isn't it fascinating that in adolescence we are taught not to tease? Now I am telling you that teasing is a basic concept for great sex. In marriage, teasing is seductive, exhilarating, and intimate. Remember to honor your own personality and femininity as you create your own brand of alluring power. You may never sing and dance and wear garter belts, but it is amazing how even the introvert can learn to be playful and erotic. Remember, proactive initiation plays a dynamic role in turning him on.

Tantalize him by telling him in the car on the way to dinner what you hope to do later on that night with him. The sexual tension will build during the course of the evening. While making love, your teasing comments will be met by increased arousal and excited orgasms.

REBEKAH'S WELL OF WATER

As a sex therapist, I have always liked the Old Testament characters of Isaac and Rebekah. Genesis 26:8 states that he was "showing endearment" (NKJV) to his wife, Rebekah, in an intimate sexual manner so that King Abimelech knew they were not brother and sister. Out of fear, they had been trying to pass as siblings, but Isaac and Rebekah couldn't keep their hands to themselves. Earlier when Abraham sent his chief servant to find a wife for Isaac, the servant prayed to God for a sign of an open, giving woman: "Behold, here I stand by the well of water, and the daughters of the men of the city are coming out to draw water. Now let it be that the young woman to whom I say, 'Please let down your pitcher that I may drink,' and she says, 'Drink, and I will also give your camels a drink'—let her be the one You have appointed for Your servant Isaac" (Gen. 24:13–14 NKJV).

Proverbs encourages husbands to drink sexual water from their own springs and rejoice in the wives of their youth (Prov. 5:15–19). Sometimes you may feel that you have exceeded Rebekah's giving behaviors and that you have watered him, his camels, and his sheep, too!

To be Rebekah with a fresh jar of water can also be a fun, exciting, and mutually fulfilling undertaking. Consider the following suggestion for activities that can enhance your lovemaking. Enjoy your one-flesh companionship. Men, though predictable, are not always easy to live with sexually. They are wired in some seemingly crazy ways, but you can enjoy your sexual power with your husband. You have a wonderfully refreshing well of water; teach him to drink deeply.

Focusing on Your Husband's Body

Because men are usually more easily stimulated physically and visually, couples neglect to focus attention and energy on the husband's body. Your husband may feel uncomfortable at first, but throughout the loveplay, keep your hands on him. It should not be a focus on his genital area. Hold and caress and stroke his body. You will probably find he ejaculates less quickly as you touch and hold more.

Both men and women can be very uncomfortable at first with hugging and touching if their families were not physically demonstrative and they have not practiced both giving and receiving physical nurturing. These are skills you and your mate need to learn to be great lovers.

Don't let your husband get away with focusing only on your body! Reread Chapter 9 on sensuous massage, and help him learn to enjoy back rubs and facials. Use some scented lotions and expand his repertoire of experiencing sensuality. Practice five-minute embraces and don't neglect caressing during intercourse. Holding his testicles lightly or massaging the prostate or reaching down and placing your index and middle finger like scissors at the mouth of your vagina to grasp his penis going in and out can all bring extra delight. Assertively insist on nurturing him physically. Like so many things in life, as he tries it, he will like it.

Special Stimulation

Making love to your husband's penis is crucial to turning him on. The penis is a part of your husband's anatomy that he is proud and protective of, but it is not fragile. Rapid and firm strokes are usually more stimulating. Develop a rhythm and pressure that he enjoys.

Orally stimulating the penis is very exciting for most men. Remember that fun sex is based on keeping sensitive to your own and your partner's needs and enjoyment sexually. Although the Bible is neutral on oral sex, many women are not comfortable with it. Some say that they are turned off by the secretions or they are afraid the husband will slip up and climax during the process. Sex is a partnership with trust and cooperation. Your husband can prevent himself from climaxing, or he can warn you so you both are ready. Take a warm washcloth and wipe off the penis before engaging in oral sex. Keep tissues handy. In this and other exercises, try them and you may find you truly like them or can relax with them for pleasuring your mate. Never berate yourself, though, if you choose not to engage in some sexual behavior. Lovemaking is much more than one method of erotic arousal.

In oral sex, probably your mouth and lips are not strong enough to give sufficient stimulation for building toward an orgasm. The fun is more in the teasing and the intimacy of his entrusting his penis to your mouth. Manually stroking the shaft while focusing on the head of the penis with your mouth can bring real enjoyment, because greater sensation exists in the head of the penis. Shield your teeth with your lips pulled over them as you orally stimulate with tongue, lips, and mouth.

Try these methods. Place the head of the penis in your mouth and suck like a vacuum as you pull it out of your mouth; repeat the process. Or stimulate the penis with licking motions lightly and firmly around the ridge and over the top with the head of the penis in and out of your mouth; wrap your hand firmly around the shaft of the penis to retain the blood in the head as you do this to increase excitement. Or tease the underside of the penis with flicking motions of your tongue or gentle sucking. The underside of the penis is very sensitive, especially on the line of skin that runs vertically up and connects at the ridge on the head of the penis.

In intercourse, practice your Kegel exercises with your mate's penis in your vagina. That can be arousing for both of you. Allow him to feel your PC muscle enclose and tighten on his penis. Let him do this with just the head of the penis as he gently thrusts into the mouth of your vagina and you tighten the PC muscle. Play and experiment—sex is fun.

Sexual Flooding

Many husbands dream about being ravished by so much sex that they couldn't stand more. At a time when you are feeling relaxed and rested—it may have to be on vacation—tell your mate that he is free to initiate sex whenever he desires and that you will be disappointed if it is not very frequent.

Help him out by planning some sexual sessions that appeal to his specific visual orientation. Place him on the bed, or wherever, and let him get aroused with some anticipation as you get your props (for example, lingerie and music) ready. Then overwhelm him with sexy apparel, sexy movements, and sexy sights of your body clothed and nude. Plan exciting surprises of your own during this time. Create a flood of sexual activity.

His Exciting Climax

Men and women experience differing types of orgasms. Some are a gentle rush, some are a fizzle, and some seem like huge waves that build and crash to the shore. Men experience greater and more satisfying orgasms with increased arousal over a period of time. Some researchers think this might have to do with a greater accumulation of semen that gives a stronger feeling of ejaculation; or it may be more psychological. It helps if you haven't had sex in a few days or you've teasingly built up tension prior to lovemaking.

Talk with your partner and discuss how he can enjoy a stronger experience of climaxing. Utilize the techniques discussed in this chapter. Tease him manually and orally as you help him build up close to an orgasm, but don't allow him to fall over the edge. Keep him on an exciting plateau; approach and back off, then approach as you increase his pleasure and excitement.

The prostate is located inside the body, with the external pressure point located between the scrotum and the anus. Take a finger or thumb as your husband gets aroused and gently stroke with pressure the area at the base of the penis behind the scrotal sac. Let him direct you as you find the exact spot and desired pressure and rhythm that feel most exciting. You can experiment and see if this increases orgasmic enjoyment for your husband. It may at least give pleasant stimulation to a new area.

Part of the secret is focusing on the orgasm and at the point of climax releasing the pent-up tension with force as the wave crashes. Encourage your mate to make loud noises and exaggerate the muscle tension and spasms. He can use his PC muscle to expel the ejaculate with gusto. Refuse to let him be inhibited. Vary the climaxes by the positions of intercourse you use as well as the occasional external climax from your manual stimulation. Tension buildup and strong release are exciting parts of making love for both of you.

Power Positions

Be sure to read the chapter on creative positions for intercourse. While enjoying intercourse, remember your husband's penchant for looking and touching. Learn to flaunt your body as you exercise your power to turn him on; encourage him to caress and explore. It is an intensely sensuous experience for him to run his penis or a finger over your clitoris, gently down to your vagina, and slowly into it—the warmth and moistness of your unique femininity is very arousing. You have tremendous power with your femininity—exercise it during intercourse. Most women, as they get comfortable with their capacity to be seductive, find themselves aroused by this ability.

Another turn-on for a man in intercourse is for him to know you want and need him thrusting inside you—throw in a little playful admiration and flattery, too. You will be surprised how excited he will get when you say, "You are so big, I need you right now!" or some variation on this theme. Your husband will be stimulated by the fact you need him. Maybe throw in a "King Kong had nothing on you," to build his ego. Have fun and be playful.

Nurturing Mini-Moments

If you initiate a quickie, unless there are other problems, your husband will rapidly make it a mutually enjoyable experience. Men relish these quick jolts of sexual connecting, and you will keep him smiling by initiating them quite often—a special sexual dessert for him in an otherwise great sex life. The unexpected surprise and thoughtful attention are very arousing and nuturing to his soul.

Men may appreciate this more than women, but many wives have come to greatly enjoy the quick dessert, too. Others just enjoy nurturing their mates and seeing the flood of excitement created by a 3:00 A.M. encounter. Remember how much power you have and the quickie will certainly confirm it. Short, refreshing drinks from Rebekah's well can be amazing.

May you have courage, spontaneity, zest, love, and a whole lot of fun as you turn yourself and man on. The rewards of learning new skills are great. Take a walk on the male side of life. You will find yourself enjoying your sexuality a lot more and your relationship reaching new depths.

Time Out: With a female friend, discuss the messages you have incorporated into your sex life and where they came from. Look at your father's and mother's attitudes on sex, your childhood, your high-school years, your first sexual experiences, any traumas, and your marriage. Which attitude(s) will you choose to alter? Discuss with her the concept of female power, how your desire is real but different from your husband's, and the difference between nurturing sex and duty sex.

CHAPTER FIFTEEN

Passionate Lovers

A NEWLYWED FRIEND SHARED with me, "I've never felt this in love. I can't get enough of her, and sex is awesome. I hate that this can't last. Could I bottle this passion and save it for later in the marriage?" I started feeling defensive and wondered if I had become a testimonial to old and tired love after these many years of being married, and he thought I needed a long drink of the excitement he was going to bottle. I also knew this was a common mistake, believing passion thrived only with the new and unusual. I hastened to inform my friend that in my fifties, I felt even more in love and sex was an even deeper enjoyment of intimacy than in those first years. Oh, granted, some of the chemicals that my body churned out in the initial romance have diminished. But true passion has evolved to richer levels.

FALLING DEEPER IN LOVE

Hollywood would have us believe that love is this magic chemistry that mysteriously happens when we meet "Mr." or "Ms. Right." We can then soar off on the wings of love into an eternally blissful marriage. If we should lose the passion, we can never recapture it and probably we just haven't found that right person and need to keep looking. Many people live their lives seeking romance like a mystical, often fruitless, quest for the "Holy Grail." Nothing is further from the truth. True love, with romance, is right at our fingertips, available to all. It has to be maintained, of course—and it can be reclaimed.

I remember a couple I was working with who stated that they did not feel in love anymore. I quickly replied, "I would examine your intelligence if you felt in love. As mean and ugly as you have treated each other the past few months, it's a wonder you can be in the same room." Chemistry can come and go, but passionate lovers have learned certain skills that can keep the "feeling in love" consistent and deepening.

1. Filling the Love Tank—Trying Smarter, and Not Harder

I find the concept really valuable that each of us has a love tank, or a love bank in which mates make deposits with strategic loving deeds, or deplete by negative behaviors. Let's face it—some days and weeks we withdraw a whole lot more than we deposit. Part of great sex builds on a full love tank and feeling emotionally close, by having done for us the things that make us feel loved. We need to learn to be *strategic* in filling up the love tank, or our efforts will accomplish nothing. The bottom line is, some actions score points and some don't!

It's sadly ineffective, but we often practice on our mate what makes us feel loved or sexually aroused, hoping it will turn him or her on too. We check the air pressure in the tires and fill the gas tank, when our mate really just wants to sit in the parking lot with us instead of going for a drive. I remember the wife who was wondering why her husband was walking around naked all the time. I told her it was because he wanted her to walk around naked more and he was thinking this behavior would make her excited. She related how partially clothed was much more sexy to her.

Do you really want to turn your partner on and have some great lovemaking? *It isn't how hard you try but whether you are wisely pushing the right buttons.* Are you speaking his, or her, love language? Passionate lovers learn what their mates enjoy and then remember and incorporate those things. If he speaks German, you learn a little German. If her language is French, you learn some French, no matter how difficult it is or how little sense it makes to you. When we are understood and our needs strategically attended to, we feel more in love and erotically inclined.

2. Traditions, History, and Hanging Out

The thrill of the chase and quick rewards get the adrenaline pumping. It's not as easy to repeat something for years, until it gains great meaning and becomes a tradition. "Starter marriages" characterize this unfortunate phenomenon of our society: no staying power or value for history. You give marriage a year or two probation period, but cut your losses quickly if it doesn't go well. Deeper, consistent love, which is built on truly knowing someone over time, can't grow in a starter marriage. True intimacy is indeed building up a *shared history with fun traditions.* This is also true of a great sex life. That fun repository of sexy memories and bedroom traditions isn't developed on the honeymoon. Favorite positions, fantasy turn-ons, tender touches on a familiar body take hours and years to grow.

So often in marriage, we try to find those small windows of quality time to balance out too many commitments. Intimacy withers if all that is given are small doses of quality time. Real companionship "hangs out" and "wastes" time together. A church newsletter (of so many years ago I've forgotten the source) profoundly touched my life with an article on "wasting time with God." I was too busy to waste any time, but the article stressed that Sunday morning alone and little snippets of quality time would never build true intimacy with our Creator. Likewise, great lovemaking over the years will be based on knowledge, history, and feeling bonded. Creating fun sexual traditions will take some quantity, not just quality, time.

3. Physical Affection and Attachment

It is common knowledge that a baby needs to trust and attach to his caretakers in infancy, or he will have real difficulties bonding with other people in later years. Babies need to be touched, cuddled, petted, and paid attention to in order to bond. The idea of attachment applies to adults and marriage too. A mate must let his or her walls and defenses down and let the partner into personal and private space. The first task is to become nondefensive and naked. Then we can learn to *crave* being near our partner and let the other fill up much of that need to be attached to another human being. Many marriages have never bonded because each partner is off in his or her own world or walled off, instead of attaching with physical affection to the sweetheart.

Physical affection is an important part of this ongoing process. Maybe you grew up in a home that was nondemonstrative, with little touching. Hugging, kissing, and holding hands don't come as natural to you as to your mate. Mates need to learn both the importance and the "how-to" of touching. In a counseling session, I prescribed for one wife (who grew up in an "unattached" home) that every time she got within five feet of her husband, she had to go touch him.

Great romance and intimate connection don't begin with sex. Feeling warmly attached through trust, commitment, and *touch* produces fun lovemaking. This is similar to the old adage that "embers re-ignite when placed in close proximity." Can you remember how quickly a fire dies down when the embers are spread out? How quickly they flame up when pushed back together? Emotional and physical warmth and tender emotions with our partner are similarly re-ignited with physical closeness.

So, you want to "feel in love" and enjoy "gourmet" sex? Learn to *keep your hands and body in close proximity* to your mate—not sexually, but attending to and connecting. This does not mean you are joined at the hip or pawing at each other—rather, you are creating a God-designed "one-flesh" bonding of your hearts and souls through physical touch.

4. Thoughtfulness, Surprises, and Tender Connecting

Couples often look at me with surprise in the counseling office when I give them this homework: "I want you to go home and for the next two weeks, I want you to be nice to each other." I think this advice startles and resonates with them because it's a simple concept; but they know they have been neglecting this important skill of every great marriage. They often come back feeling more in love when they have intentionally returned to doing the small, loving gestures that are the glue in intimate relationships—asking if the partner wants something since they are already in the kitchen, courtesy calls home, compliments and tender touches. Thoughtfulness and choosing to be nice spill over into wanting to connect sexually. It's not much fun sleeping with the enemy.

One fun type of thoughtfulness is surprises. Surprises tell our mates that we thought of them when we weren't with them and that they are important to us. It truly isn't the cost but the attentiveness and time that score points, especially with our wives. Taking time to call, getting a baby-sitter, or remembering to buy a small gift truly contributes to our feeling loved.

Romantic sexual surprises are meaningful too. These creative innovations say to our sweetheart, "I thought of you and your pleasure. I'm stretching to reach out beyond myself to nurture you." One wife, knowing what aroused her husband, went out and bought a complete outfit of lingerie for her own private striptease.

Chemistry doesn't usually strike randomly—remember how unselfish and nice you were in those dating days and recapture some of that. These little acts of self-sacrificing love are the brush strokes that paint a beautiful picture of commitment, romance, and passion in your mate's heart.

Time Out: Plan a surprise for your mate that will truly convey in a way that he or she cannot miss: "I love you and I thought deeply about what could bring a smile to your face."

5. Three-Dimensional Intimacy

Falling deeper in love and experiencing moving sexual intimacy demands that lovers bring body, soul, and spirit together. In the Garden of Eden, these three parts (of God's image in us) were comfortably joined, not different and distinct. We have distorted the whole, especially pushing the body into being a separate object.

Body and soul. Sit across from each other nude and gently place a hand over each other's heart, and in the quiet, feel life pulsing in the body of the one you love. Close your eyes and sense the closeness that is being allowed by a person who needs and loves you. Place a hand on a breast or testicles but remember that this isn't an erotic object—this is your lover's tender body (and heart) that he or she chooses to share only with you.

Body, soul, and spirit. Look deeply into the window of the soul, the eyes, and communicate love with no words spoken. Eye-to-eye sex is special and it doesn't have to be with constant eye contact. It is a state of mind and heart that makes our lover truly present with us. Snuggling into each other's emotional and physical space turns distance into a warm tenderness. Whether eye to eye, voice to ear, or hand to face, we are together creating sensual pleasure and erotic arousal. This is not a sex thing; this is an *intimacy* thing. It can be done in private or in candlelight at a favorite restaurant.

Soul and spirit. Affirm verbally that you are completed in wonderful, inexplicable ways by this spiritual and physical union: "I need to be needed and long for completion. Holding you close fills me up in some deep, real way." Our lover cannot read our mind. It is remarkable how much love and tenderness we hide inside ourselves, which if we would let out would rejoice the romantic soul of our mate. Write down and practice some of these affirmation statements: "When I hug you for a minute or more, the world disappears"; "I don't know why you adore me, but I am glad God gave you to me"; or "When you are inside me and hold me tight, I feel we blend into a oneness I can only feel but can't describe."

We must be convinced to our core that falling deeper in love does not depend on the unpredictable, transient whims of chemistry. Rather, romantic love can be re-ignited with thoughtful, self-sacrificing strategies. Put into practice wasting time together, being nice, and passionately experiencing three-dimensional lovemaking.

THE PERSONAL DISCIPLINES OF PASSIONATE INTIMACY

I've got some good news and some bad news. The bad news? Dynamic intimacy and fantastic lovemaking come at a great price and elude most of us, because we are too *immature* and untrained. A deeply passionate relationship doesn't just happen because you love each other. Now the good news: specific disciplines can be practiced over time that will help us create mature, exciting intimacy—and if we ask, God will teach us these disciplines. "No discipline seems pleasant at the time, but painful. Later on, however, it produces a harvest of righteousness and peace for those who have been trained by it" (Heb. 12:11 NIV). God's professional lovers must learn from Him and incorporate His heart of intimacy. Passionate lovers realize a great sex life is based on the following disciplines they learn from their Creator.

Unconditionally Committed

I love the analogy that marriage is like a submarine. If you keep the escape hatch open and try to submerge, you will surely sink. Great relationships and sex lives thrive on unconditionally being there for that other person. The prophet Jeremiah declares God's commitment so vividly: "I have loved you with an everlasting love"; "I will make an everlasting covenant with them: I will never stop doing good to them" (Jer. 31:3, 32:40 NIV). Commitment is intrusive and makes life-changing demands, but without the total surrender of deep commitment there can be no true intimacy—especially sexual intimacy.

In order to open up to intimacy, one must feel safe. God is consistently trustworthy, and He gives His children the ability to practice this same steadfastness. Real love casts out fear.

In great marriages, no one leaves or abandons the other, because mates are in a covenant relationship for a lifetime of lovemaking and supportive companionship. This trustworthiness provides a foundation for an ever-deepening vulnerability and the ability to be totally naked and unashamed.

How do we practice this discipline? (1) True lovers promise the long-term commitment necessary to learn skills of sexual intimacy. We will do whatever it takes, including counseling. (2) Committed lovers also demonstrate an acceptance that is unconditional. New sexual behaviors are easier to attempt if the partner does not fear being ridiculed or rejected. Many mates have shut down when stretching out of their comfort zones has brought laughter, criticism, or continued dissatisfaction. (3) Remember the line of the old song, "Just call my name and I'll be there"? Availability and a constant presence despite personal stressors anchor commitment. It doesn't take rocket science to see how feeling safe and unconditionally supported encourages each of us to blossom into an erotic and intimate lover.

Confidently Secure, Then Wildly Adventurous

Tim loved the way Jackie allowed her friends to be his friends and covered up his shyness. She often initiated lovemaking and made him feel less insecure. They came to counseling because Tim's feelings of inadequacy had caused Jackie to lose respect and become tremendously dissatisfied. He didn't realize that it takes two whole people to make a whole relationship. The scriptural injunction—"each one should test his own actions. Then he can take pride in himself, without comparing himself to somebody else" (Gal. 6:4 NIV)—encourages this type of personal wholeness. Every mate who *wants to be a passionate lover* must practice the discipline of growing up and *becoming a confident person*.

Genuine self-esteem is based on accepting God's verdict that each human being is "fearfully and wonderfully made" (Ps. 139:14 NIV). It is not pride but godly self-awareness to know one's strengths and spiritual gifts. Romans 12:3 encourages, "Do not think of yourself more highly than you ought, but rather think of yourself with sober judgment [a realistic assessment], in accordance with the measure of faith God has given you" (NIV). In this confident awareness and wholeness, lovers express their needs and choose to risk deeper intimacy and new behaviors.

A great question may be, How do your personal spiritual gifts make you a better lover? Are you even self-aware enough to know your gifts and natural talents? Tim didn't. Everyone is a great lover waiting to blossom if we build on our personality strengths and abilities. This may be the servant's heart of running that bubble bath, or the assertive planning for a getaway, or the gentle sensitivity to recognize the need for a nap.

God wants all men and women to embark on their own unique adventures—journeys only they can take with relationships only they can build and enjoy. Every morning this discipline can allow us to thank God for a new day and a new adventure with Him and our spouse. What intimacy is created if we discipline our heart and mind to accept our adventurous nature and risk the unusual and new! God is there, thinking "outside the box" because His thoughts are not our thoughts. He is inviting His children into an exciting and dangerous experience of closeness and fulfillment. This certainly applies to a great sex life.

There is nothing sexier than men or women who are comfortable in their own skin and can confidently launch into new adventures in wild and unique ways. Lovemaking can reach new dimensions of freshness and passion. You may be like the wife who took up belly dancing to her husband's delight; maybe your crazy style involves organizing a trip to Tahiti. Making love in the car or bringing one of your wife's fantasies to life may be your way of seizing the day (*carpe diem*). Confidently unleash the wildness within you.

Time Out: Think through a mutual adventure that would bring out feelings of anticipation, excitement, and living a little on the edge. Plan through how you could make this happen. Discuss what in your marriage will keep you from embarking on this adventure and how to overcome these blocks. With God's help, take some risks and create some passion.

Emotionally Passionate

My granddaughter continually amazes me with her uninhibited expressions of awe at the world around her. Christmas lights make her yell, ice cream gets her excited, the kitty brings squeals of joy, and discomfort produces cries of pain. Her feelings come out immediately, whether in a church service or awakening in the middle of the night.

An ancient Greek philosopher said that "the passions are the winds that fill the sails of our souls." God gave us feelings to understand and enjoy, in passionate relationships, something of who He is. Expressing feelings and becoming emotionally passionate are dear to God's heart. Think of David and Peter, who were men of such passions and loved by God. David danced naked before the ark and Peter jumped into the cold water so he could swim to shore to be with Jesus. As adults, this ability to live comfortably and joyfully in our feeling state seems to get lost— to our great detriment. I would never swim to shore, because I am careful and logical. I would not risk being cold and wet for a few hours in order to be with my Lord for a few extra minutes.

Take a ride on the wild side of feelings and bring them back into your bedroom. What a fun discipline to practice. Dance joyously at a wedding as you do the Hokie Pokie, ride a roller coaster with your mouth screaming wide open, jump into a cold lake on a hot summer day. Risk stronger feelings in your love life and you will be amazed how your partner is turned on by a passionate person.

Mysteriously Creative

Our God is a God of mystery, romance, and endlessly creative variety. Should we expect anything less in our own relationships, marriages, and lovemaking? The prophet Jeremiah wrote in amazement, "Yet this I call to mind and therefore I have hope: Because of the LORD's great love we are not consumed, for his compassions never fail. They are new every morning" (Lam. 3:21–23 NIV). Each day we can create a new relationship with our Creator—and also with our human lover and mate.

I think that women more than men enjoy romanticizing and desire some creative mystery in their lives. One client whose wife desired more mystery and romance went out and bought a mask and a cape to surprise her. They both got a real laugh when he burst into the bedroom with nothing else on, but she was looking for something a little more profound.

God indeed creatively thinks outside the box and revels in a personal, unique relationship with millions of people at the same time. What romance, as He intimately creates growth and meaning for each of His children. Creativity is a divine trait that God imparts to humans and it is so essential to the vibrancy and vitality of true intimacy.

Sexual intimacy can particularly lead us into the unexpected, creative, and novel, and allow us glimpses into the Almighty. Risking new experiences, remembering to do what romantically attracted us in courtship, and creating fresh adventures are all a part of this discipline. Creating sexual surprises is certainly a part of it. I am amazed at how lovers come up with the unusual when unleashing their romantic side. One husband arranged a complete weekend, from talking to his wife's boss about picking her up from work early, to sexy lingerie and her bags packed, to a surprise spot (which he had scouted out) they had never been to. Women love that mysterious, unpredictable, creative person—leaving them to wonder, *Who is that masked man?*

Sensuously Celebrating

God created pleasure and gave humans the intentional ability to celebrate with body, soul, and spirit. Sensuality is His gift, and Christians above all people should be able to celebrate, as they utilize all of their five senses. The Song of Solomon depicts a sensual, sexual celebration: "My lover has gone down to his garden, to the beds of spices, to browse in the gardens and to gather lilies" (6:2 NIV).

Sensual celebrations and the ability to party are not about simple indulgence. Celebration is about sharing with others and gathers momentum with the connection of souls. It is centered in tuning in to God's heart. The discipline of romantic celebration involves joy and lightheartedness. Like so many of the disciplines, it helps join body and soul in experiencing an intimate connection.

Sexual celebrations create this same personal excitement by reaching out to enjoy our one-flesh lover. Though the childlike traits of playfulness and uninhibited vulnerability are present, celebration is an adult activity. True romance and sensual celebration take adult experience and feelings of love and Eros, of bodies and hearts resonating in sexual tension and release. Learn to truly party as you tune in to the heart of your Creator and your spouse.

Totally Present

A husband complained that his wife was so distracted she had asked if they were out of diapers—during the height of their lovemaking! She said he wasn't much better. The previous night at a tender moment, he had exclaimed those endearing words: "Oh no, my mom's visit starts tomorrow." They were praying that God would help both of them bring their hearts, minds, and bodies into the bedroom to mutually enjoy their love life. Jesus encourages us to live each day and moment in a full and thorough manner. "Therefore do not worry about tomorrow, for tomorrow will worry about itself" (Matt. 6:34 NIV). An early church father, Jean Pierre de Cassaude, said it so beautifully as he encouraged every Christian to carefully honor "the sacrament of the present moment." It is exciting and tremendously romantic to be fully present and available to another person, with no distractions or preoccupations. Just the two of you there in that moment.

Practicing this discipline with Jesus' help gives us glimpses into the supernatural throughout our daily living. To be totally present for our mate and our lovemaking can create amazing discoveries in intimacy. However, this focus requires the mental discipline to rebalance our priorities, to say no to conflicting demands, and to reprioritize the truly important segments of our life. Romantic love does not come in a jar that can be opened whenever we please. Rather, like a beautifully maintained garden, it requires time, energy, and mental discipline.

Being truly present is a marvelous but difficult exercise in intimacy. Tuning out the rest of our life (especially children and job) and focusing in on the "now" with our mind, heart, and body are such valuable aspects of lovers becoming erotic and intimate. Eliminate distractions and center in on your mate's body and soul. Revel for a few minutes in this closeness. Wow! The bedroom can offer many great examples of "the sacrament of the present moment."

Erotically Adored

Years ago when I started dating my Cathy, had you asked me one of the things that was so appealing, I would have quickly responded, "She totally adores me." I desired and so valued from a human partner what God feels for those He loves: "I have summoned you by name; you are mine" (Isa. 43:1 NIV). David so often reveled in God's love as well: "I trust in God's unfailing love for ever and ever" (Ps. 52:8 NIV).

I could also have added that she unconditionally accepts me and finds me so sexy. These are critical aspects of the discipline of erotically adoring someone. In real love, a person can come to be naked and exposed physically and emotionally and feel comfortable. Looking through the eyes of love creates an adoration of the person that transcends wrinkles, cellulite, and human foibles. If you are a "breast man" and your wife has a smaller build, then you become lovingly aroused by nipples and contour—not size. If your husband doesn't have a hairy chest or deep voice, then you adoringly enjoy sensual hands and an empathetic tone.

Are you adored and able to adore? One of my friends relates that at parties he will look across the room and wink at his wife. She will light up because he has so constantly told her, "You are the sexiest one here and I'm lucky to have you." Now just his wink conveys that message of adoration.

My hope for you in discovering passionate intimacy is the same as that of Scripture: "And this is my prayer: that your love may abound more and more in knowledge and depth of insight" (Phil. 1:9 NIV).

CREATIVE LOVEMAKING

Making love is much more than just getting nude or rushing into intercourse. Loveplay can lead "nowhere," can even keep your clothes on, and can include intimate nurturing, teasing, and relaxation. Remember the key axiom of this book:

GREAT LOVEMAKING = AN INTIMATE COMPANIONSHIP + A MATURE LOVER

Intimate, wise lovers know how to create and enjoy a variety of atmospheres, attitudes, and behaviors in their sexual connecting within their covenant companionships. Incorporate variety into your intimate passion and see your lovemaking flourish. You may combine a couple of these ideas or enjoy them separately. Remember the importance of uninterrupted privacy, effective timing, a sensual setting, and keeping an open invitation to make love.

1. Gourmet Marathon

Perhaps the most precious gift mates can give each other is time. If fifteen minutes is fun, an hour can become truly sensual. With gourmet lovemaking, all five senses are emphasized, with much creative variety. Lovers can vary the tempo from intense to languid. Intercourse and orgasms will be included at various times along the way, but intimate connecting of all kinds is the course du jour. Gourmet marathons may start with intimate eye contact and conversation at a restaurant and include the evening date night or it may be that Sunday afternoon delight. Hanging out for hours as lovers is quite awesome!

2. Quick Encounter

I love the quick jolt that the Free Fall gives me at Six Flags Over Georgia—what a ride. On a hot summer day to stop at Baskin-Robbins and get a Daiquiri ice-cream cone. Wow! God created us with nerve endings, an important feelings center in our brain called the amygdala, and an enjoyment of adventure and romance. No wonder mates enjoy the spontaneous fun of sexual quickies. To indulge in immediate arousal and gratification is hilarious and uninhibited. I think God, in His playfulness, laughs with us.

I used to state that quickies were more of a "man thing" with our need to live on the edge and be wild at heart. But women confronted me when I said that and stated that they too enjoyed that spontaneous romp and an unexpected climax in the daily routine. Now, I don't think any of us would live daily on the Free Fall or at Baskin-Robbins, but what a treat now and again. What are kitchens for anyway, or the bathroom with a locked door, or that reclining car seat, or the kids leaving the house with Grandpa for an ice-cream cone?

3. Playful Romp

Great lovers know how to revel in their child ego state (Chapter 2). Children are so fascinating as everything becomes a toy or a game, with play reigning supreme. When is the last time you got nude and chased each other with a squirt gun or rubbed lotion all over your bodies? Adults forget how to frolic and tickle and squeal with delight. Lovemaking can include much lighthearted laughter and simple fun. Play may be more necessary than passion sometimes.

I often prescribe as homework for couples that they take showers together. They can soap each other up with a lot of touching that is not intensely erotic, but playful. Props can be fun, like a shower and soap or feathers or food or Crisco oil. Romp and play!

4. Erotic Volcano

Have you ever thought of why God created orgasms as a part of sexual lovemaking and what they represent within His economy? It is more profound than simply a release of tension and increasing the likelihood that we will procreate. I think He wanted to give us a profound experience of what can happen when the body and soul combine to give us focused sensuality and feeling—much as we can internally resonate with music and worship. A candlelit bedroom or a deserted beach can increase the ambiance for this passionate explosion.

It is fun to deliberately build passionate feelings and create orgasms that feel like Mount Saint Helens going off—either one partner at a time or somewhat mutually. Some of this is having enough of a prelude and a teasing, erotic setup. Then it is focusing in on personal arousal and allowing the sexual tension to increase with rapid friction, as you approach orgasm and then back off, enjoying the build up. (Note: Partners giving the pleasure increase their mate's arousal by mirroring his or her approaching climax with empathetic groans of pleasure, tense muscles, and heavier breathing too.) Finally, hang on the edge with muscles tense and holding your breath—and then truly abandon your inhibitions and surrender to the explosion. Help your mate experience that erotic volcano.

Time Out: I stated at the beginning of this section the importance of uninterrupted privacy, effective timing, a sensual setting, and keeping an open invitation to make love. Go through the first four types of lovemaking and discuss together timing, setting, and what would make the invitation to this type of sexual connecting most inviting to you.

5. Teasing Prelude

God gave us as male and female the ability to be very seductive to our mate. This doesn't have to lead anywhere, or it may be part of a prolonged buildup. Sexy talk and suggestions on the way to or from running an errand may be a part of it. Some deliberate nudity or teasing touches with twenty minutes to get to church could fit the bill. The adage holds true that "the best sex starts in the kitchen" with flirtation, compliments, strokes, whispering in your spouse's ear—follow-through isn't necessary. It's playmates and lovers "browsing among the lilies" and giving and enjoying our personal vineyard.

In passionately intimate marriages, erotic sexuality permeates the atmosphere and relationship. Teasing helps keep the concept of lovers, not roommates, on the front burner. I am so touched when I see that couple in their eighties who are still coy and seductive with teasing lover's touches. These little advances and unexpected approaches keep the monotony and predictability in check and add a needed lightheartedness.

6. Nurturing Release

In Chapters 11 and 14, we discussed that sometimes a husband, or especially a wife, will not want as much involvement in lovemaking. She, or he, is open to sex to feel close and honor the mate's desire for sexual connection and release. I really laughed in one of my counseling sessions. The wife was saying that sometimes she didn't feel like having an orgasm but enjoyed nurturing him. The husband was being such a gallant lover. He insisted that he reciprocate and bring her to a climax or she might resent his having all the fun. Finally, fed up with his logic, she turned to him and said, "What is two minutes of my time?" Between my laughs, I looked at him and said, "A little quick aren't we?"

It may also become a mutual, nurturing release with each partner enjoying an orgasm. There won't be any volcanoes but each basking in the relaxation of sexual connection with very limited expectations. It is important that mates learn to receive as well as to give sexually. This can be lovemaking at its receiving and giving best, even at 11:00 P.M. on a Wednesday evening.

7. Fantasy Enrichment

Remember that our mind, with imagination and mental imagery, is the most crucial sexual organ for great lovemaking (see Chapter 7). We create a whole repository of sexual memories in a lifetime together that can be very stimulating and bonding. The reminders can come in various ways. It may be sitting together and reminiscing, or sharing a flashback during lovemaking; it can be a whole style of making love with provocative or loving reminders of treats to come or times already enjoyed.

I am reminded of one couple whose lovemaking tradition is Friday night. From Wednesday on, the fantasy and reminders of the evening to come flow through their personal e-mails. Lovers need to occasionally act out that fantasy with the Hawaiian shirt and the smell of suntan lotion on a dreary January evening. Use your imaginations to create an ideal lovemaking session in conversation and then enrich your love life by bringing facets of it into reality. The mind and emotions can so marvelously pull us out of the ordinary and into the magic world of imagination and romance.

8. Connecting Companionship

Sometimes sex just needs to be warmly comfortable. Your mutually favorite position and the old tried-and-true caresses fit the bill. Massaging tender and intimate areas like face and tummy or giving each other a full body intercourse hug fills that inner longing. It may get a little vigorous or it may stay quite gentle with slow hands. Best friends love to laugh and be together—this sexual connecting just makes it even more special. Making love can cement that special bond, making us more aware that sex is the by-product of the real deal: an intimate companionship.

Passionately bonded partners are captivated by such a variety of feelings: excitement, comfort, intoxication, warmth, joy, and passion. Remember to grow up, try smarter, and risk new behaviors. God calls us to a sensual feast, as we continuously fall deeper in love with our covenant companion.

CHAPTER SIXTEEN

Body Image and Feeling Sexy in Lovemaking

IN A MAJOR STUDY, TWO-THIRDS of the women said they were affected sexually by one or more aspects of their body image. "Most women suffer from unrealistic expectations about how their bodies must look and must continue to look."[1] As I mentioned earlier in the book, one of my female colleagues once asked me, "Why is it that women's breasts come in only two sizes: too big or too small?" Our culture especially bombards women with so many unrealistic expectations and stereotypes of what is sexy—no wonder more women than men are afflicted by poor body image and a lack of sexual self-esteem. But men can get caught up in the cultural stereotypes as well.

The cosmetic surgeons are kept busy making breasts bigger or smaller, enlarging penises, removing wrinkles, eliminating sags, and liposuctioning off fat. How we feel about ourselves definitely affects our ability to relax and enjoy making love with abandon and pleasure. Great lovers have grown to be comfortable and confident with their bodies and sexuality.

In this chapter, we'll start out by considering the concept of body image. You will seek to better understand how you feel about your body and explore where some of your values and ideas originated. Then we'll discuss how to create a more positive body image and become a more secure lover. This can mean a difficult journey into forgiving and accepting yourself and working through your shame and disgust. Finally, you will discover the importance of building empowering attitudes and self-affirming behaviors, as you remain forever sexy.

BODY IMAGE

Where do we learn about ourselves and what is sexually attractive? How do we develop a body image, both positive and negative? Many women and men dislike their physical features, while others flaunt them; and many older women and men are often intimidated by youth. Yet God made each of us unique. It's a shame that we have to categorize and label. So, how do you feel about yourself?

Exploring Self-Perception

We generally form our attitudes about our body from the people and ideas around us. Look at the following list. How have these influences affected the way you think and feel? Take particular parts of your body and sort through how each one has affected the way you perceive yourself. Think about your feet, your legs, your chest, your mouth, your hips, your thighs, your body shape, and your genitals.

- The media—television, movies, videos, songs, books, newspapers, and magazines
- Parents and family—family values, comments, body shapes, interaction with opposite sex/interaction with same-sex siblings, parents, and grandparents
- Peers—friends, schoolmates, work associates, opposite-sex influence, and same-sex influence
- Church and religious beliefs—sermons, comments, type of dress and conduct, and biblical interpretations
- Significant adults—Scout leader or youth minister, teacher, neighbor, boss, and friend of family
- Dates or romantic interests—group dating, individual dates, boyfriends/girlfriends

Which of the above affected you the most in your attitudes about your body? Where do you think the people who have influenced you acquired their attitudes and values? I laughed with one of my clients, who had been at the pool with her kids all summer, as she shared one of her new insights. "I have come to realize that there are no perfect bodies," she said. And it's true: your body gives you and your mate pleasure regardless of whether it is "perfect."

Trace the silhouettes in Figure 16.1 on a separate sheet of paper.

1. Using crayons or colored pencils, color the appropriate silhouette in the way you feel about your body. Light, happy, favorite colors could represent the parts you like about your body. Darker colors or colors you dislike can shade in the parts you are unhappy with and wish you could change.

2. Now color in the silhouette of your mate, showing the parts of his or her masculinity or

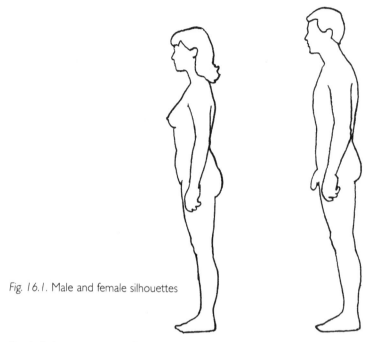

Fig. 16.1. Male and female silhouettes

femininity you notice first, the aspects of the body that affect your attraction and sexual reaction.

Why do you like the parts of your body that you have colored positively? How did you get the feedback that they were strong points? Who influenced you to dislike the parts of your body you see as imperfect or unacceptable? Observe the silhouette of the opposite sex. How did you come to find those characteristics appealing or sexy? Would it help you enjoy your mate more if you broadened your repertoire of arousing physical attributes? Think of one physical characteristic of your mate that could become very exciting if you chose to notice it more.

Talk over and process this exercise with your mate. Discuss the manner in which you have colored in your silhouettes. Start with yourself and explain what you like and dislike about your body image; then, tell your partner how you think these opinions evolved and how your mate can help you improve your positive body image. Discuss the opposite-sex silhouette and how men and women differ in their appreciation of physical characteristics. Remember that body image and acceptance/appreciation of yourself has a ripple effect. They can influence your posture, the way you walk and portray yourself, your smile, the way you laugh, voice tone, some favorite mannerism, and even how you utilize and enjoy some of the body parts. It is time for some healing and affirmation.

Pick three things about your mate that you sometimes notice and enjoy but seldom point out. Tell him or her about those three things. You might pick aspects of the opposite sex that usually go unnoticed—a body part such as hands or lower lip or calves or earlobes; possibly a

Time Out: Tell your mate three things you truly enjoy about his or her physical appearance and body image. Now brag on yourself. Yes, you must compliment yourself! Do not disagree with what your partner said. Accept the affirmation by adding to what was said about the three characteristics. You might further expound, "My smile is appealing; I like the way my eyes light up," or "My pubic hair is sexy; I like the curly thickness of it." Real change occurs when you receive and enjoy affirmations.

chuckle, a wrinkle of the forehead, or a pose the other assumes that brings you real pleasure.

A final exercise in exploring your self-perception and body image helps increase your self-acceptance. Psychological research shows that proximity and exposure create acceptance and attraction. Let me explain. If you ride on an elevator with a stranger every day for a week (being in the same proximity and being exposed to seeing him), you begin to accept and like him. We can apply this idea to eggplant, which is a vegetable I do not like. If I did want to like eggplant, what would I do?

Proximity and exposure mean that I would need to buy several of them and leave them around my house so I would see them every day (exposure) and be close to them (proximity). It would be helpful if I picked them up and held them as I noticed their texture and beautiful color. I might cut one open and examine it further or cook it but not eat it. The more I was around eggplant, the more I would accept and even start liking them. Being familiar with something builds acceptance and attachments. That also happens with your body.

An excellent place to start this process with your body is in the tub or shower or in the bedroom when you are dressing. You usually are nude but probably unobservant. Start to notice your hands, stomach, thighs, feet, and other parts of your body. Do not make any judgments; simply observe the skin texture, hair, wrinkles, and proportions.

Now schedule in some time specifically for observing (exposure and proximity) your body. Stand in front of a full-length mirror and look at yourself. If it is too threatening at first, do the observing with a towel or clothes on, but it is important to progress to the nude. Start with the top of your head and slowly go down your body to your feet. Turn around and observe the backside, using a hand-held mirror if needed. Notice what you are seeing, but detach from your usual knee-jerk reactions to your body. Close your eyes for a minute and try to picture in your mind what you are seeing. Tune in to your feelings as you do this mirror exercise.

(Note to reader: Some women may have flashbacks during this exercise. Those with abuse backgrounds may encounter negative memories. If this happens, stop the exercise for the moment and come back to the present. Allow a few minutes to contain the flashback as you sit and reflect on its possible significance. Processing these feelings and flashbacks with a wise friend or professional counselor may be helpful in understanding what is happening. You may want to totally stop or continue the exercise more fully clothed.)

After your first mirror session, ask yourself questions to help you sort through your attitudes about your body. How do you emphasize or hide parts of your body? How does your body image affect your sexuality and lovemaking?

Continue with your observation and mirror sessions over the course of several months. You'll see how interesting and affirming it is to see your self-acceptance and personal appeal grow with exposure and proximity. But negative attitudes may also need disputing.

Disputing Negative Images

Certain ideas of Albert Ellis and the rational-emotive school of psychotherapy are useful for disputing negative images of yourself. One very interesting device is the *A-B-C-D* way of viewing life and the concept of a rational and an irrational way of living life.

A = the activating event
B = personal belief system
C = the consequence of an event
D = disputing the irrational part of the belief system

You have been observing yourself in the mirror, and you have seen your thighs. This is the activating event *(A)*, and this information then passes through your mind and attitudes and belief system. Your belief system *(B)* thinks larger thighs are not sexually appealing. The consequence *(C)* of the activating data running through your belief system results in more self-hate and the refusal to be nude unless the lights are out or you are lying flat in bed. Another person looks in the mirror and sees the heavier thighs *(A)*, but the partner loves it and finds thighs, with their connections to bottoms and legs, very sexy. The positive belief *(B)* creates a happy ending with a nude parade around the bedroom, not worrying about thighs, and ending in making love *(C)*.

It is not the activating event, but your rational or irrational belief system that creates the positive or negative consequences. Sometimes mates set themselves up to be victimized by their poor body images and belief systems. I remember the young couple I was counseling and the wife who said she could understand how her husband would not be turned on by her small breasts. I asked her if her husband had said anything—praying he had not (husbands can inadvertently make comments that take years to live down)—but fortunately he hadn't. She related that on her honeymoon night she had fearfully told him he might not be excited by her flat chest and that it had often made her feel less feminine. I immediately told her she had set herself up to be victimized. If she had said, "Look at these breasts—what beautiful contours, and these nipples are to die for," he'd have believed that too and felt privileged to have such a shapely wife.

God created each of us unique and special—a rational belief system, based on the opinion of the Creator of the universe. How does this belief system get distorted with women thinking their hips are disproportionate and men believing their penises are an inadequate size? How do we come to conclusions about one thing being more aesthetic than another? An especially troubling belief revolves around the idea that *one* right body shape exists for each sex. For women, it is an hourglass with a slim waist, and for men, it is a wedge with broad shoulders.

Please let go of your idea of any perfect bodies. Better yet, let go of the idea that there is any ideal body image you must measure up against. Women especially must recognize that they contribute to their own insecurities and feed the negative thoughts and feelings about their bodies, as they buy in to the cultural icons of fashion magazines, television, and movies (five-foot-ten and one-hundred-ten pounds). Women must intentionally resist embracing these supposed ideals, because women are masters of comparison. How can you not follow with the inevitable put-downs and inferior feelings about your body if you focus on the icons, which vary from year to year? We need magazines with normal women in average and plus sizes as women seek out alternative models to embrace. You *do* make the choices as to whether you accept and see yourself as sexy and attractive.

You can give and experience sensual pleasure regardless of body size and shape. You are worthwhile and sexy because God created you that way. Think about the *D* part of this technique and the need to search out and dispute or change irrational, ineffective attitudes. Go back to your silhouette and pick out two areas that you dislike about your body. Try to learn some ways to dispute your irrational, self-denigrating thinking:

1. Search out the rational truth. The truth, if you will believe and act on it, has a way of setting you free. Where did you come up with the idea your _____ is too big or too small or ugly? Were your sources wise and accurate? What is God's opinion? Do you have a wise friend to consult with?

2. Create positive self-statements. You have many messages in your head that you need to erase. One great way to do this, once you have identified the truth, is to create a positive statement that counters the false belief: "My thighs are sexy and uniquely mine"; "My stretch marks are a reminder of my wonderful children and my maturity—I am a better lover than I used to be"; "My penis is the right size to create tremendous excitement and passion in my wife"; "My nude body is sexy and able to experience such great pleasure." List your statements and repeat them often as you change your belief system. Say them to yourself with conviction as you look at yourself in the mirror or record them on tape and play them back while dressing in the morning.

3. Use mental imagery. God has given you the marvelous ability to imagine how something could be. You can imagine an activating event (walking across the bedroom nude) and bypass your current irrational beliefs as you imagine positive consequences. This is a great way to dispute your old belief system and advance the possibility for positive consequences. Imagine looking in the full-length mirror and accepting and appreciating what you see. *Imagine what your silhouette would look like if God colored it.* Imagine your eyes, voice, and waist being seductive and arousing your mate.

Keep working on disputing irrational thoughts and beliefs. You, not the activating event, create the consequences of what happens in your lovemaking and body image. It is also important to understand God's opinion of you and to affirm that.

Affirming a Positive Body Image

God created every person uniquely individual, and sexy in his or her own right. The psalmist David said that God knew him even before he was born and carefully made him a unique creation in his mother's womb: "I will praise You, for I am fearfully and wonderfully made" (Ps. 139:14 NKJV). Your body is fearfully and wonderfully made and God hopes you will accept and agree with His opinion.

God did not intend for you to feel compelled to measure up to some arbitrary standard: youthfulness is sexy and older bodies are unappealing; slim is bad but hippy is worse. He affirms your body and wishes you could, too.

Do you have a difficult time complimenting and affirming your own sexiness? The following exercises can help. Ladies, I know that you are shaking your heads and thinking, *A man must be writing this chapter.* Granted, it would probably be easier for you to learn Russian than change your body image. But let God and your husband and your own desire to feel less self-conscious and more secure help motivate these changes. Please persist through to a healthier self-perception and more sexy lovemaking.

1. Stand in front of the mirror and start with the top of your head and make affirmation statements about every part of your body: "This is my hair, and it is great hair"; "This is my nose, and I love my nose"; and "These are my legs, and they support me well." When you get to your genitals, name each part as you affirm even the body parts you cannot see. Proceed to your feet.

2. Get a sheet of paper and write on it the same affirmation statement twenty times until your knowledge starts to connect with your feelings: "My body doesn't need to be perfect to enjoy sexual pleasure"; "If I believe my body is sexy, it is"; or "My penis/vagina is marvelous, and I love the excitement it gives my mate." Think up more affirmation statements that will heal your damaged body image and your inability to feel sexy.

God also holds you accountable to help your mate be the most secure and confident lover possible. You have a tremendous opportunity to help your partner feel great about his or her body. It is not always natural to give compliments generously to another person, but that should be one of your goals with your mate and your children. Lavish praise and affirmation on your partner. This is tougher for some men to do than for most women. Men may tend to be less self-disclosing and more one-dimensional in what they enjoy. That is, men often separate the *body* from the personality and a loving relationship, which can make them very critical.

Your mate will be much more involved and feel more sexy, knowing that you admire and appreciate his or her body and sexuality. If you exclaim over arousing nipples, cute legs, seductive eyes, gentle hands, and an overwhelming penis or vagina, making love will blossom. *Continual* compliments as you see your mate step out of the shower or while you romp around the bedroom will pay great dividends. You have the power to make a real difference in your mate's self-image. There is one hitch, though: you have to learn to take compliments and believe what your mate says about you. You have to allow your mate to affirm you and increase your positive self-image and the way you think about your own body.

Insist that your mate learn to take a compliment and feel affirmed. Ask for an acknowledgment of compliments given. Keep giving affirmation statements until they sink in and become belief. Husband, be prepared for this to take a long time—probably a lifetime—with your wife, who, after all, is a woman.

Time Out: You and your mate do this at the same time. Get pen and paper and write a short paragraph bragging on your partner as the most fantastic lover ever. List all the physical characteristics you love, personal appeal and charm, the activity that really arouses you, and so on. You may want to try it on a weekend away so you can fall into bed together and enjoy the exciting ambiance created by the affirmation as you share your lists.

ADJUSTING ATTITUDES AND FEELING SEXY IN LOVEMAKING

Couples must learn to talk openly about sex as they readjust their attitudes. How can you bring your lovemaking into a more sexy and erotic place? Try the following!

Affirming Sexiness

In any relationship it is good to start with what you are doing right and what feels good. What are your existing strengths and positive points? You can then rest secure and confident in the fact that there are many ways in which you already have a great sex life with a foundation on which to improve. As you do this, you will also begin to identify some of the changes in attitude and behavior that need to take place.

Time Out: Create at least a half-hour window of uninterrupted time and share with your mate what you enjoy about your lovemaking. Describe what you are aroused by and how different things turn you on. Share what makes you feel sexy and what creates passion and excitement. Name things you find sexy in your mate, and say how much you are looking forward to making love together for a lifetime.

Identifying Old Fears, Messages, and Irrational Beliefs

There are many common fears about lovemaking: letting yourself go, losing control, making a fool of yourself, making noises or appearing silly, being inept and clumsy. Identify what you are afraid of and where these fears came from.

One wife realized that her fears were based upon a variety of old messages: "Nice girls are very careful about being overtly sexual"; "Never make a fool of yourself—it is safer to be seen and not heard"; and "If I'm embarrassed or made fun of, I'll just die." Her greatest catastrophe was to lose control of herself and make a real fool of herself. She dreaded that her husband might find her inadequate and make a critical comment when she was opening up a very personal part of herself—her sexuality.

One husband who was reluctant to initiate new things in lovemaking identified how critical his father had been whenever he did chores around the house. The worst thing that could happen to him was looking dumb and lacking the requisite skills to be good at something, so he seldom took risks unless he could practice privately and perfect his skills before trying them out. He realized he did not completely trust his wife and feared that she might be critical and he wouldn't measure up. His core irrational belief seemed to be: "If I make a mistake, I am a failure."

Time Out: Zero in on one part of your lovemaking that is uncomfortable for you. What is the worst thing that could happen? What do you fear your mate might think or say? What is your core irrational belief that needs to change so you can become comfortable? Dialogue and learn to trust.

Disputing and Changing Irrational Beliefs

As a couple, work on disputing and changing some of the old messages and irrational fears and beliefs affecting your marriage. As each of you listens and shares gently and respectfully, you will be pleasantly surprised as you feel more trusting and in love. Intimacy is built upon honest sharing and nurturing each other. Your attitudes will begin to get readjusted in advantageous ways as your relationship grows.

Time Out: Dispute your irrational beliefs by helping each other make up positive statements that are more in accord with God's ideals in lovemaking: "I am human and will make mistakes, and this is a natural part of learning"; "I can look foolish and still be accepted and loved"; "God wants me to enjoy my feelings of pleasure and be wild and abandoned in my lovemaking." Repeat these statements back and forth to each other. Try practicing the ones designed for your mate; they will be helpful too, and may uncover some more of your irrational beliefs and core fears. Look your mate in the eye and offer affirmation in areas of core fears (for example, "I love you and you do not need to fear looking stupid with me").

Try behaviors that will make you violate your irrational beliefs so you have to deal with the fears. Affirm and support each other in what can be scary and uncomfortable behaviors (for example, simulate an orgasm with wild abandonment, make love trying three new behaviors, practice kissing). Together you can realize that no catastrophes occurred, and you are growing and changing personally and sexually.

SKILL BUILDING

Each partnership has areas of lovemaking that could benefit from new and better skills. An ability to communicate about sex and the freedom to try new things without embarrassment and fear of failure really help in implementing these changes. To overcome insecure lovemaking, carefully evaluate your sex life and pinpoint specific areas that need to be addressed. Technique is not the be-all and end-all, but feeling knowledgeable, experienced, and confident bolsters overall sexiness. Remember to relax and play as you try these new behaviors.

Time Out: Step away from your fears and defensiveness and carefully assess your sex life. Think through the way your average lovemaking session progresses. Brainstorm together and pinpoint the exact areas you would like to improve: initiating, foreplay, kissing, intercourse, easier orgasms, slower ejaculations, smoother birth control, mood setting, greater variety. Go to Chapter 4 and read through the McCluskey Lovemaking Cycle for more ideas of areas to consider modifying and improving. Focus on one or two specific areas and plan some specific changes. Then try some new behaviors, remembering it takes time and practice to incorporate these changes.

Other needed skills in a great love life are healing the past and not hanging on to present hurts. We are human and make mistakes that can damage sexy lovemaking. The skills of confession, repentance, forgiveness, and making amends are invaluable and are developed in Chapter 26.

I'M OKAY—WE'RE OKAY

It's a crazy dynamic in a relationship—you can get on either a positive or a negative roll. Insecurity and inadequacy feed on themselves and grow worse. Believing you are sexy, or not, becomes a self-fulfilling prophecy. Confidence and greater skills create a platform for launching a couple into an even better sex life.

Sexy Attitudes and Behaviors

Which comes first: the attitudes or the behaviors? Do you initially need to think you are sexy and then build a repertoire of sexy behaviors? Or do you practice sexually stimulating behaviors and from these actions derive increasing confidence and a sexy attitude? You can't eliminate either the attitudes or the behaviors. They go hand in hand. Inadequate knowledge could hamper the most positive attitudes of feeling sexy. An inferior, self-conscious perspective could hinder great technique. The truly sexy couple has to work on both.

There is a fundamental rule for staying confident with lovemaking in an intimate marriage: the truly sexy couple is *forever changing in both attitudes and behaviors*. Life is constantly in flux. The forever-changing couple is characterized by openness, flexibility, the ability to take risks, a zestful enjoyment of life, and the gracious ability to forgive and live with the messiness of a real relationship.

Forever Sexy

Inhibitions, misbeliefs, lazy ruts, and poor body image won't create a forever-sexy couple. Get on a positive roll and keep it up for the rest of your marriage. Concepts like truth, sexiness, admiration, playfulness, frequency, and power must conquer embarrassment, timidity, control, naiveté, and boredom. "I'm not very sexy" must be disputed and countered in your mind and behavior. God has given you a wonderful body and an awesome relationship—make love with vigor and confidence.

CHAPTER SEVENTEEN

Women Becoming More Easily Orgasmic

I WISH I KNEW YOUR STORY. You may be a newlywed and have just started on the journey of exploring your sexual sensations and becoming orgasmic; you might be a little disappointed that sexual arousal hasn't fallen into place more easily, because you find your husband very sexy. Maybe you have been married for years and have felt very frustrated that the pleasure of a climax has always eluded you. Somehow stimulating your clitoris doesn't produce the desired results.

Anxiety and frustration have possibly crept in as an unfortunate sexual saboteur and made the existing sexual problems worse. Anxiety can become a real killer of sexual arousal. Instead of relaxing and enjoying lovemaking with sensuous abandonment, you worry about the process and are upset that you are not orgasmic. Too much focus is now on you, and you are trying too hard to achieve a climax.

Let me reassure you. You can overcome this hurdle like so many women before you, and you are definitely not alone! Women commonly face this issue. God has given you the body, mind, and sexual feelings to be orgasmic—you just have to learn the skills.

UNDERSTANDING ORGASMS

Perhaps you are wondering if you have experienced an orgasm. Sometimes during lovemaking you do feel tingling and physical excitement. But if you wonder, you probably haven't. A climax includes muscle contractions and sensations that are usually easily recognizable. The pulsing and tingling you feel in your vulval area are probably strong arousal that precedes an orgasm, but not the actual climax.

The Nature of an Orgasm

The sensation of an orgasm begins with a pause in time as if your body is on the brink. Then occurs a rush of delightful feelings and sexual sensations centered in the clitoris but experienced throughout the pelvic area and, if an intense climax, throughout the body. These sensations are immediately accompanied by muscle contractions in the pubococcygeal (PC) muscle, which can be felt in the vagina and uterus. An average orgasm will be three to five contractions, and an intense, extended one may be twelve or more.

Women greatly differ in their descriptions of their climaxes. As a woman becomes more acquainted with her PC muscle and vaginal contractions, she may describe the experience as pulsing and contracting sensations. Often it is described as a flooding or warm, shivery, tingling feelings that begin in the genital area and spread throughout the body. Sometimes it is likened to an explosion or a wave sweeping over the body with an abandonment to the bodily sensations.

Tuning In to Body and Mind

Orgasms are a reflex like a sneeze; they don't occur through willpower. The reflexive action of an orgasm is created by tuning in to (1) your body and (2) your mind. The body has to receive stimulating friction to the erogenous zones, with a special focus on the clitoris, in a manner that feels erotic to the woman and builds adequate sexual tension. This will include a rhythm and pace that usually increase in intensity as the climax is approached and achieved. The *mental*, though, is the usual culprit. It is not easy erasing some girlhood messages, overcoming skill deficits, and becoming openly erotic and sexy. Focusing the mind on sexual arousal and allowing sexual tension to build are skills learned through practice.

The rest of this chapter contains three specific programs that mates can work through to help the wife become more easily orgasmic. The first program the wife accomplishes on her own as she becomes orgasmic with self-stimulation, learning about her sexuality and responses. Some wives prefer involving their husbands from the beginning in the arousal process, and that is effective too. For some women it is easier and less threatening to begin the skill building alone and then share with their husbands. In the second program the wife and her husband incorporate her new knowledge into her becoming orgasmic in their mutual lovemaking, with her coaching him in becoming the primary stimulator. Finally, in the third program, the wife can learn to be more easily orgasmic during intercourse. (Note: It may be helpful to read Chapter 16 on body image as a prelude to doing this work on becoming orgasmic.)

BECOMING ORGASMIC WITH SELF-STIMULATION

The following plan contains five steps. Please take the time to carefully complete each—if you skip ahead, you can sabotage the process.

It may be important to turn to Chapter 11 and read the first few pages on pleasuring. I make a distinction between isolating masturbation that excludes your mate and pleasuring yourself as a part of furthering your mutual lovemaking. Touching or stimulating yourself may occur during lovemaking because of convenience (for example, a position of intercourse where the wife can more easily stimulate her clitoris); may be employed to learn about your personal sexual sensations and the ability to become orgasmic (this chapter); or may be used in demonstrating to your mate what feels good as you coach him into being a skilled lover.

Some women prefer having their husbands stimulate them in these exercises. That is fine and you can bring him in to participate in steps three and five, as you complete steps one, two, and part of four on your own.

As you begin these exercises, please release yourself from a focus on orgasm. Allow your mind and body to enjoy pleasure and focus on the immediate sensations. Learn, grow, and enjoy your body and sexual feelings with increased fun and excitement. Allow yourself to delight in building sexual tension.

As you work through these exercises, block out at least *three* thirty-minute to one-hour sessions per week. This will take planning and perhaps even arranging a baby-sitter, but you will become frustrated if you do these steps sporadically. It will take time and focused attention to make changes, so structure in enough time and privacy. These months will pass quickly, and in addition to becoming orgasmic, you will enjoy many spillover benefits in your attitudes toward yourself, sex, and making love.

Step One: Self-Exploration

Exploring your attitudes. Before exploring your body and genitals, start this journey by exploring and understanding your attitudes about your body and sexuality. Many women find reading Chapter 16 on body image a helpful prelude to doing the work on becoming orgasmic. Take at least a week with three sessions to sort through your attitudes about sex and yourself. It would be helpful to take a pen and paper and write answers in a free-flowing style; writing makes things more real and connects your head with your feelings.

Session One:

1. How was the topic of sex treated in your family? What messages were conveyed concerning nudity, reproduction, menstrual cycles, and the different roles of boys and girls? Were you allowed to discuss sex, and were your questions answered?

2. Were your parents affectionate with each other? with you? What do you think their personal attitudes were toward sex? How did your siblings affect you sexually?

3. What place did your religious convictions and church involvement have in developing

your sexual values? Which messages do you think were helpful, and which were negative in your sexual development?

4. What part did your peers and friends play in the formation of your sexual attitudes?

Session Two:

1. What are your earliest sexual memories in which you realized that boys and girls were different? Your earliest memories of experiencing genital pleasure? Are these memories positive or negative?

2. What are your memories of sexual experiences in elementary school? Did you play doctor or expose/touch your private areas?

3. What happened as you approached puberty? As you began menstruating and developing breasts, how did you feel differently about your body?

4. When did you begin dating, and how did that affect your attitude toward yourself and your femininity? Did you have any sexual encounters in your dating experiences? Where and under what conditions did they take place? Were they enjoyable, awkward, pressured, or fun? What was the most confusing and troubling part in this process?

5. When did you begin touching in the erogenous zones? Was it arousing? How was your first time with intercourse? How did it develop from there as a part of your sexual activity?

Session Three:

1. If you were picking two positive and two negative experiences that affected your sexuality as you entered marriage, what would they be?

2. How did the sexual relationship between the two of you develop before you were married? What activities did you engage in? Were they comfortable? Did both of you have an active sexual desire? Who initiated? Were there any traumatizing events?

3. How were the honeymoon and the first year of the marriage sexually? Was there a time in the beginning of the marriage that sex changed in any way?

4. If you could make three changes in your sex life right now, in addition to becoming orgasmic, what would they be?

Exploring your body. This part of the self-exploration step is becoming familiar with your body and its sensuality. You will need a private, comfortable place to practice, body lotion or oil, and a hand-held mirror. It would be better to have an hour for each session and repeat each session twice or until it becomes comfortable.

Session One:

1. Sensual touching is an important part of sexual enjoyment and arousal. Lying back or

propped up on the headboard of the bed with pillows, gently begin with your face and head and slowly work down your arms and hands and torso and legs to your feet. Use lotion as you desire as you lightly rub and sensitively explore all the skin of your body within your reach.

2. Go back to several of the more sensitive areas (breasts, stomach, thighs) and now practice different types of touching: soft, firm, long, slow, rapid, changing directions, using fingertips and palms. Just enjoy and focus on the sensations it creates in your body.

3. You now have a better understanding of the types of touch and areas that are most sensitive. Close your eyes and focus on these parts of your body as you enjoy the sensual feelings. Experience the tingling and warmth and stimulation you are able to produce in your skin and nerve endings. Don't worry if it feels more uncomfortable than sensually enjoyable at first.

Relaxation exercise: A part of becoming orgasmic is relaxing and eliminating anxiety. You will feel very tense or anxious sometimes in going through this process. Take in a deep breath through your nose and hold it a second or two, then slowly let it out through your mouth; repeat. You may need to actually calm your mind for a couple of minutes and take a break. Lie back, get comfortable, and go to a place in your imagination that is soothing and safe (perhaps a favorite place in nature). Gently breathe in and out as you put yourself into the scene, feeling a breeze, or the mist from a relaxing waterfall, or whatever sensations are a part of the scene you imagine. Let your body and mind calm down. It may help to consciously relax your muscles as you lie back and go limp—allowing the tension to subside as you calmly breathe and feel safely comforted for a minute or two. You will occasionally need these relaxation breaks if anxiety builds.

Session Two:

1. Lie down or prop up or sit comfortably so that you can easily see your genitals with your hand-held mirror. Begin with the pubic hair; then explore your inner lips and how they meet at the clitoris. Examine the clitoris and pull the clitoral hood back. Find the opening of the urethra. Pull the lips back and carefully examine the vagina. Notice colors, contours, skin textures, and shapes.

2. Write a description of your genitals. What do they remind you of in shape and texture? Look over your description. What is negative? How could you phrase it more positively?

Session Three:

1. Begin with your nipples and proceed to your genital area and carefully explore, only this time pay attention to sensations and what area is most sensitive to the touch. Use your mirror as you look and slowly touch and caress each part, paying special attention to the vagina and the clitoral area.

2. Lie or sit back comfortably, and this time close your eyes as you focus on the feeling in your genital area. Stay in the present experience as the nerve endings relay to your mind what feels most sensuous and pleasurable. The goal at this point is not to stimulate or build tension

but to discover the pleasure points of your erogenous zones and the types of touch that feel best.

Step Two: Kegel Exercises

Kegel exercises can sensitize the genital area. These exercises involve the PC muscle, which surrounds the opening of the vagina and anus, and is one of the muscles that contracts during orgasm.

Why bother with the PC muscle? This is an excellent way to tune in to your genital sexuality as you progress toward orgasm. It increases sensation in the pubic area and the vagina, which can increase your pleasure. These exercises can be easily practiced throughout your marriage, and many women report an increase in the intensity of their orgasms with a strengthened PC muscle.

Turn to Chapter 14 and practice the three different types of Kegel exercises listed there. It would be helpful to practice them in ten-minute sessions two to three times a day for a week.

Step Three: Self-Pleasuring

These two sessions concentrate on stimulation of the clitoris—the organ that helps produce orgasms. Some wives may involve their husband in step three, where you have him do the stimulating and coach him on what feels good. Don't start with the clitoral area as you enjoy your increasing understanding of your body. Sensuously begin by rubbing other parts of your body (breasts, thighs, and so on) that you have discovered are sensitive and produce tingling sensations.

Remember, this is not the time to try to produce orgasms, but to relax and focus on your sensations. They may seem mild at first or not the kinds of feelings you expect would lead to a climax. Please do not worry about arousal, but experience whatever sensations are there as you slowly blossom in your ability to enjoy stimulation. Allow yourself to appreciate all your feelings without overanalyzing or resisting them.

You will want to have some oil or lotion for lubrication. Eliminate distractions so you can focus entirely on your body and its feelings. Don't worry about what you should feel, but feel free to stop to relax when needed. You may want to try each session three or more times (allow about thirty minutes each time) as you learn about your bodily responses and encourage the sexual tension to build.

Session One:
After you have done some sensual warm-up, focus on stimulating the clitoral area. Remember, the clitoris has three parts to it: the clitoral hood formed by the inner labia, the

glans, which is pealike in size and under the hood, and the clitoral shaft, which extends back from the glans toward the pubic mound. Women vary in whether they want direct stimulation on the glans or more indirect on the shaft or edges of the labia.

This step continues the exploration as you try to find the right touches, rhythms, pressures, and places to increase pleasurable stimulation. Move from place to place in the clitoral area as you enjoy erotic sensations. Some touches will feel more arousing, and you'll want to repeat them.

Session Two:
Do some warm-up stroking of your body as you relax and focus. Utilize the knowledge you have acquired on stimulating your clitoris, and in this session concentrate more on repeating the touches, pressures, and locations that felt best. The glans can become more sensitive with arousal, and you may want to continue a given rhythm but not as directly. (When aroused, the shaft becomes hard and can be felt under the skin as if you are rubbing across a small cord.) Continue to experiment as you find a rhythm that can begin to build sexual tension.

This session focuses on building excitement. Again, don't worry about orgasms, but enjoy the feelings. After your session, lie back and relax with some deep breathing as you inhale through your nose and exhale through your mouth.

Step Four: Renewing the Mind and Fantasy

The most powerful sex organ of the body is our mind. Unfortunately, it can record both positive and negative sexual messages. This step works with your mind to erase ineffective sexual programming and replace it with positive statements and create romantically stimulating fantasies. The first session focuses on positive self-statements. The second session develops erotically stimulating fantasies and allows you to relax control as you delight in your sexual feelings. Each part of this step will take at least a sixty-minute session.

Session One:
Create positive self-statements. There is power in affirmative self-statements and positive thinking. We are encouraged in Scripture, "Whatever things are true, whatever things are noble, whatever things are just, whatever things are pure, whatever things are lovely . . . if there is any virtue and if there is anything praiseworthy—meditate on these things" (Phil. 4:8 NKJV). Use the following self-statements to create your own list of at least ten positive affirmations:

- The negative things I learned about my body and sexual feelings as a child no longer apply to me as an adult, married woman. I am learning new feelings.
- I enjoy the way my body is sensuous and gives me pleasure.

- God created lovemaking and orgasms for my enjoyment.
- My breasts, clitoris, and vagina make me a woman, and I appreciate being a woman. They bring a lot of pleasure to me and my mate.
- I've started my journey to becoming orgasmic, and now it is just a matter of time.
- I know other women who enjoy their bodies and sexual feelings, and I am no different from them. I can enjoy my sexuality with my husband.
- My genitals are beautiful and respond delightfully to sexual stimulation.
- I feel the part of me that was controlling and uncomfortable with sex starting to change. I am more feminine and sexy than I have ever been.
- I am not trapped by my growing-up experiences and deficits. I am a marvelously sexual woman, and in an exciting way I now control my sexuality.
- There is nothing sinful or unnatural about me. I rejoice in my body and its sexual feelings.

Here are four important ways to implement the affirmation statements you create in your sixty minutes of practice and in future sessions:

1. In the privacy of your bedroom or bathroom, stand in front of a mirror, look yourself in the eye, and state them with conviction.

2. Take the three that you especially want to emphasize, and write each on a sheet of paper at least ten times. Writing somehow helps connect a statement from the head to the heart, and you start to believe it.

3. Use a cassette recorder to record your affirmation messages over and over again, for about ten minutes of listening. Relax and get comfortable and listen as you let them affirm and change your attitudes.

4. Get in a place where you feel comfortably supported and relaxed (chair or bed). Now take a deep breath and slowly let it out as you practice some of your relaxation exercises. Mental imagery is important to athletes as they visualize success. Do the same and imagine yourself achieving your goals in your affirmation statements.

Session Two: Fantasy is a significant part of sexuality. In this sixty-minute session, you will try three different exercises to increase your ability to fantasize and enhance your erotic arousal. Women can truly enjoy fantasy and can be visually aroused by erotic symbols. Romantic and sensual imagery can enhance sexual focusing and physical stimulation—increasing the possibility of that reflexive orgasm. You may wish to read Chapter 7 on keeping fantasies between the lines and enhancing lovemaking. If you wish to include your husband, you can have him join you in parts two and three.

1. A fantasy doesn't have to be explicitly sexual to be erotically arousing. Women usually create more ambiance and relating in their fantasies. Get comfortable and relax as you create in your imagination a warm and romantically sensual scene with your husband. Imagine him

holding you gently and whispering to you how much he loves you. He is softly caressing you in a setting that you find very sensual (Hawaii, a hot tub, the Ritz honeymoon suite). Now try lightly touching or sensually holding or moving your body as you focus on this romantic scene.

2. Now proceed to more explicit sexual fantasy, and pleasure your clitoris as you use your imagination to simulate lovemaking scenes with your husband. If you include your husband for stimulation, don't let him be a distraction from creating your mental imagery. He can be a quiet participant as he stimulates your body under your coaching. You can share the fantasies with him later or during if you desire. Picture sexual activity and arousing interaction as in romance novels. Discover and create images that are sexually exciting for you as you allow your mind to augment your body's response. It may help you to increase your knowledge of fantasy by talking to a friend who is more comfortable with her sexuality, or by reading some of the other chapters on making love.

3. Complete your fantasy session by developing a complete, ideal lovemaking session with your husband. Bring the romantic sensuality and some of the specific images into the lovemaking as you (or your husband) caress your clitoris and body. This is imaginary as you progress through romantic settings, touches, and types of sexual interaction. Let your imagination take flight and picture him and yourself in stimulating sexual touches, intercourse, and increasing arousal. Your mind can build a repertoire of sexually arousing images that excite and increase sexual tension—and give some sexy potential to future playful romps.

Step Five: Building Tension

The last step is designed to help you achieve an orgasm if you have not already done so. You may have to practice each of these last sessions many times over several months. You may want to rotate through sessions one, two, and three as you practice your affirmation statements and relaxation exercises before each session. Remember that an orgasm is a reflexive action. Allow your body, fantasies, and pleasurable feelings to take over.

Session One:

An orgasm occurs as you relax, focus on feelings, and the sexual tension builds in your mind and body. Start with an affirmation statement or two and get relaxed, then (you or your husband) begin stimulation of your clitoris in the ways you have found that build tension. Make a special point to concentrate on your sexual feelings as you tune in to your body and give in to your growing arousal. Enjoy some fantasy to help you focus and increase arousal. Keep a steady, continuous stroking in a rhythm that is arousing, and don't stop even if you feel a tingling or warm feeling. Remember, an orgasm is the contracting of the PC muscle, and you may be on the verge of an orgasm and need to keep the stimulation going all the way through to the actual orgasm. Don't exhaust yourself, but play and enjoy this continuous stimulation for a half hour.

Session Two:

In this session, you simulate an orgasm. The physiological and other signs of arousal may be described as "orgasmic triggers." They are a part of and can actually help produce a climax. At an orgasm: your body will increase muscle tension in your legs, thighs, stomach, and arms; your breathing will become heavier and more rapid; your pelvis may rock or thrust up to meet the stimulation of the clitoris, and there will be other writhing motions of the body and a desire for more rapid stimulation; your face will contort with pleasure and excited grimaces; and your noises and verbal exclamations increase, and you express sexual arousal with squeals, excited moans, and "wows!" Practice each of these separately before role-playing your enjoyable and exciting orgasm. You may want to do this exercise alone and then with your husband.

Session Three:

Combine sessions one and two as you relax, focus your feelings, and begin to build sexual tension by stimulating the clitoral area. As the tension mounts, more vigorously stimulate the clitoris and begin to incorporate some of the orgasmic triggers. Tense your muscles and allow your breathing to become heavier. Rock and express verbally and nonverbally your growing excitement. Keep the tension growing, but don't exhaust yourself. Stop after thirty minutes.

Women ask about using a vibrator as an aid in increasing stimulation. I discussed vibrators in Chapter 6 as a prop that some couples used and enjoyed, while others feared their use could create sensations the husband could not duplicate. In becoming orgasmic, I would start without the vibrator, but you may find it a useful tool in helping you to experience that first climax—to initially know what an orgasm is like. I also know some women, perhaps with nerve damage or needing intense stimulation, for whom a vibrator is the preferred means of creating orgasms in lovemaking. If you are having a difficult time triggering that reflexive climax, a vibrator may be helpful.

As you rotate through these last three sessions, keep practicing your Kegel exercises and incorporating affirmation statements as you change your attitudes. If an orgasm has not been achieved after three months of steady practice, you may need a sex therapist; or if you are guilt-ridden over previous events you may need to work through these issues with a counselor. You may have been raised in a very sexually repressive home or church setting and need to sort through this for healing. Personality-wise you may need control or anxiously try too hard; or your marriage may have produced some scars if your husband in his frustration pressured you for sex. Many women have been victimized by sexual abuse, and these traumas may especially require some professional help to resolve. These roadblocks may need some work before or in conjunction with this growth program.

Becoming Orgasmic with Your Mate

This section develops your husband's stimulation of you to an orgasm. This process will be very exciting and bonding as you share your orgasms with your mate. If you have involved your husband in the process already, then you have accomplished your goal of becoming orgasmic together.

This will not always go smoothly but that's okay. You've come a long way. Practice some of your affirmation statements and don't *work* at these changes—laugh and play at them. It takes a sense of humor and a lot of creativity to implement sexual changes and learn new skills. You will make mistakes and will feel silly and will lose some of the erotic charge as you teach him to create the stimulation and rhythms that you require. You also will enjoy the process as you pair new excitements and experience many connecting moments sharing your newfound ability.

Implementing Change

Talk through each session with each other before setting out to accomplish it. What will be tough to do and why? How can you overcome these barriers to progress and not sabotage the process? Each session should be repeated at least twice, and do your own improvising as you move toward your goal.

Session One:
Begin this session by both being nude and doing some gentle, connecting massage of each other's bodies. Let the wife get into a comfortable position. Each may feel self-conscious—this exercise will take trust to let your mate into your private world of sexual arousal. Be a teacher and allow questions within limits that don't destroy focusing and building arousal. It may be helpful to save questions until after the first session or to do more teaching in a repeat of this session

Wife, now demonstrate your process in pleasuring yourself to an orgasm. Go slow if needed. Feel free to pleasure yourself to an orgasm with your mate farther away, more indirectly observing. Perhaps it would be easier to allow him to quietly come in and observe, as you maintain your focus, after you have begun self-pleasuring. Set a thirty-minute time limit and enjoy the pleasuring and shared experience without worrying about orgasm; this is a learning and teaching experience. Let him observe only—no touching yet. It may help you to be less self-conscious and to desensitize by simulating an orgasm for your mate as you employ the orgasmic triggers. Don't fake it, but tell your mate what you are doing. Repeat this session until you are able to achieve a climax with your mate present.

Session Two:
This session creatively coaches your mate on bringing you to an orgasm. Begin by doing your own pleasuring, and allow your husband to be an active participant as you teach. One excellent technique is to place his fingers over yours or your fingers over his. Help him learn

to duplicate the strokes, pressures, and rhythms that you use to build sexual tension. If your arousal decreases, switch to stimulating yourself closer to an orgasm or right to the point of your climax beginning and then quickly switch to him stimulating. The gymnastics of this teaching may be amusing as you rapidly pull these switches off, but you are playing and learning together.

Limit these sessions to a half hour as you build to an orgasm with your mate. Husband, learn from her. Keep your hand and fingers loose as she guides the motions, and try to approximate the type of stroking and procedures your wife enjoys. You can improvise and expand your techniques later. It can be exciting for your wife if you, her husband, mirror her sexual arousal yourself, with muscle tension, heavier breathing, verbal and nonverbal excitement, and more rapid movements.

Enjoy and play at this session until you as a couple have coached and played through to an orgasm with the husband stimulating. Don't get discouraged after several attempts. You are aware that the tension is building, and you will break through. Practice affirmation statements and keep enjoying the process.

Session Three:

This session expands your repertoire of methods for creating orgasms. It also begins your journey of becoming multiorgasmic as it encourages you to achieve two orgasms.

1. Husband, get comfortable with your back supported in a sitting position on the bed and your wife sitting between your legs, leaning back against you. (See Chapter 11 and the pleasuring positions.) Use your hands to caress and massage her face, back, and outer arms and legs. Progress to her breasts and genital area as you begin arousal. As you advance to direct clitoral stimulation, proactively utilize what you have learned from your wife in the past sessions. Don't worry about an orgasm, but enjoy nondemanding genital pleasuring. If after twenty minutes she hasn't achieved a climax, move on to part two of this session. (Once you have achieved an orgasm, move directly to part two.)

2. Take a few minutes to cuddle and kiss and delight in your sexual closeness. Husband, get into a sitting position and let your wife's legs straddle yours, genitals to genitals, as she comfortably lies back. She will not have lost all of her arousal but use lubrication as needed. After getting an erection, stimulate her genital area with your penis, using it to arouse her as you focus on her clitoris. Let your penis become a tool for pleasuring as you gently but vigorously build her sexual tension toward an orgasm. As she gets closer to a climax, briskly increase the rapidity of your wrist and arm movements.

Wife, coach what feels best because your genital area will already be sensitive and some touches will feel better than others. Lie back and focus on your sexual feelings and let yourself build again to a climax. In time you may desire many orgasms in a single session—and maybe not. After climaxing, feel free to have your mate continue to stimulate you to another orgasm if you so desire.

BECOMING ORGASMIC DURING INTERCOURSE

It is fun to enjoy sexual variety and be able to share sexual excitement and stimulate a climax in different ways. Experimenting and working at becoming orgasmic during intercourse for playful and intimate reasons sounds great.

Helpful Techniques

Here are two techniques that can help you achieve the goal of being more easily orgasmic during intercourse. The first includes direct clitoral stimulation and the second focuses on vaginal stimulation. Most wives do not have orgasms during intercourse without direct clitoral stimulation.

Session One:
1. Apply direct stimulation to the clitoris. Self-pleasuring by the wife during intercourse is sometimes more easily accomplished than the husband's trying to apply friction, but certain positions of intercourse give better mobility. The wife-on-top and scissors positions allow the husband to more easily apply manual stimulation. The clitoris may be particularly sensitive during intercourse and may need more indirect stimulation.

The wife might have to pleasure herself to an orgasm initially with the husband's penis in her vagina and then switch to the husband's stimulation as it progresses. As you move into intercourse and more rapid thrusting, don't worry if the husband cannot always contain himself. Chapter 21 gives helpful tips to prevent premature ejaculation and you can practice some of them.

Allow your mind to make this an exciting, erotic experience. Sensitize your mind and pair arousal with his penis as you eroticize this thrusting type of friction. Let it ignite sexual intensity for you as you enjoy intercourse. You are becoming orgasmic with penis thrusting but maintaining clitoral stimulation as needed. This is one way of becoming orgasmic during intercourse and begins sensitizing you for the next step.

2. To increase sexual stimulation without caressing the clitoris directly, sensitize the vagina and train the mind to focus on different erotic sensations than just clitoral arousal. Center feelings in the vagina, with the clitoris only receiving indirect pelvic stimulation. As the vagina and vulval area are sensitized, they can build sensual tension enough to trigger an orgasm. Utilize some clitoral stimulation, but more sporadically, to increase arousal.

The orgasmic platform is the most sensitive part of the vagina (the outer third) with greater nerve endings in the PC muscle. Tightening the muscle during intercourse can create vaginal stimulation that helps build toward orgasm.

Session Two:
This exercise pairs vaginal stimulation with sexual tension and more easily achieving an orgasm through vaginal stimulation alone.

1. Begin intercourse with a position that allows you to practice PC muscle squeezing and experience pleasure with your orgasmic platform as well as stimulating the clitoris. Stimulate the clitoris to build to an orgasm, and switch to vaginal thrusting alone at the point of climax. Again, use your mind and imagination to picture your husband's penis and thrusting producing the orgasm in an exciting fashion.

2. Continue building clitoral arousal and switching more quickly to intercourse, until you are able to build all or most of the sexual tension needed to trigger an orgasm with vaginal stimulation alone. If tension subsides occasionally, include some clitoral stimulation and then switch back to vaginal alone. Enjoy the feelings and focus on your climax as you allow all the orgasmic triggers to be present. Allow more and more of the arousal to be through intercourse, and allow the climax to be triggered with penis thrusting.

3. Some positions of intercourse will give more stimulation of the clitoris, which can be helpful. Experiment with what position can give more indirect clitoral stimulation, perhaps with legs tightening together. One that sometimes helps is an override position with the man on top, but higher up so the pubic bone is hitting more of the clitoral area. As with any new learning, the more consistently you practice, the more likely you are to master the skill.

As you build greater sexual enjoyment and practice new skills, please don't lose sight of making love playfully with eye-to-eye intimacy. Becoming orgasmic, alone or with your partner, can become a quest that consumes your lovemaking focus. The goals should be pursued with playfulness as you enjoy the trip regardless of the destination. Keep in mind that orgasms are reflexive actions, and you simply set the stage for them to occur. If you have still not broken through to a climax alone or with your mate, keep trying the suggestions of this chapter. It takes time. You also might consider finding a competent sex therapist and getting some extra help. Relax and let your lovemaking be much more than just orgasmic.

CHAPTER EIGHTEEN

Sexual Desire and Frequency

(WITH MICHAEL SYTSMA, M.S., AND DEBRA TAYLOR, M.A.)

FRUSTRATIONS OVER SEXUAL DESIRE are the most common presenting problem that brings couples into sex therapy or marital therapy for sexual issues. In a survey of more than two thousand Christian women, the National Study on the Sexuality of Christian Women (NSSCW), almost one in three of the married women reported experiencing difficulty feeling sexual desire.[1] Contrary to what people often think, men struggle with this issue too. In our practices, wives often initiate therapy complaining of their husbands' lack of interest in sex, wondering if their men are gay, having an affair, or if they themselves are not attractive. Usually, none of these prove to be true.

So many problems in counseling and sex therapy do not have one simple cause. Sometimes medicine seems a lot neater: "Oh my, an appendicitis! Let's take this appendix out." With sexual issues, there are often five or six contributing factors and all must be taken into consideration. This complexity makes resolving problems of low sexual desire a real challenge. Often both partners uniquely contribute to the problem with multiple, multilayered causes. Instead of providing a cookie-cutter approach to addressing problems of low sexual desire, this chapter will explore what sexual desire is and then suggest a number of areas and interventions to consider.

DEFINING DESIRE

One of the serious difficulties in treating desire disorders is that there are no agreed-upon definitions of sexual desire in women or in men. If we can't define *desire,* then how can we understand when there is a deficit that needs treatment? Frequently, responses used to measure desire are more characteristic of male sexual desire, such as the presence of sexual fantasies, genital responses (such as erections, clitoral swelling), or more aggressive initiating. Recently, changes have occurred in the definition of sexual desire disorders as we move away from traditionally male definitions. Especially for women, desire can often manifest itself as a willingness to be sexually engaged rather than by active sexual initiation.

Normal Sexual Desire

Couples struggling with desire issues often have unrealistic expectations of what "normal" sexual desire and frequency should be. Many men use their own sexual desire as the standards their wives must meet. Others pull from the standards of friends, media, or culture. Historically, the church has added another standard, teaching that women (and often men) should not have sexual desire. Now our society says that husbands and wives should expect consistent sexual desire and demand sex with great frequency. When couples fail to meet the standard they have adopted, they often feel inadequate or negatively judge their mates. Yet, none of these standards are accurate.

The way the media have depicted sex has added a great deal of pressure to many spouse's lives, and false expectations to men's and women's minds. In media sex, bodies are perfect and no one is ever too stressed, too tired, or too ill to engage in it. Partners are always eager, no discussion is needed, no one struggles to become aroused, no one objects to the mess, no one has to find a baby-sitter, no one has to set the mood, no one is affected by her menstrual cycle, and everyone has fantastic orgasms. With these expectations ingrained in each of us, a real sexual relationship in the real world will most likely produce feelings of inferiority and dissatisfaction. One or both partners begin to wonder, "What is wrong with us?" when in fact their sex life may be quite normal.

Gender Differences

A helpful first step for couples who are struggling with sexual desire or frequency problems is to educate themselves about the differences between male sexuality and female sexuality. Husbands and wives will rarely (if ever) have the same level of sexual desire, or express it in the same way. Most experts and studies conclude that men seek out sex more frequently and think about sex more often. However, men have sexual desire problems also. Although men generally have a more apparent and assertive desire, it is a myth that men are always testosterone driven or that they can instantly get erections. Men too get their feelings hurt, are turned off by angry or controlling wives, feel incompetent, fear intimacy, focus their energy into their work, struggle with letting moms be lovers, and have sexual wounds. They also are more likely to be involved in pornography and masturbation, which siphons off sexual energy.

The complexity of sexual desire in women cannot be underestimated. Many elements can sabotage a woman's sexual desire: her physical health, energy level, whether or not she is depressed, the ages of her children, hormones, breast-feeding, how she feels about her appearance, how she perceives her marriage partner, how she feels in her other relationships (friends or extended family), how distracted she is by other concerns, whether or not she has been sexually abused, how her family of origin viewed sexuality, any medications she is taking, whether or not sex has been or has become painful—physically or emotionally. All of these factors and their interactions combine to create, enhance, or diminish a woman's sexual desire.

Sexual desire can be thought of as having several different types: assertive, receptive, and blocked desire. Sometimes the problem in not inhibited or blocked desire, but actually understanding various types of desire with their gender differences. Assertive desire is more typical of male desire, while receptive desire is more typical of female desire. Often couples believe both partners should crave and seek out sex with their partner (assertive desire). An interestign observation on assertive desire is that the partner may have already been thinking about sex and often comes to the lovemaking ready to go. This type of desire initiates and seeks out sexual adventure and connection with more of a physical drive.

Many wives are relieved to find out that being open to sex, enjoying the closeness it can bring, and getting involved after initiation (receptive desire) is more typical of women. Sexual thoughts and arousal may come to the wife after engaging in lovemaking, with an internal response of "I wasn't thinking of sex tonight but, wow, this was a good idea." With greater understanding and wisdom, we can get beyond false expectations and relax with our own unique type of desire.

Assertive and receptive sexual desires often come in different flavors. A more feminine variety of assertive desire occurs with alluring desire. This is typical of the wife who enjoys the feminine power of her body in enticing and turning her husband on sexually. Alluring desire is enhanced as mates accept their God-given sexiness in being created uniquely male and female. A flavor of receptive desire emerges as nuturing desire. This again may be more characteristic of females and comes to the forefront when a mate may not want lovemaking for him or herself, but wants to give fulfillment as a gift to the partner. This differs from "duty" sex that is more a chore than a "nurturing desire" with mutual participation with different levels of sexual involvement (see Chapter 14 for further development of these two concepts).

It is also important to realize that "low" sexual desire can be a relative and arbitrary term. Often couples come to therapy (or remain in an unproductive, ongoing argument without coming to therapy) for a "low desire" problem, when in fact the "low desire spouse" has normal sexual desire. Most couples experience desire discrepancy—one of the partners has high normal desire and the other has low normal desire. Because our culture continues to push the idea that everybody should want sex and want it "a lot," and because early in a relationship there is usually strong physical attraction and higher sexual drive, many couples begin marriage with ignorant and unrealistic expectations of what their sex lives "should" be like in a normal marriage.

HOW DESIRE GETS DAMPENED, AND IMPROVED

We have separated the various ways that sexual desire can be dampened or blocked, as well as improved, into five categories. We are trying to make the complicated interactions of inhibited sexual desire more understandable; we know it isn't this simple and that these categories spill over into each other. However, these categories give you an overview from which you can begin to seek out appropriate help and make changes to further your journey into more satisfying sexual desire and frequency.

1. Body Busters and Boosters (written with Dr. James Childerston)

Body busters are physical problems that can negatively affect desire and sexual performance. The human body with its blood vessels, nerves, hormonal and brain chemistry is so wonderfully complex. Sexual desire can be negatively and positively affected in so many ways, both directly and indirectly. For example, indirectly a medication may inhibit erections and decrease the desire to have sex and face another failure. Directly, hormones and other medications decrease the body chemicals and reactions that create desire.

(Note: Important information on body busters and boosters can also be found in Chapter 20, "Sex After Forty-Five"; Chapter 21, "Common Male Malfunctions"; Chapter 22, "Common Female Difficulties"; and Chapter 23, "Making Love When You Have a Disability.")

This section will focus on biochemistry and medications that can affect sexual desire in our bodies. All medications and drugs have side effects and most have sexual side effects. For instance, alcohol is a depressant, and although in small amounts it may decrease inhibitions, in larger amounts alcohol markedly suppresses sexual arousal in both men and women. Another example would be a common cold remedy like an antihistamine; it dries out sinus passages—and the female vagina as well, making sex less comfortable and desirous. Talk to your physician and pharmacist about the possible sexual side effects of the prescription and over-the-counter medications you take. The following sections may help you recognize medical and hormonal factors that need to be discussed with your doctor.

Medications. In trying to understand the effects of drugs on the sexual process, let's take a look at a simplified explanation that describes how sexual desire, arousal, and pleasure occur in our body.

The brain is our most important sexual organ, and sexual activity is initiated and controlled in the brain by a number of chemical messengers (neurotransmitters, peptides, and hormones) that communicate through nerve cells called neurons. Neurons have thousands of receptors to receive the chemical messages much like a lock would receive a key. As a neurotransmitter fits into its specific receptor, a cascade of actions will then occur and the body will respond accordingly. Some of these neurotransmitters encourage excitatory responses ("turning on," or arousal) and some will result in inhibitory actions ("turning off," or relaxation).

There are dozens of neurotransmitters, many of which we know very little about, but three types of neurotransmitters are very influential in our sexual physiology: norepinephrine, dopamine, and serotonin.

Norepinephrine is the key chemical in general physical and mental arousal. It works like a battery current that must be activated in order for the rest of the sexual mechanism to ignite and operate. Norepinephrine enhances desire and arousal in that it produces an alerting, focusing, orienting response (similar to the fight-or-flight response), as well as regulating blood pressure. However, this kind of stimulation causes a constriction of the blood vessels in the periphery and can interfere with erection. Basic responses like hunger, thirst, and emotion—as well as sex—may be caused by norepinephrine release.

Dopamine is the pleasure chemical in the brain and is the primary neurotransmitter involved in sex drive, attraction, desire, arousal, response, orgasm, and satisfaction. It makes us feel good. This may be why cocaine and amphetamines are so addicting and pleasurable, in that these drugs stimulate dopamine receptors.

Serotonin functions to restrain excessive excitation and decrease anxiety and aggressiveness. It helps to regulate mood as well as functioning in sleep, wakefulness, temperature regulation, and feeding behaviors. It helps make people *nicer* and functions as a balance to norepinephrine and dopamine. However, in so doing, it can inhibit arousal and orgasm.

Arousal begins when the dopamine-activated brain sends a message to the genitals that sexual activity is possible. Norepinephrine is involved in this nerve transmission down the spinal cord to the pelvic area and genitals. Serotonin plays a role helping people be nice to each other so that sex may be possible and in controlling the sexual urges so that the sex is not destructive or overly aggressive.

The sex hormones (estrogen, progesterone, and testosterone) have a profound influence on the neurotransmitter actions that mediate sexual behavior, and account for the intricate modulations of sexual arousal, functioning, and pleasure. Dopamine and testosterone are symbiotic in that they tend to stimulate each other's release; serotonin and estrogen also function in a similar manner with each other. A proper balance in the brain and body of these and other neurotransmitters and hormones is necessary for desire, arousal, and orgasm to occur—and anything that interrupts the cascade of signals and reflexes in neurotransmission can cause sexual dysfunction.

Medications can serve as sex busters or boosters depending on the type of impact they have on neurotransmitters and hormones. Commonly prescribed medications and drugs of abuse can cause changes in sexual functioning; they include, but are not limited to, antiandrogens, antiarrhythmics, anticancer agents, anticholinergics, antihistamines, antihypertensives, diuretics, hormones (for example, corticosteroids, progestins), illicit and nonprescription drugs (such as alcohol, cocaine, nicotine, amphetamines, marijuana), opiates (Demerol and Methadone, for example), and psychotropics (such as anxiolytics, anticonvulsants, antidepressants, antipsychotics, sedatives/hypnotics, or stimulants).

Obviously, not everyone will experience sexual difficulties as a side effect of taking these drugs, and the dysfunction can vary in severity depending on the individual, the particular medication, the dosage, the number of medications prescribed for that individual, and his or her particular medical condition. Every drug has certain chemical mechanisms of action that can influence any or all aspects of sexual desire and activity. Some drugs will have mixed effects and/or impact the nervous system differently (centrally versus in the periphery). There is no simple, or "cookbook," approach to this incredibly complex process.

In examining the impact of medications, there are a number of sexual problems that can result. These effects can be the direct result of the chemical mechanisms the drug has on the body, or the sexual side effects can be indirect in nature in that they result from some other drug side effect. The most common sexually related effect of medication is diminished desire, which applies fairly equally to both sexes. The next most frequent direct sexual side effect is erectile difficulties, followed by orgasmic difficulties in both males and females. The most common orgasmic dysfunction in women is delayed orgasm. Symptoms of gynecomastia (breast enlargement), lactation, priapism (painful, sustained erection), dyspareunia (painful sex), infertility, and hypogonadism are less frequent, but still quite disturbing when they occur. Females can experience lubrication difficulties and menstrual disorders, which can interfere with sexual appetite, function, and frequency. Certain drugs can induce states of psychosies, which can initially manifest as hypersexuality.

It is also important to recognize possible indirect sexual side effects that result not from the chemical properties of the drug, but from some other drug effect, such as sedation, changes in mood and energy levels, weight loss or gain, body image, and so on. These indirect effects can make a person too sleepy, too unhappy, too tired, or too confused for sex to be appealing or possible. These effects may be the result of neurological factors (for example, headaches, dizziness, pain, analgesia), physical levels of comfort (constipation, dryness, nausea, indigestion, rash); they may be endocrinological in nature (such as alterations in insulin metabolism or thyroid function), or a function of vascular problems (arrhythmias, headaches, or vasoconstriction, for example).

The antihypertensives—the medications used to control high blood pressure—have the highest incidence of interfering with erections and ejaculations, as well as having some impact on libido. This is because these drugs tend to block the norepinephrine activity necessary for sexual activation—trying to calm your overactive system down, not add to your excitement. The angiotensin-converting enzyme (ACE) inhibitors such as captopril (Capoten), lisinipril (Zestril, Prinivil), and enalapril (Vasotec) appear to have fewer sexual side effects than many of the other antihypertensives.

Antiulcer medications tend to block histamine, which is excitatory. Cimitadine (Tagamet) is the most sexually toxic because it interferes with testosterone metabolism. Ranitadine (Zantac) and famotidine (Pepcid) appear less likely to have this side effect. Cold and allergy medications include antihistamines (such as Benadryl) and decongestants (such as Sudafed). Antihistamines can cause sedation and problems with lubrication; decongestants can cause sympathetic stimulation that can interfere with erections.

Psychiatric medications can also interfere with sexual function. The antipsychotic drugs block the overactive dopamine receptors that are creating the psychosis, but dopamine is necessary for the sexual process to occur. The newer antipsychotics like olanzapine (Zyprexa) or risperidone (Risperdal) appear to have a lower incidence of sexual dysfunction.

The antidepressants have the highest incidence of inhibiting desire. They can also be associated with ejaculatory problems, erectile problems, and occasionally, pain with ejaculation. The serotonin selective reuptake inhibitors (SSRIs) like fluoxetine (Prozac), paroxetine (Paxil), sertraline (Zoloft), and citalopram (Celexa) are the worst offenders because they work to increase serotonin. A potential benefit of the side effect of delayed ejaculation is the use of these medications in the treatment of premature ejaculation. There is a decreased incidence of sexual difficulties with nefazadone (Serzone), mirtazapine (Remeron), and fluvoxamine (Luvox). This is especially true for bupropion (Wellbutrin) because it stimulates the release of dopamine and norepinephrine and not serotonin.

Hormones. Besides the interaction of medications, hormones themselves are critical players in sexual desire. Almost 50 percent of the women in the NSSCW cited Premenstrual Syndrome (PMS) or menopause as affecting their sexual desire. The most common symptoms of PMS are anger, anxiety, bloating, breast tenderness, clumsiness, depression, difficulty concentrating, emotional sensitivity, fatigue, food cravings, headaches, and insomnia. A few of these symptoms in any combination tend to inhibit sexual desire.

As a woman goes through the process of menopause she may experience increased depression, emotional instability, hot flashes, irregular periods, memory lapses, skin breakouts, and vaginal dryness or pain. Each of these, or any combination, will usually decrease sexual desire. Pregnancy, childbirth, and nursing disrupt a woman's usual hormonal cycle. Besides the fatigue and stress associated with pregnancy and nurturing an infant, couples need to be aware that the hormone shifts that regulate pregnancy and nursing can prompt dramatic changes in sexual desire. These changes are normal and can last for weeks or months after childbirth or weaning.

Hormones are also a critical variable in sexual desire for men. Testosterone and other androgens play a large role in sexual desire by engaging the circuit in the human brain that prompts us to seek out sexual activity. If testosterone is abnormally low, individuals will experience a decrease in sexual desire.

Boosters. Encouraging exercise and generally healthy behavior (sleeping, eating, stress management) can dramatically change testosterone levels for some men, improving sexual desire. Healthy eating and exercise can help wives with their body image, which has many indirect effects on sexual desire.

Hormone replacement therapy can be effective with certain women and men in alleviating some of the physical problems that indirectly affect sexual enjoyment and desire, as well as boosting desire. Despite recent media reports, however, adding testosterone or other hormones is not a "quick fix" for most people and has potentially damaging side affects. (Hormones and hormone replacement therapy is discussed more thoroughly in Chapter 20, "Sex After Forty-Five.")

In general, when possible, it is best to adjust the dosage or change the medication rather than add another one to offset the side effect of the first drug. With drugs that decrease or affect desire, however, adding an adjunctive agent may be possible in many cases. Concern should be given to the possibility of additional side effects or drug interactions. The following are possible adjunctive agents:

- A low dose of bupropion (Wellbutrin), 75 milligrams once or twice a day can be added to counter the SSRI (antidepressants') side effects.
- Viagra (50 to 75 percent response rates) is contraindicated in those with cardiovascular disease or those taking nitrates but helps with erectile difficulties and confidence.
- Cyproheptadine (Periactin) can be taken in doses of 4 to 12 milligrams, one to two hours prior to intercourse.
- Dopamine-stimulating drugs and psychostimulants Amantadine (Symmetrel) (100 to 200 milligrams once a day), Lisuride, Bromocriptine (Parlodel), Dextroamphetamine (Dexedrine), and Methylphenidate (Ritalin) have all been used with varying success.

As always, talk to your physician about current information and how these tips might help or interfere with your treatment.

2. Emotional Toxins and Antidotes

Positive emotions are so vital to exciting, passionate sexual arousal. Other feelings can be quite toxic to sexual desire, as they have serious negative impact on our personal and relational well-being.

Depression. Depression is a powerful emotional toxin. Research consistently shows a strong connection between depression and low sexual desire. Some of blocked desire is physical, due to changes in neurotransmitters when we're depressed. Some of it is also the effects of depression—loss of energy, mood changes, loss of interest in enjoyable activities, and irritability are all symptoms of depression and affect sexual desire and frequency. As negative as the depression itself is, we have already discussed how antidepressants often have an inhibitory impact not only on sexual desire but on sexual arousal or orgasm as well, further complicating desire.

Loss and grief. Grief has a tremendous impact on intimacy in general and lovemaking in particular. One husband in counseling wondered what had happened to his sex drive. In exploring recent losses, he had lost his dad to cancer and a friend to a car accident in the past year. Any serious loss can cause a person and couple to feel numb, angry, isolated, and sad. This can certainly contribute to depression and loss of energy and libido.

Fear. In a culture that adores the successful and ignores those who struggle, fear can be a very restricting brake on sexual desire. Feeling fearful can be difficult to accept, requires courage to explore, and effort to change. Fear evidences itself in varying toxic ways, but three common categories include:

1. Debilitating fears: The fear of pregnancy or the agony of infertility can undermine sexual relationships; the fear of appearing inadequate or incompetent can quickly dampen sexual initiative; the fear of aging and its effects on the body can cause one person to try to be a sexual athlete and another to give up. Fear puts unrealistic expectations and debilitating anxiety on mates, sabotaging lovemaking.

2. Performance anxiety: Men can be particularly sensitive to sexual pressure. If a man has an episode of erectile difficulty—due to exhaustion, stress, alcohol, or medication—he may become overly concerned regarding future erections. Sometimes this causes a decrease in desire, in anticipation of being unable to maintain an erection. If a man has difficulty with rapid ejaculation and his partner becomes frustrated or angry, this can cause him to pull back from sexual interaction to avoid her reaction. The fear of failure in his own eyes, or his wife's eyes, is enough of a deterrent to cause a loss of desire to even try.

This general condition of being apprehensive and uneasy produces sexual performance anxiety, which creates the phenomenon of spectating. This means mentally being "up on the bedpost," watching what is going on rather than enjoying the process. If you are anxious about having a climax or getting an erection, anxiety usually ensures that you won't. Being relaxed, playful, and focused in the present are important in combating performance anxiety.

3. Fear of intimacy: Negotiating the physical aspects of sex is one thing; negotiating the emotional impact of sex with another can be far more intimidating. As a relationship moves past the excitement of a new partner, individuals who are afraid of intimacy or who have never learned to negotiate deeper intimacy in themselves or their relationships may lose a desire to engage sexually when deep emotion is needed to intensify the sexual experience. We have found this especially true of some men who cannot move beyond the thrill of the chase to build intimate trust and vulnerability in ongoing marital relationships with a mate who knows them at their best and worst.

Anger and resentment and hurt. It is not much fun trying to make love to someone you dislike and resent—sleeping with the enemy. You have to resolve the anger before you can draw closer to your mate. There is a saying in marriage therapy that "sex is the first thing to go and the last to come back" in an angry, conflict-ridden relationship. This may not be true for every couple, but overall it fits. Anger and resentment distance lovers and disrupt companionship. God designed making love to involve the total person—body, mind, and emotions.

Below anger and resentment, deeper feelings often exist, creating the anger. Try to understand anger by hyphenating it. Is it angry-hurt or angry-disappointed or angry-afraid? Hurt and other negative feelings are land mines that explode into anger unexpectedly. Disappointment and hurt come when expectations and needs are not met satisfactorily—when you feel neglected or taken advantage of. They can crop up when you believe your sexual initiative is snubbed or not valued, or your mate seldom initiates and you feel unattractive. When you are disappointed and hurt, you feel you are constantly walking on eggshells and don't know what to expect. All sense of a nurturing partnership is gone, and sex becomes unappealing or not worth the risk.

Guilt and shame. Guilt often results from a violation of personal sexual guidelines and values. Shame is feeling defective or inadequate about your deeper self in some way. Guilt and shame can be legitimate in helping couples to stay within God-designed sexual boundaries. It can also be false and destructive, impairing a healthy sex life. Unfortunately common among Christians, falsely shameful and guilt-ridden beliefs about the meaning and purpose of sex can increase or decrease sexual desire in an individual or his or her spouse. Distorted beliefs like "sex is dirty" or "unholy" or that sex is a way of using or being used will understandably decrease desire.

The antidote of a healing emotional connection. The most enjoyable part of sex to 90 percent of the married women in the NSSCW was closeness: physical closeness, emotional closeness, or both. Cuddling, caressing (see Chapter 9 on massage), and expressing loving feelings for each other does wonders for overcoming the negative feelings mentioned previously. Even guilt and shame can disappear with an accepting hug and "I love you."

LAUGH! Not only do couples who struggle with sexual desire discrepancy frequently stop initiating physical affection and emotional closeness, they also tend to become so discouraged or angry that they begin to focus on the negatives in the relationship. This surfaces all kinds of negative feelings. Couples should focus on the positives in their relationship, as well as finding other ways to bond and enjoy each other while working through their desire problems. As Scripture says: "A cheerful heart is good medicine" (Prov. 17:22 NIV).

Laughter affects brain chemicals positively, gives perspective, and helps create connection between partners. It's a great antidote to many of our discouraging emotions. When down, hurt, anxious, or angry, couples need to find ways to share nonsarcastic, nonderisive laughter, explore fun activities, and intentionally create humorous experiences with each other. This will dramatically change your outlook and feelings.

3. Personal Brakes and Accelerators

How partners initiate sexual activity—sights, sounds, smells, words that are said (or not said), location, time of day, pace, and a host of other factors—can be thought of as brakes or accelerators. The book *Secrets of Eve* presents a detailed list of common brakes and accelerators in women, some of which will be developed in this chapter. Be advised that what is an accelerator one day might be a brake the next day. While this can be frustrating, it is especially common in women and often due to hormonal shifts that occur throughout the day and month.

One valuable exercise is to explore brakes and accelerators for each stage of the lovemaking process. Simple models like McCluskey's (Chapter 4), where the sexual process is broken down into four stages (atmosphere, arousal, apex, and afterglow), can provide the structure for discussion on internal and external inhibitors and enhancers of sexual desire. Take the time to explore brakes and accelerators for each stage with your spouse. Some of the common brakes and accelerators are as follows.

Fatigue. One of the surprising discoveries in the NSSCW was that lack of sexual desire was not the most frequently cited sexual difficulty. Forty-five percent of the married women said their greatest difficulty was finding the energy for sex. Children contributed to the depletion of energy. Over half of the mothers with children living at home reported "finding energy for sex" was difficult.

Although many husbands somehow find just enough energy to desire and have sex even though they are exhausted and sleep deprived, women do not. Usually the more exhausted a woman feels, the less she desires sex and the less she enjoys sex. When four hundred women were asked to describe their ideal sexual experiences, about 10 percent specifically wrote about their need to be rested or relaxed; some even wrote about napping as a part of their ideal sexual experience (*Secrets of Eve*).

Busyness and stress can cause or add to fatigue. Having privacy and minimizing stressors are vital aspects of managing your sexual environment. The luxury of focusing on each other in a private time together does not come easily. Couples have to learn to streamline their lives and practice stress management as they leave work at work and say no to new commitments. They have to make deliberate choices, set priorities, and guard their time to combat the saboteur of busyness (see Chapter 19).

Issues of attractiveness and body image. Two-thirds of the married women in the NSSCW specifically identified their body image and weight concerns as impacting their sexual desire. Ninety-five percent of American women cannot measure up to our culture's current ideal female body (the thinnest 5 percent of a normal weight distribution). Women are masters of comparison, which leads to insecurity, body loathing, anxiety, depression, and a belief they are not attractive to their husbands. Poor body image and our culture's ideal of thinness lead women to feel depressed and to develop eating disorders. Eating disorders, hormone imbalances (which can be caused by eating disorders), and depression all decrease sexual desire.

Our culture's nearly impossible standard for beauty is taking a toll on men as well. Lifting weights and being sculpted are becoming male ideals—beyond a healthy focus on fitness. Men can also buy into an unrealistic stereotype of what is masculine and attractive.

Need for control. You may be a perfectionist and need to structure life so it remains organized and neat. Husbands (and some wives) want sex at such inopportune times. Sex can be messy and out of control—by nature a little wild and crazy. It can be difficult to surrender to pleasurable feelings. Some people, especially women with small children, can struggle with pleasure seeming frivolous—it just doesn't fit in the schedule!

Some people pride themselves on their ability to keep calm and controlled regardless of what is going on around them. Active lovemaking can make a person feel overwhelmed and internally "out of control." If letting go is one of your personal brakes, read some of the earlier chapters on enhancing pleasure in lovemaking.

Sexual addiction, masturbation, and homosexuality. Though not always primary causes, these three factors should be explored when sexual frequency and desire seem absent. Sexual addiction is when a person compulsively uses sex to alter his or her mood to escape pain or create pleasure (see Chapter 28). When lovemaking is not intimate, the spouse may sense something is wrong, only to discover Internet pornography and addiction. If a mate, for a variety of reasons (greater control and pleasure, habit, self-nurturing, fear of intimacy, laziness), frequently masturbates, this obviously will have to change to increase sexual desire and frequency with the partner. Masturbation detracts from passionately intimate marriages (see Chapter 11).

Sometimes a person has struggled with homosexual feelings and thoughts throughout his or her life. This individual married because as a Christian, he or she wanted to be straight and not gay—hoping that with marriage the feelings would change. Sometimes initially the homosexual feelings do change because of the newness of the marriage and the novelty of intense and frequent sexual activity. The attraction to and love of the mate can also spill over into the sexual relationship. As time goes on, though, the homosexuality reemerges and must be dealt with. (Chapter 29 further develops the possibility of making changes and realistically working toward sexual desire for the mate.)

Traumatic sexual experiences. Sometimes we limit sexual trauma to violations like rape, incest, or unwanted physical touching. A better definition of *sexual abuse* is anything that disrupts healthy sexual development, bringing distortion and inhibition to personal sexuality and married lovemaking.

Estimates are that one out of three women have experienced a traumatizing sexual event by the age of seventeen, and the statistics for men are not much different. It may be a pushy boyfriend, an uncle who makes crude gestures or comments, beginning menstruation without adequate information, or a guilt-evoking same-sex experience. It may be date rape, a terrifying or confusing molesting occurrence, being made sexually aware at too early an age, an abortion, or a sexual encounter with a person in power, such as a pastor, teacher, or boss.

Traumatic sexual experiences often require professional counseling in order to heal. Some events may already have been recognized and resolved, but there may also be unrecognized incidents tying up emotional energy and blocking present lovemaking. Sexual traumas sabotage comfortable and intimate sexual relating until resolved. (Chapter 24 carefully explores this topic, with suggestions for healing.)

Accelerators. What are some of the accelerators for great lovemaking and overcoming sexual desire difficulties? Commonsense remedies can help, such as napping on the days of lovemaking, complimenting your spouse's body, making a point to daydream positively about sex with your spouse several times each week, and learning to relax control in other areas of your life first, before trying to tackle sex. Turn to Chapter 4 on Lovemaking Cycles and discuss with your spouse what gets in the way of creating atmosphere, arousal, and deeper sexual connecting. Change those turn-offs! Get therapy and heal traumas, addictions, and broken areas of your life. You may be surprised at what you can personally do to restore desire.

4. Relationship Bombs and Builders

The interpersonal dynamics within your marriage relationship are often the *most important factor* in dealing with loss of desire and lack of frequency. A couple's companionship can be a microcosm of what happens in their sex life, and vice versa. Even if the relationship isn't the direct cause of low sexual desire, the resulting marital conflict often intensifies the lack of desire. Traditional marital therapy techniques of teaching forgiveness, assertiveness, communication skills, and conflict resolution skills, as well as working through control issues, are all important when addressing the relational issues affecting sexual desire.

Though it may seem indirect, going to a marriage class or working with a therapist to make needed changes may be what your sex life needs. Here are some common relationship issues that can get in the way of having the needed desire for a great sex life.

Conflict and control. It is not true that men are unaffected sexually by hurt feelings, anger, and conflict. It may be true that they compartmentalize their angry or hurt feelings more easily and allow their sexual desires to overcome the effects of a fight more quickly. But men dealing with desire issues often state their inability to be turned on when their wives are frequently frustrated and screaming. If they feel one down, incompetent, or controlled, these continued power struggles and unresolved fights have a negative impact on their libidos. Wives are no different with their desire being negatively affected by husbands who are self-centered and angrily dominating.

Extramarital affairs and other distractions. Affairs are prevalent and have destructive impact even in Christian marriages. Infidelity destroys trust, honesty, and committed playfulness, which are vital to inspired lovemaking. Other distractions can adulterate or contaminate intimacy, including children, addictive hobbies (such as exercise or renovating your house), and aging parents. Managing yourself and your environment are powerful aphrodisiacs.

Inertia. An object at rest tends to stay at rest and dig a deeper rut, while one in motion will stay in motion. This law certainly applies to a sex life too. If a couple makes love once a month, it is easy to slip into once every three months. A slowing sex life settles into more sluggishness and embarrassing awkwardness. Initiating becomes difficult and lovemaking ceases to be convenient. Earlier chapters offer some solutions to this problem. Sometimes the solution is like entering into a cold lake on a hot summer day—you simply have to grab your nose and jump. Sometimes the issue is more involved and will need some of the other interventions mentioned in this chapter.

Polarization. As a couple wrestles with adjusting to differing levels of sexual desire, often each person begins to polarize: one partner feels they have sex "hardly ever" and the other believes they have sex "all the time." One mate will feel emotionally neglected and the other will feel sexually deprived. This conflict and exaggeration in perception leads to further conflict, feelings of rejection, and fear (that the spouse is unfaithful, that the other is no longer attractive). This can prompt destructive arguing, accusations, and further hurt or hostility. It is interesting that when polarization occurs, mates live in each other's debit column and focus on shortcomings. A negative pattern develops, which further inhibits sexual desire.

High desire versus low desire and control. In addressing problems of sexual desire, the spouse with the least desire will be in control of the sexual relationship and often the partner's mood. A spouse who is withholding sex or using a lack of desire to punish the spouse can be especially damaging. Of course, the one with higher desire can react like a person in the desert without water and become obsessive and controlling in his or her own way.

Using lack of desire to punish a spouse is not a dominant motivation in most cases of low sexual desire. Many individuals truly dislike the control their low desire burdens them with. If you do use a lack of desire to punish your spouse, know that you are exacerbating the issue and will likely compound it with additional problems.

If you are the high-desire spouse, don't give up, escalate problems, or withdraw from your mate. Examine yourself to see if you have become pushy, judgmental, or preachy. Find ways to keep addressing the issue of sexual desire respectfully, while the low-desire spouse must find motivation to keep a personal focus on the issue and to keep sex on the front burner. Each spouse should find tasks they can be working on. Focus on yourself, and changes you are striving for—don't blame your spouse for what he or she isn't doing.

Relationship builders. Relationship bombs *can* be defused and a passionate desire rekindled or built. How do you rev up a sex life where the relationship and desire have come to a screeching halt?

1. Start with rebuilding the companionship, and do some playful, nonsexual activities together first. If possible, plan a vacation and include time for connecting and conversation. Learn to truly listen to each other and to talk effectively together. Make sure you are actually understanding what your spouse is saying and vice versa. Once you have learned these skills, put them into practice and make them a part of your daily life together. Learn to use skills of conflict resolution, how to engage in light conversation, and how to share. Identify feelings,

take risks to self-disclose, learn to accept your partner and yourself, ask for what you need, and refuse what you do not want. If there are deep-seated issues that have stalled your marriage and sex life, talk them through. If you cannot talk them through on your own, get counseling.

2. Increase your nonsexual touch and physical affection. Oxytocin is a peptide secreted in the brain that flows to various parts of the brain and throughout the reproductive organs of both men and women. It rises in response to touch and promotes touching. Oxytocin also promotes bonding between lovers and between parents and children. It sensitizes the skin to touch, spikes at orgasm, causes uterine contractions during orgasm and labor, increases sexual receptivity, increases penile sensitivity, and speeds ejaculation. Oxytocin effects are increased by estrogen, which has led researchers to hypothesize that oxytocin may be especially important in sexual desire in women.

Unfortunately, as couples struggle with sexual desire issues it is not uncommon for them to withdraw from each other and cease touching. Hugs, massages, and intimate kisses fade into relationship history. Without touch, oxytocin production falls, as does the bonding in the relationship, lowering sexual desire even further.[2] Learn to nurture and be nurtured with physical touch. Put your head in your spouse's lap and enjoy gentle caresses, hug while rubbing each other's back tenderly, rub each other's feet, lay in each other's arms—produce that oxytocin!

3. Create separateness and togetherness in a solid companionship. Blocked lovemaking often evolves into a serious relationship problem. Learn to be close and depend on each other as well as create individual hobbies and downtime. Make time for each other and encourage time for individual pursuits. It takes two whole people to make a whole marriage and sex life.

4. Make love more frequently. It may take some effort and a few failed attempts to get back to a more consistent sex life. Start with sensual massage, tune in to sexual sensations, and then include a lot of loveplay, nude hugs, and showers together before attempting intercourse. As with jumping into cold lake water, eventually you must hold your breath, psych yourselves up, and jump into having intercourse. Go into it with no expectation other than breaking the ice. Orgasms aren't necessary. Choose to make love.

5. Environmental Hazards and Healers

Sexual desire can also get blocked and dumped on by our religious and family values, societal myths, and factors out of our control. These various "environmental hazards" must be comprehended, disputed, and healed.

Expectations and myths. Some women expect sex to be a lot more romantic and less animalistic (physical) than it turns out to be. They may wish that perspiration, secretions, and odors were not associated with being aroused. They may be disappointed that their husbands aren't the knights they appeared to be in dating days. The husbands may not be very playful or they may be rough, insensitive to their wives' needs for romance and ambiance.

Many men are disappointed and angry that their wives' sexual interest decreases after the initial courting or "honeymoon" stage of marriage. Some men are surprised to discover that they are uncomfortable with their wives' sexuality after a baby arrives. Being a mother and being sexy seem to be two opposing concepts. Psychologically, when this sabotaging attitude is pushed to the extreme, it is called the Madonna-prostitute complex: moms adore their babies, but wanton women long for sex. This and other expectations are obviously crippling. Search out these false beliefs and work to erase them from your mental tapes.

Parental models. Your parents teach you about sex and relationships. They model the ability (or inability) to be affectionate and affirming, openly and subtly imparting values to you about sex and trust and self-esteem. Your relationship with your primary caretakers in growing up has an ongoing impact on your current sexual relationship.

Those parents who set poor boundaries and engaged in affairs or promiscuous liasons destructively influenced your sexual development and present desire. Someone may also grow up thinking something is wrong with sex because discussion of the subject was avoided in the home. Someone else may have trouble trusting others because the relationships in his or her family were emotionally unsafe and caused a fear of intimacy.

Life stressors. This can be a long list that can vary according to the stage of marriage. Early marital adjustments and conflict with roles are stressful. Children bring exhausting physical and emotional work as well as joys. Aging brings special challenges, and illnesses, injuries, and medications take their tolls. Caring for the younger generation and the older generation at the same time can be overwhelming. Each life stage may bring anxiety and fear as well as fatigue and relational conflict.

Pregnancy. Pregnancy causes massive shifts in hormones and structural changes in a woman's body. Both men and women can be broadsided by unexpected and unpredictable feelings and attitudes about becoming parents, the impending changes in the marital relationship, and the wife's changing body shape. While some men find a pregnant woman sexy, others are repulsed. Most women already are challenged in the area of body image, but some women struggle excessively with feelings of being "ugly" or "fat," and fears regarding their husbands' reactions to their pregnant bodies.

Topics related to pregnancy can decrease desire also. Some husbands have to work through seeing the birth of a child and separate the birth canal and bleeding from the vagina and lovemaking. Couples must also examine how confident they are in their birth control. After permanent measures, it is fascinating how some couples describe an increase in desire and frequency. More complex are couples who have experienced miscarriage. Often these couples desire children but also fear pregnancy will lead to another painful miscarriage. The resulting internal struggle can decrease sexual desire.

Infertility and medical problems. Struggling to get pregnant and then perhaps experiencing a difficult pregnancy can throw buckets of cold water on your sex life. Unless you have been through infertility, it is impossible to imagine how consuming the process can be. Christian faith can help you see hope and comfort in the midst of trials and tribulations, but the physical exams and sex by the calendar and on demand take a definite toll on your lovemaking. (See Chapter 25.)

It is important to remember that most illnesses, especially chronic illness, take a direct or indirect toll on sexual desire also. Pain and pain medications can decrease libido and frequency as well. (See Chapter 20 on aging and Chapter 23 on disabilities.)

Religious and societal prohibitions. Sex is a gift from God, but you couldn't prove it by one young woman raised in a Christian home. Sex was never talked about and was treated with such hesitation and avoidance that she was afraid of it. She confessed that if bananas had been given the same treatment, she would never allow a banana in her home today. She was ashamed of her desires in high school, and she tried to repress what she considered lust or sinful feelings. She never was helped to work through effective values; she was simply told to remain a virgin. Later she came to realize that her understanding of sexual sin was not based on Scripture. In the meantime, she had tuned out most sexual cues and was afraid of her sexual sensations. Just because she got married did not mean she could turn her mind back on and instantly be sexy.

So often couples hope that desire is a switch that will automatically be flipped to let the sexual desire flow once married. Unfortunately, sexual desire and comfortableness are more of a rheostat that is slowly turned up after marriage. Overcoming the environmental repression and skill deficits many experience will be a process and not a switch.

Skill deficits. As you and your mate explore your lovemaking, you may discover some definite skill deficits. Men don't know all about sex. Curiosity, playfulness, a willingness to learn and experiment, and a trusting companionship can go a long way in overcoming a lack of technical ability. Both of you can humbly and playfully pick up new skills as you learn from each other.

In addition to technical knowledge (positions, anatomy, effective friction, for example), other skills needed include character traits (enthusiasm, curiosity, a humble openness) and relational skills (effective communication, gracefully initiating and refusing sex, romance, time). All are needed for increased sexual desire and great lovemaking.

If sexual desire has been squelched by environmental factors, what can bring healing?

Undertake renewing your mind. Through reading this book, you may have discovered you possess many unrealistic expectations, distorted messages from growing up, and poor attitudes. Begin to restructure and change these thoughts and beliefs. Some of this is done by understanding the erroneous messages and challenging them with truth. Do a lot of positive self-talk. You might say, "Relax . . . you can do it . . . it's okay . . . enjoy . . . play at it." Create affirmation statements: "God created sexual pleasure"; "I am capable of change"; "If I enjoy sex, it does not mean I will lose control"; "Sex is fun, and I don't need to feel guilty anymore."

Practice these change statements by writing them over and over, saying them out loud to your spouse or to a mirror. Slowly, you will restructure your thinking, and your new attitudes will begin changing your feelings. This will take time but will be worth the effort as you actually begin looking forward to making love.

Pray! Many of you have experienced the healing power of prayer or the bonding nature of praying together and building your common faith. Sexuality and sexual expression were God's idea and His gift to us. When we encounter sexual problems, we need to turn to God for help, hope, and healing. Couples *need* to pray, individually and together, for the growth and health of their sexual relationship.

Blocked sexual desire is truly a complex puzzle. Many times mates may be asking for the unrealistic in their spouses, selves, or marriages. Sometimes the issue is education. Learn about normal sexual desire and understand gender differences. Keep an open mind and do not blame low sexual desire on any one issue. Instead, study your unique and complex web of issues that complicate blocked sexual desire. Be sure to consider the body busters, emotional toxins, personal brakes, relationship bombs, and environmental hazards. Attack the problems from a variety of fronts as you seek out solutions. You may need professional help to resolve these dilemmas, but be courageous and assertive in not settling for blocked desire and unsatisfying, infrequent lovemaking.

Reverend Michael Sytsma, M.S., is a husband, father, licensed professional counselor and ordained minister in Lawrenceville, Georgia. He is cofounder and faculty member of the Institute for Sexual Wholeness. Michael is also founder of Building Intimate Marriages, Inc., and is currently completing his Ph.D. in Marriage and Family Therapy at the University of Georgia. Michael can be reached at michael@sexualwholeness.com.

Debra Taylor, M.A., is a licensed marriage and family therapist and certified sex therapist in private practice in Ventura, California. She is a wife and mother and is also a cofounder and on the faculty of the Institute for Sexual Wholeness. Debra is coauthor of Secrets of Eve: Understanding the Mystery of Female Sexuality *(Hart, Weber, and Taylor, 1998). She can be reached at* debra@sexualwholeness.com.

CHAPTER NINETEEN

Staying Lovers in the Children Years

(WITH CHRISTOPHER MCCLUSKEY, M.S.W., AND RACHEL MCCLUSKEY, B.A.)

ALMOST NO BOOKS OFFER PRACTICAL ADVICE OR PREPARATION for love-making during pregnancy or after children. What a shame that a large segment of married people stumbles along to figure things out as best they can. Much confusion and many pitfalls could be avoided with a little knowledge and preparation.

Let's set the stage. At the start of the children years, younger marriages often find couples still adjusting to new roles, struggling through the loss of independence and privacy, and blending their lives together. Deeper financial security exists farther down the road, with expensive items like a house and cars being a huge drain on the present budget. The husband and wife may still be launching careers, especially his, with hopes of her being able to stay home at least part time. The husband's lack of availability hurts, as he attempts to create more income. Those who marry or have children later may have fewer financial or career pressures, but other issues, like time and energy, can come into play.

The bottom line? Pay attention that the baby may be a catalyst to bring to the surface or compound already-existing stressors on intimacy—as well as adding new ones. Your sex life will need wise protection and loving encouragement in those times of marriage when huge adjustments and stress attack it. The children years more than qualify.

The hallmark and central task of a marriage in these years becomes achieving maturity. This requires huge doses of self-control flavored with creativity, love, and playfulness. Maturity can be characterized as learning to postpone immediate pleasure for long-term gain (delayed gratification), living comfortably with ambiguity and mess as solutions are discovered, and proactively learning needed skills while capitalizing on your strengths.

I want to encourage readers that though the children years are a time of disciplining your lives along with your sexuality and lovemaking, they are also a time of growth and of expanding the sense of "us." A couple must not give up on the pursuit of passionate lovemaking, but must become more flexible, seizing opportunities despite the mood, and at times must settle for a quickie rather than nothing at all. This chapter will develop five practical areas that can help parents protect and enhance their sex lives during these demanding years.

SEX DURING PREGNANCY AND AFTER CHILDBIRTH

Couples have some real fears about having sex during pregnancy. Let us first list some commonsense advice:

Sex During Pregnancy

- Consult your physician and follow her or his suggestions. Your body and pregnancy are unique and may need special guidelines (for example, if you are prone to miscarriages).
- If there is any bleeding or change in condition, immediately seek medical help.
- Unless there is nausea or complications, most couples can enjoy making love throughout the nine months.
- Sexual intercourse is possible right up to the last week, unless your physician advises otherwise. Refrain from intercourse when labor begins or when your water breaks.

A couple's sex life during pregnancy will often reflect the frequency and level of enjoyment prior to pregnancy. If a couple has a low frequency of lovemaking before pregnancy, they may stop completely during these months. Many women report a normal desire for sex or even an increased arousal with the hormonal fluctuations of pregnancy. During the first trimester, some women experience problems with morning sickness, which dampens desire. In the third trimester, especially near the birth of the baby, the mother-to-be will feel big and tired and awkward. These feelings will slow sexual desire and activity.

Different concerns that can squelch lovemaking during pregnancy need to be actively addressed. One couple worried that the baby was hearing everything they did and had to do some attitude adjustment. A more common concern is that the baby may be hurt. Consult your physician for reassurance. Both the mucous plug in the cervix and the amniotic sac protect the baby from semen or infections in the vagina. The baby is suspended in its own protective environment (amniotic sac and fluid), which is a shock absorber. It doesn't hurt to be active, but you as a couple should be gentler as time goes on. Another way to overcome the factor of pregnancy in your love life is to employ more comfortable positions of intercourse. The rear entry with spoons, the crosswise position with legs scissored, the edge-of-the-bed position—all are effective during pregnancy (see Chapter 12).

Another common difficulty in pregnancy is body image. A woman can feel very unsexy as she gains weight and her stomach distends. Some men find themselves more excited by their wives' bodies, while others find difficulty being aroused, which can reinforce her fears of being unattractive. Though the wife's breasts can be tender and sensitive, the changes in them can also be exciting and arousing to the man. As the pregnancy progresses, both of you may be eager for the wife's body to return to normal. This is a great opportunity to allow lovemaking and sexiness to extend beyond body shape and size. As you age, you will both need this skill more and more, and it is a wonderful opportunity to grow your sex life beyond the purely physical plane. Don't stop making love; broaden your understanding of it.

If you struggle with body image, you may want to go to Chapter 16 and pursue some healing. Everyone has flaws, and if you make them the focus, you will destroy your ability to truly enjoy and be aroused by your mate. Wife, let your pregnant body symbolize femininity in a beautiful, sexy manner. Do some self-talk. Husband, affirm her in ways that you haven't in the past. She needs it now, with varicose veins and a tummy that will probably never be as flat again.

Sex After Childbirth

Husbands, I would encourage you to observe the wonder of your child being born, but be aware that fallout can occur. Seeing the baby exiting the birth canal and covered in blood can impair your view of the vagina as erotic for a while. You may have to fantasize this through as you shrink the image to black and white and let it recede in your memory. Erectile difficulties and decreased desire are not abnormal during this time of readjustment.

It is also helpful for those with sexual traumas to be aware that pregnancy and childbirth can trigger emotions and flashbacks that may have to be worked through in therapy, or at least talked through with the mate. These can impair sexual desire until they are resolved.

After the birth, breasts have become milk containers rather than something erotically arousing, especially for the wife. The body is more of a baby-servicing machine than an enticing vehicle of lovemaking. There is pain after childbirth, with the vagina and vulva swollen and perhaps surgery stitches and scars. It will take time and healing before certain positions and activities are comfortable again. Parts and places on the female body that once were stimulating may now be irritating.

Loneliness can pervade the life of the husband and wife. She may be used to a career and much adult stimulation, and this has abruptly stopped. She may fear the vulnerability of being dependent on him financially. He misses her having time for him, and misses seeing her dressed for work each morning with her hair done and makeup on instead of the nightgown without a shower. Many of the things that once cued both of you sexually may now be in short supply.

Although intercourse is usually restricted during the first couple of months, this can be a time to reconnect emotionally, reprocess a difficult childbirth or the triggering of sexual trauma, and dream about your future as a family. It can also be a time to work through the apprehensions of the new roles and responsibilities that parenting will bring. More time for baby means less time to talk and work through the marital conflicts that arose while adjusting to a new way of life. Although it is often difficult to make love when a conflict is not yet resolved, it can actually become a beautiful way to say with your bodies, "I am yours even through the hard times, and I commit myself to sticking this out."

Fatigue can become overwhelming and the little time you do have together can quickly disappear with tending to the needs of a colicky baby or the bedtime routines of small children. Couples sometimes go months and months without any level of sexual frequency after the first or second child. This may be unavoidable, but the following ideas may at least help considerably.

KEY INGREDIENTS OF A GREAT SEX LIFE AFTER CHILDREN

Many of you reading this section who already have children are saying, "Who cares about a *great* sex life—how about any at all, or even a mediocre sex life?" In the Lovemaking Cycle (see Chapter 4), Christopher McCluskey stresses some of the key ingredients for creating quality lovemaking. Among these are privacy, energy, time, and initiation—all of which are hard to come by in the children years, which emphasizes the importance of planning ahead and being creative. Two other factors that can enhance the lovemaking of your child-filled marriage are simplicity and a willingness to live with imperfection.

I remember one marriage conference at which I was waxing eloquent about God giving marriages natural aphrodisiacs (see Chapter 6). I reminded couples that a vacation was a great example of when we often practiced needed skills that were aphrodisiacs, like intimate time alone and anticipating lovemaking. One couple in the audience raised their hands and told me, "Obviously you have never taken a vacation with three children under the age of six. We made love once in the bathroom and the three-year-old was pounding on the door throughout the last half of our intimate experience."

Certain foundational elements of a fulfilling sex life are always important but very difficult to achieve with children in our lives. Let's consider the following six ingredients as they came to be applied in the lives of Alex and Jenny. They have four children: John, 3, Rebecca, 5, Al Junior, 8, and Krista, 10. They have been married fourteen years and love and respect each other. It's a good marriage, but their sex life has taken some real work to maintain and enjoy in the children years.

Privacy

The privacy that Alex and Jenny missed was not just finding those moments alone to make love. They often longed for that connecting as lovers that they seemed to enjoy hourly on weekends before the children. They weren't prepared for the pervasiveness of children at first, and now with four, it was even harder.

It took Alex and Jenny a while to understand the importance of getting away from everyone and focusing on each other. Sometimes this was one hour at Starbucks or a walk in their neighborhood. Creating a baby-sitter network was crucial, and Jenny's mom was so helpful on those occasional outings.

They also took advantage of any private moments like time in the bathroom or waking up early in the morning when the children were still sleeping and they were fresher. Fortunately they could both be morning people. They attempted in these private moments to meet Alex's need for physical connection and activity as well as Jenny's desire for emotional closeness with some plain old cuddling.

Energy

Alex was always more high energy than Jenny, and now with the constant drain of the children, her energy was lower than usual. She had little left over and it became a quest for both of them to help her find the additional energy to make love. No easy answers presented themselves, but they fought through for more help for Jenny. Two children were less draining than four, so they would divide and conquer, with the oldest children sometimes going to a friend's house. A portable crib made it easy on family and friends to keep the littlest ones for a few hours when possible.

Time

Alex and Jenny both hate to be scheduled and prefer sex to be more spontaneous. It was tough for them to come to the conclusion that there were optimal times and that often, if they didn't make love then, they might not for days. They worked around the kids' schedules with new rituals and romance. A cup of tea together after bedtime routines as they sat near each other on the couch became a wonderful ritual. Much-needed conversation and loving looks shared at the end of another day became a way to connect even without being sexual. They tried to go to bed together and share a few words and an embrace before exhaustedly falling asleep.

Initiation

Like many facets of a great sex life, even initiating is not as simple with children. Right after Al Jr. was born, Jenny scared Alex by telling him that she had not thought of sex in six weeks. With two babies in diapers, all her energy was put into mothering. They both decided to be more uninhibited and assertive in their initiating. They would grab those sudden moments of both being in the bathroom at the same time, or of the kids becoming mesmerized by a new videotape.

Simplicity

Simplifying one's lifestyle is not easy. Alex and Jenny had to learn to say no to new commitments and make their "no" stick. They avoided complicating relationships, and Alex actually changed his job to lessen stress. They worked to set better boundaries with her parents concerning weekly visits. Jenny streamlined household chores and got the older children to help as much as possible. Choices were constantly made to create a gentler lifestyle that could include lovemaking. Some things had to go, others were put off, and corners were cut as *simplify* and *streamline* became their operative words.

Imperfection

A wise mentor once stated, "If a job is worth doing, it is worth doing poorly." Often in these years the choice is between not doing many important things at all, or completing them imperfectly. Jenny, even more than Alex, struggled with accepting second best and being comfortable with loose ends. She had to learn that if there were six household chores needing attention, two or three of them would have to be done halfway or quickly.

Alex accepted a B grade rather than an A in his graduate course and helped Jenny dust the visible places before company came over. Pizza got ordered for supper some nights, and the kids skipped baths occasionally, as Alex and Jenny slowly progressed beyond their discomfort with loose ends and learned to live with ambiguity and imperfection. They kept an eye on their big goals: a home with love and time for each other. Some of the lesser goals could be neglected.

TRAINING TIPS FOR PARENTING

The natural parent doesn't exist. Oh, people may have maternal or paternal tendencies to love and nurture, but parenting is overall a learned skill. Begin with the following ideas, read, and talk to fellow parents as you share wisdom, because a great sex life depends on your parenting and disciplining abilities.

Discipline

Enforcing bedtimes. Enforcing bedtimes is tough. Rewards and loss of privileges work well with older children, but for the very little ones—eighteen months through four years—no reward (or sometimes even punishment) is more powerful than the fear or loneliness a child may experience in the solitude of a dark bedroom. "Mommy and Daddy have someone to sleep with, but I'm all alone." This is where rituals and routines—stories and bedtime prayers—make bedtime a time to look forward to rather than dread. Sometimes a cassette tape made by Mommy or Daddy talking to the child provides the much-needed distraction as the child tries to focus on all the good things being said about him or her.

Naps as family rituals. If one of the staples of lovemaking during the children years is quickies and seizing opportunities, then nap times can be crucial. Schedule them in—especially on Sundays after church.

Limiting Activites. Discipline involves saying no to extracurricular activites and peer involvement at times ot protect marital intimacy. These preteen and teen years can occupy every minute with demands and erratic schedules. Some parental selfishness may be needed for lovemaking to exist—much less flourish.

House Rules

Respecting a locked door. Teaching privacy and the need to knock on a locked door is important. Even with the door locked, the wife can struggle with focusing and letting go without worrying about interruptions. It slowly becomes easier after the children are trained better and the locked door can be trusted. Sometimes moms, even with their feminine susceptibility to being distracted, are able to get back into the lovemaking after an interruption. Other times the mood is completely broken and the couple simply needs to get up and agree to resume later.

I am reminded of the parents whose child wanted a peanut-butter-and-jelly sandwich and the parents were trying to train him to wait while they were in the bedroom. Dad saw a piece of bread being forced under the door and jumped up—knowing the peanut butter and jelly was soon to follow.

Mommy and Daddy time. Friends of mine trained their kids to allow Mommy and Daddy to have a few minutes together after the evening meal, while the children played by themselves. This can be taught in various ways as children respect that parents need private time personally and together as a couple. One of my clients remembers when he was a teenager and Mom and Dad sent him and his sister into town for a movie so they could clean the garage. They returned to find Mom and Dad grinning and laughing, but the garage had not been touched. Now that they are both married it is a family joke, and they will sometimes kid their parents that they hope they can keep the kids because their own garages really need cleaning.

PRACTICALLY PROACTIVE

I remember one of my country clients who I could tell was not very impressed with counseling. After his first session, he looked at me and slowly drawled, "Dr. Rosenau, you ain't told me nothing my momma didn't tell me." And I quickly replied, "And if you were doing everything your mama told you, you probably wouldn't be here." Part of the following suggestions you could get from your mama or a close friend. The problem is that we do not practice "proactive practicality"—to the huge detriment of our sex lives.

Common Sense Suggestions

Create a support network. An interesting question I ask on marriage retreats is: "You've been given five thousand dollars to improve your sex life. How will you use it?" So often those with children will tell of increased baby-sitting, flying parents in for weeks at a time, and vacationing all alone. This area demands practicality and creativity for lovemaking to survive. If family or surrogate family is around, negotiate regular time if possible. Take another teen or two to the beach so your kids have companionship and you can relax.

Accept that life is forever altered. Many things that you once took for granted may now be much more difficult to have in your life. One of these is time alone—time to pray, take a walk, and regain your perspective; time to read; even time to go to the bathroom. Your children will often be with you, and it can become quite a task to plan your errands and grocery shopping around a nursing schedule, naps, and potty breaks. Then preteens and teens become constant disruptions with their active coming and going. But the difficulties and frustrations are *good things.* They are what life is really made of. They cause our spiritual weaknesses to surface and challenge us to grow and mature in love. Remember that this is only for a *season* of life. One day you will reap the fruit of having been there to mold their frustration into patience or their unkind response into an apology. Once your children are grown you will never again have the same impact you have on them in this stage.

If you are trying to live as though you don't have any children, you will completely miss this season of life. Adjust your expectations. Change your pace to match that of your children and get rid of the things that keep you from doing so. Look for new and simpler ways to fill your soul—ways that take less time and don't require leaving home so much. Pray for perspective and learn to yield rather than fighting to hold on to your old lifestyle. God will bless you with a much richer one.

Creatively adapt to the ages of your children. An infant, a five-year-old who can crawl out of bed, and a teenager will make different demands. The infant and the teen will create sleep deprivation. You won't outlast the teen, so go to bed with the family rules of not leaving the house and lights off at a certain time. Summers create real challenges. Adolescents can respect locked bedroom doors and understand Mom and Dad are lovers, as parents discreetly create space for date nights and time alone together. Remember some of your best talks with your teen may be between 11:30 P.M. and 2:00 A.M. Keep flexibly adapting the rules and guiding that growth into maturity—always realizing that your marital companionship is the foundation for your children feeling secure. Nurture and protect your irreplaceable marriage.

Budget the money. Everything from diapers to car seats to food to colleges drains your finances. It is important to find good deals, pinch a penny, and to swap child care. My friend Karen sends her preteens to a friend's house for a week during the summer and keeps their three boys for a week in exchange. This is basically two weeks of camp for the boys. Sometimes swapping child care is even more important during the infant years. Romantic dinners at home may allow you to save up for an overnighter every once in a while. Sending those teens to the movies or camp can be a wise investment.

Plan for regular times together. Couples who don't make time alone will have difficulty staying emotionally intimate. This does not mean a couple needs to go out on the town, eat at a restaurant, or spend the night at a nice hotel. Although these are wonderful events, for most couples in this season of life it is not practical or affordable most of the time. Nursing mothers during the first year have a difficult time being away from the baby for more than six hours due to painful engorgement that develops. Expressing milk every four hours doesn't work for every mom—and it's not exactly a sexual turn-on. Plan time together in the everyday routine; early morning breakfasts, an early shower together, nighttime tea before bed, even lunch together in the middle of the day if your schedules allow it.

When you do have a night out alone, avoid spending this valuable time watching TV or renting a movie—these allow no time for communication and emotional intimacy. Plan weekend mini-vacations, or full vacations with another family with children the same age. This allows for on-site swapping of baby-sitting so each couple can take private walks or have dinner out. (Remember that you will likely be so tired that the first hours or day of the alone time will need to be regrouping and rest time before the sexual fun and intimate connecting begin.)

Maximize those quickies. In Chapter 15 we ended the chapter with various types of lovemaking and encouraged couples not to overuse the quickie. In the children years of fighting for time and privacy, however, this may be a real staple of your love life. Just be creative with the quickies and include some cuddling with the climaxes.

Utilize technology. Thank God for cell phones and the ease of keeping in touch with teenage baby-sitters. Monitors help in allowing comfortable times on the deck or in the family room, with children tucked safely away in their beds. Portable cribs and a variety of easy-to-use baby products save time and create mobility and ease for childcare. Time and support are key ingredients for augmenting lovemaking in the children years.

Those Gender Differences

Mom is distracted and Dad is focused. Research is showing that women can multitask more easily than men, while men focus on the job at hand. The downside of Mom's attending to many details manifests itself in a difficulty to leave the concerns outside the bedroom and tune in to lovemaking. Wives will be more easily distracted by children and not excited about making love if a little one is about to burst through the door. Husbands can have more of that task focus and be ready to finish making love while the baby cries.

Mom wants to be emotionally connected and Dad wants physical interaction. Moms get more physical touch with constant childcare than dads do. Fellow sex-therapist friend Michael Sytsma tells of the female client who strongly stated, "My body gets sucked on, climbed over, pawed at, slobbered on, and hugged to death. The last thing I need is my husband to start doing the same when he climbs into bed at night." The husband has to be sensitive to this as he reminds himself that this stage of marriage takes mature delayed gratification and self-control. The wife can also keep in mind that her partner may feel more love and deep connection through sex than through any other avenue.

A friend told me of the time she was pregnant and really wishing the loose step on their front porch was fixed so she wouldn't lose her balance. She came home one afternoon with groceries and realized that her husband had fixed the step. She felt very much in love and sexually interested in him at that moment because of his act of thoughtfulness. I was laughing at a friend who told me his wife was feeling very attracted to him as he paid attention to their daughter. He told me, "If this is what makes my wife frisky, you can imagine how much I have been playing with my child recently."

Assertive versus receptive sexual desire. In Chapter 18 on sexual desire, the idea of different kinds of desire was developed. Women often have what we call "receptive" or "responsive" desire, which isn't as hormonally driven or apparent. On a busy day taking care of children, they may never think of sex. But that evening, if approached early enough, the wife might think, *Hmm, I can get into this tonight. What a pleasant ending to the day.*

The partner with the more apparent, initiating desire will think of sex more often and desire greater frequency. This is often the husband, who has been contemplating sexual activity all day and is ready to jump his tired, distracted wife when he bursts through the door. This will definitely take some negotiating and self-discipline on both partners' parts to postpone and compromise and engage.

Applied Maturity

Practicing self-control. The many traits of being a mature adult are not always easy or fun, but they do make for a more joyful and meaningful life. Children in their childishness can't always postpone immediate pleasure to achieve a future goal. Parents, as adults, come to realize lovemaking will have to be postponed at times. The wife's fatigue will take precedent over sexual playfulness. These choices also occur throughout a great marriage with periods, yeast infections, and illnesses. Sexual pleasure doesn't disappear. One young husband complained that he only had so many times to make love over the next fifty years and he was losing some valuable chances during these children years. Obviously some maturing was needed.

Living with mess and ambiguity. A couple with a four-month-old shared with me the story of their wedding anniversary. She was so romantic with a special dress and careful planning for a wonderful evening. You know the rest of the story. Their son had colic and they spent the entire night with a crying baby. Maturity teaches us to live with the less than perfect and think on our feet and improvise. Lovemaking will get challenged, but the creative couple persists through the alligators to the other side of the swamp, and occasionally climbs up on a cypress stump and makes love there.

Get over the disappointed expectations. Not all grandmothers will be grandmotherly and want to be with the grandchildren a lot. A wife won't feel very sexy with milk dripping from her nipples. Your mate will not always be as romantic as a parent as he or she was when dating. You can't fix up the nursery the way you wanted because you can't afford it. Life goes on and it is actually pretty wonderful. Sex hasn't disappeared, and you will still feel quite sexually attractive sometimes. The less frequent passionate connecting becomes more enjoyable and appreciated.

Seek out advice and therapy. Mature couples confidently seek out needed resources and help.

GIFTS FROM MOM AND DAD

In being parents and working on also having a sex life, there are things that both the husband and wife can do for each other and the relationship.

From Mom to Dad with Love

Create energy for sex. It is not easy, but if Friday night is an optimal time for making love, then taking a rest during the day can be very helpful.

Stay sexy. Nursing bras and nightgowns are a necessity if you are not bottle feeding, but treat yourself and your husband to a few new pieces of lingerie, even if they are a few sizes larger than you hope to return to someday. Taxiing teens is easier in sweats but a nice dress and makeup is great occasionally too.

Keep the lines open. Be sure to communicate with your husband about anything that hurts, as well as what feels good, as your body recovers from pregnancy and delivery. Many things may not feel like they once did, but your husband won't know this unless you tell him.

From Dad to Mom with Love

Pitch in with quantity parenting. So often dads try to spend quality time with children as they play and read, but there is a great deal of quantity time in raising children with chores like grocery shopping, diapers, baths, monitoring their play, getting up in the middle of the night, and chauffering to activities. Moms need help with this quantity parenting and not just the quality time together.

Make love without ceasing. The Bible tells us to pray without ceasing; we need to make love without ceasing too. Oftentimes the best way to make love is not necessarily engaging in sexual relations. It may be in giving of yourself and pouring yourself into the relationship in more practical ways. Fixing the front porch step, unloading the dishwasher, bathing the kids, cleaning the toilets—maybe *especially* cleaning the toilets. These are activities that are making, growing, and expressing love.

Pamper her. This can be as simple as bringing her a cup of coffee or making her favorite snack. Buy her an outfit that is not "mommy clothes." Watch the kids so she can read a magazine in the bathtub or spend some time on a hobby.

From Dad and Mom to the Marriage with Love

Choose to give each other real attention. It may be that some people limit their children because they fear not having enough love to go around. Husbands can begin to feel neglected emotionally and lonely for hugging and cuddling time. Wives can feel that all they do is give and can resent not feeling special, missing those little nurturing gestures. Again, you will need that time away from responsibilities and the children, especially the infants or teens as you focus on romance and each other.

Prepare for and anticipate some "tantric sex." Within the tantric ideas of Eastern religions, a single act of lovemaking might be prepared for over the course of an entire month. With children, passionate times together may require that same amount of special preparation! Plan some of these times into a special weekend or when the little ones are at Grandma's.

Make romantic dinners at home. You cannot replicate life before children, but this does not mean that romance has to fly out the window. Create romantic dinners at home after the children are in bed, so you don't have to rush home from a restaurant and ruin an expensive dinner by responding to an emergency. Early mornings and late evenings can allow for some atmosphere in which to stay lovers.

At the risk of sounding pedantic, who said the really important things in life did not come with a price? Being great parents and growing a fun love life will take mature choices and much self-discipline. The cornerstone of these children years is indeed maturity, but what an awesome reward grows out of this process.

Christopher and Rachel McCluskey were immensely helpful in writing this chapter. They are the parents of five children (so far!) and have coauthored a forthcoming book by Baker/Revell Publishers on sexual intimacy. Chris is a certified sex therapist and cofounder with me of Sexual Wholeness, Inc. He does Christian life coaching and marital enhancement by telephone from the couple's farm in Missouri. He has produced an excellent videotape, Coaching Couples into Passionate Intimacy, *which can be ordered through his Web site at www.christian-living.com.*

CHAPTER TWENTY

Sex After Forty-Five

(WITH JAMES K. CHILDERSTON, PH.D., AND CAROLYN SUE CHILDERSTON, B.A.)

SO MUCH OF MAKING LOVE depends on our attitudes. Some couples think sex will drastically change when they reach forty-five or sixty-five, and for them it does. Other mates know life changes with age but determine to continue to enjoy making love. They gracefully adjust to change and create an active and meaningful sex life.

But often, people lack the necessary and explicit information about how age-related changes will impact them. We have found that if they are adequately informed, older adults are generally open to change, especially if they are presented with clear possibilities and wise choices. The old adage should be altered; the truth is that "old dogs learn more tricks" because we have the wisdom to know you don't get different results trying the same thing over and over—implementing something new is the only solution.

As couples age together, it is vital that they learn to partner through this process so that sex not only continues to be a celebration, but a true reflection of their genuine intimacy and love. How beautiful to see a mature couple holding hands, exchanging glances, and more deeply in love and sexy after all the years.

Both men and women struggle with the aging process and their sexuality. Though it shouldn't be true, our culture discriminates against the aging person. A man's ego is affected by performance. Concepts like strength, stamina, production, and physical prowess are valued. A man will naturally get concerned as he experiences aging and normal changes in sexual performance. He may wonder about his erection not being as firm and about taking more stimulation to achieve it. In youth he could look at a nude body and instantly get firm. Occasionally now he is impotent, he cannot experience an ejaculation, or his aching back and muscles prevent some activities. He begins to question if he will continue to enjoy sexual pleasure and be able to bring true enjoyment to his partner.

A woman may experience even greater discrimination than a man and have difficulty with her self-image. A female friend once told me, "Men are allowed to age gracefully with graying hair a sign of maturity, but women just get old." It is a distorted and very limited way of thinking to believe that only the young are beautiful. This is putting too much of attractiveness into tight skin and firm bodies. A wise definition of beauty includes tolerance, wisdom, character developed through suffering, enjoyment of life, the eyes and the voice, achievements, and social adeptness. Age has a positive effect on beauty and sexiness when these qualities are considered.

In the first section, we will look at the age-related changes that a female can expect, including the transition into menopause, the influence of hormones, and psychological and personal issues that affect sexual response. The second section will address how the aging process impacts men in terms of expected physical changes, hormonal transitions, and the sexual challenges an older male may encounter. The third section will discuss how physical problems impact sexual behavior, including various disease states and medication effects. The final section explores relational changes with maturity, as environment and needs alter, and will expand on the concept that sex after forty-five can be more exciting and fulfilling than in earlier years.

AGE-RELATED SEXUAL CHANGES IN THE FEMALE

The key word describing shifts in sexual function beginning at midlife for the female is *change*. A woman may experience an increase in sexual desire or she may find desire subsides. As a result, her frequency of sexual activity may increase or decrease. She may also experience an increase or a decrease in the sensitivity of her clitoris, and her sexual responsiveness may also go up or down. A wife may find that she experiences fewer orgasms and with decreased intensity, or she may realize an increase in orgasms and a sexual awakening. It is impossible to predict how an individual woman will experience midlife sexual changes, but we can predict that what was normal before may not be now. Many women will not experience a decrease in sexual desire during menopause, but when they do it is generally due to hormonal imbalance, negative thinking, or relational problems.

As levels of the sex steroids (estrogen and testosterone) begin to fluctuate, changes may be noticed in the genitals. Dropping estrogen levels will cause the vaginal walls to thin and they will not have the same elasticity and soft padding. The vagina may shrink, with its mouth becoming narrower. Because the vagina has lost some of its cushioned effect, some women will experience urethritis (sometimes called the "honeymoon disease," it is an irritation of the urethra and bladder from the penis hitting them during intercourse). The loss of estrogen can affect lubrication, too. It may take longer to lubricate, and the amount may be less. In the past it may have taken seconds and now may require several minutes of loveplay to create arousal and sufficient lubrication. Dyspareunia (painful intercourse) is the most common sexual complaint in older women.

These symptoms of aging may diminish sexual enthusiasm and comfort in lovemaking. Couples will need to creatively address these issues for intercourse to be possible, let alone enjoyable. Intercourse may need to be gentler at first, with care taken on entry. Artificial lubrication ceases to be optional as more liberal and frequent applications are necessary to counteract some of these changes. The husband may need to be more charming and alert to what pleasures his wife so that she feels cared for and open to his sexual advances.

Perimenopause/Menopause and Sexuality

Menopause is the time in life when the female stops having her menstrual cycle and the possibility of pregnancy is over. It is defined as having occurred when a woman goes twelve months without a period. Menopause can also be "induced" when a woman has a hysterectomy (removal of the uterus and possibly the ovaries), so this process may occur earlier for some women. Menopause "naturally" occurs between the ages of forty-five and fifty-five (average 51.4 years), yet it can begin as early as in the thirties or as late as the sixties.

Perimenopause is the transition between fertility and the last menstrual period and can begin as early as age thirty-five but generally begins in the mid-forties. There may be some overlap in symptoms with regard to perimenopause and menopause, as one may notice irregular menstrual patterns, hot flashes, and night sweats corresponding to changes in estrogen levels. Other common symptoms include vaginal inelasticity and/or dryness, urinary incontinence, insomnia, fatigue, loss of concentration and memory lapses, skin changes, gray hair (or hair loss including that in the pubic area), and formication (a perception of skin crawling, a prickly feeling, or a feeling of bugs biting you). Although it has not been shown to be directly related to menopause, periodic depression and an increase in headaches are common, as well as dizziness, heart palpitations, and anxiety. If a person is predisposed to headaches, the headaches can be worse during this time. Weight gain is also common because of slower basal metabolism.

Many of these symptoms can affect a wife's motivation for sex and her self-esteem, which are so intertwined. With all of the physical changes, women need a positive attitude and crucial spousal support to cope with menopause. One point of encouragement is research that suggests women consistently feel relief when menstruation ends, and that postmenopausal women have a more positive view of menopause than do perimenopausal women. Wives do not feel they become less sexually attractive after menopause. For some the freedom can enhance sexual desire and increase frequency of lovemaking.

Hormonal Changes and Sexuality

Estrogen, progesterone, and testosterone are the chief hormones involved in the cycles of female sexuality. All three are used in various hormone replacement treatments for women, with testosterone supplementation most used with men. Levels of estrogen and sexual desire do not seem to be correlated, and libido fluctuations across the menstrual cycle do not seem to be related to estrogen levels. In fact, many women find their sexual desire increases when estrogen levels drop, because the ratio of testosterone (the strongest hormone of sexual desire in a group of chemicals called androgens) to female hormones is proportionally greater.

Estrogen Replacement Therapy (ERT) can provide relief from some of the psychological and physical problems associated with menopause, and thus enhance sexual response indirectly. Benefits appear to be related to an overall increase in well-being, a decrease in anxiety, fewer sleep disruptions (because of reduced hot flashes and cold sweats), and improved vaginal lubrication. Estrogens promote REM sleep, during which time secretions may "irrigate" the vagina. Women who do not suffer from painful intercourse (due to vaginal atrophy and problems with lubrication) will benefit little from estrogen replacement. The full benefits of ERT in relation to improved sexual desire are reliably achieved only with the addition of testosterone.

Progesterone (Provera and other brands) is utilized in replacement therapy along with estrogen in order to regulate the menstrual cycle. It may help to prevent uterine cancer by allowing cells in the uterine lining to slough off periodically in the form of a period. An increase in progesterone levels throughout the menstrual cycle has been associated with decreased sexual desire, primarily due to its tendency to reduce testosterone levels. Progesterone also has the propensity to cause depression, inhibit orgasm, and may lower DHEA (another plentiful androgen but less potent than testosterone in sexual desire, this androgen creates desire and steroid effects in muscle and hair growth). Progesterone is associated with reduced physical sensitivity, and it functions as a sedative in moderate doses and as an anesthetic at high doses. However, there are some women who may benefit from the use of a 2 percent progesterone cream, because natural progesterone can be turned into androgens and even a form of estrogen when the body needs more of these hormones. It is important to note that the body functions best when there is an appropriate balance between the sex hormones. Often, sexual difficulties or emotional instability is the result of too much or too little of one or more of these hormones.

In women the ovaries produce testosterone, with additional testosterone being derived from the adrenal steroids. Removal of the ovaries will decrease sexual desire to a certain extent, but removal of the adrenal glands may have a devastating effect on sexual desire. With natural menopause, androgen levels are positively correlated with sexual interest, but androgens alone are not sufficient for the experience of sexual desire. Testosterone treatment seems to be useful in facilitating sexual desire in a subset of women with low sexual desire, but it requires safety monitoring and there are not clearly defined dosage levels for females. However, women with higher testosterone levels report less depression, experience more sexual gratification with their husbands, and show a greater capacity to form good interpersonal relationships. Testosterone also seems to increase clitoral sensitivity.

In addition to seeing your gynecologist, you may need to consult an endocrinologist who specializes in hormonal treatment to discuss whether you may benefit from some form of hormone replacement. All women who are seeking treatment for diminished sex drive should have their testosterone and DHEA levels measured. In those women who don't seem to be able to produce enough of their own androgens, DHEA or testosterone can be given in the form of a skin cream, a gel, or a capsule. If both levels are low, it may be a good idea to try replenishing DHEA first (10 to 25 milligrams a day), because it is a precursor to testosterone and it can increase testosterone levels by one and a half to two times. The dosage for testosterone replacement for those that don't respond to DHEA is not clearly defined and will depend on the woman's individual needs and/or blood levels. The possible negative side effects of testosterone replacement in women can be extra hair growth, skin changes, and in rare cases a lowering of the voice. Testosterone can also decrease HDL (good) cholesterol levels.

Psychological and Interpersonal Issues Affecting Sexual Response

When it comes to sexual response, perhaps even more significant than the physical and hormonal changes a woman experiences with aging is what occurs in her head and in her relationships. The combination of menopause and the changing roles of an empty nest can cause some wives to come to the erroneous conclusion that they are "too old for sex." What we believe about our sexuality as we grow older has a lot to do with our sexual expectations (parents, society) and our experience with our spouse. When a society views menopause as "failed productivity" and associates reproductive ability with sexual ability, many women may believe that this is the time their sex drive is supposed to go away. But these are two separate functions and you can have one without the other. This is a time husbands struggle with accepting their own aging body and may notice their wife's sags and wrinkles. Men must be sensitive. Now especially, a wife needs affirmation of her sexual appeal, not introspection about aging bodies.

Many women may struggle with long-standing sexual inhibitions, or may have experienced sexual abuse or victimization, or may have fears about losing their attractiveness, or may be in unsatisfactory relationships. Perhaps after many years of marriage, predictability has replaced spontaneity and sex has become routine and mechanical. Sex therapy or counseling may be helpful in these situations.

So much of sex is in the head. This can be a rich time for you sexually; you have lost some of your earlier inhibitions and know more about what arouses you. Pregnancy is no longer a fear. You may have to engage in some self-talk about your sexiness as your body loses its firm-ness and its skin tone decreases. Again, maturity can be associated with greater skills and more comfortable attitudes. Older women make great lovers, but they may need their partners to help convince them of this fact.

AGE-RELATED SEXUAL CHANGES IN THE MALE

Physical Changes

As you get older, there is normal wear and tear on your body's nerves, muscles, and blood supply, which can affect sexual functioning. You may have to "ease up" on certain positions, or there may be some changes in the quality and quantity of your erections—this does not make you impotent or sexually inadequate. With a better understanding of yourself, you'll have the freedom for greater enjoyment with less anxiety. Be reassured that sex will continue to be good.

Here are five common changes a man experiences with the aging process:

1. Erections will need more direct physical stimulation of the penis. In younger years, visual or mental sexual stimuli could bring about an erection. It doesn't mean you are losing your sex-ual desire because your wife's breasts or genitals don't create the same quick reflex action. Sometimes this can mistakenly be seen as impotence because both partners expect sponta-neous reactions as in the past. When enjoying loveplay and wanting to engage in intercourse, you and your partner will have to touch and play with the penis. If while focusing on plea-suring your wife you lose some or all of your erection, it will take direct stimulation to get the penis firm again.

Like other aspects of aging, this does not have to be a serious problem. Your wife must not interpret the lack of instant arousal as a reflection on her attractiveness. It is physiological, and she can simply make a note to engage in more manual and oral stimulation of the penis. Both of you can be erotically aroused as you make adjustments and, in a loving, sensual way, cre-atively stimulate the male organ. Throughout this chapter, you'll learn that sex over forty-five can add new dimensions of sensuality.

2. The penis may not achieve the same firmness with erections. With aging, the blood supply can be diminished and the muscle valve system that keeps the blood in the penis can have leakage; the penis therefore will not achieve the same hardness as before. This change can evolve into more of an attitude problem than a real issue. The penis does not need to be extra firm; it simply needs to be hard enough to insert and thrust. This condition is made worse if one is a smoker, because nicotine promotes arterial damage in the penis as well as other parts of the body and the valve system that holds blood in the penis is even more compromised. In a sense then, smoking will prematurely age the penis.

Don't let your attitude get in the way. The firmness of erections does not make the man; it is not the symbol of a great lover. The surest way to become psychologically impotent is to worry about erections rather than enjoy the moment. During some lovemaking sessions you may not achieve an erection, or you may achieve only partial firmness. Don't worry about it. Chalk it up to fatigue and distractions, and know that the erection will come back. (You may want to read the section of Chapter 21 on working through impotence.) Your wife can be helpful in reducing your anxiety as well. Don't mentally destroy your lovemaking by worrying about firmness.

With aging, the foreskin of the uncircumcised penis may lose some of its elasticity and tighten. With full erections and intercourse, the skin may split rather than stretch as it used to. These skin tears will be small and will heal quickly, but they can be painful. Pulling back the foreskin at night before going to sleep can often prevent this condition. During the sleep cycle and nightly erections, the skin will be stretched and be less likely to split during subsequent erections.

3. The waiting time between erections/ejaculations will increase, with climaxes needed less often. Men are different from women and need what is called a refractory time to rest between orgasms. Women are multiorgasmic even into older age and can be stimulated to a climax several times in a row. When you were nineteen, your refractory period was less than a minute, but it may be a day or more as you get into your sixties. Both partners need to remember this so you don't panic or create feelings of anxiety or failure by attempting to create another erection and orgasm before the body has had enough recuperative time.

Remember that making love does not depend upon an erection or an orgasm. Enjoy each other, but if an erection is difficult to achieve, your body may be recuperating. Be creative and enjoy intimacy as you help your partner achieve her climax. If you have not climaxed and you are focusing on your partner and lose your erection, this is not a refractory period. Apply direct stimulation and the erection will most likely return.

As you age into your sixties and seventies, you may need to climax only once a week or once or twice a month. That does not mean sexual closeness with your wife two or three times a week will be impossible, but remember that this is a mutual endeavor and may also involve cuddling, caressing, and holding—not always intercourse. You should not push yourself to climax every time there is intercourse; you can have pleasant intercourse and enjoyable thrusting without a climax and ejaculation. Putting pressure on yourself to perform and achieve certain results can result in anxiety and loss of erections.

4. Ejaculation is less strong, and erections disappear more quickly. With aging, you may not feel quite as much like a volcano going off at your climax. The muscles that expel the semen are weaker, but that does not have to affect the pleasure of an orgasm. Part of feeling like it's an explosion is in your head and has nothing to do with the expulsion of semen. Here are three suggestions for building greater sexual tension that can create stronger orgasms: (1) Accumulate more semen through extended exciting foreplay and recuperating time between lovemaking, (2) let yourself mentally and physically build and focus (with your partner's cooperation) right to the edge of climax, (3) abandon yourself with an explosion of feelings, and physically and mentally exaggerate the sensations of ejaculation.

After you climax, you may find yourself losing your erection faster than in years past. Don't let that affect the afterglow as you hold each other and share closeness. If your penis doesn't stay in her vagina, caress and hug and hold as you tell her how much pleasure she brings you sexually. Learn not to worry about seepage of semen from the vagina. In the afterglow sensually and emotionally enjoy each other in intimate ways.

5. *The pleasure of intercourse can be longer.* This is a pleasant outcome of needing less ejaculation and fewer climaxes. You can last longer and even with active thrusting can pleasure your wife with added endurance. It is important to be sensitive to her pleasure needs, which may not always require longer, active thrusting.

You may want to use some positions (for example, the wife on top) that allow your wife to be more active. This is a great time to experiment and play at this aspect of making love, proving that there are advantages to growing older.

Hormonal Changes and Sexuality

Testosterone is the primary sex hormone influencing sexual desire in both males and females. Women need a smaller amount for sexual desire compared to men, who have higher levels of testosterone produced by the testicles in addition to the adrenal gland. However, this does not mean that men always have a higher sexual desire, because this hormone is also utilized to masculinize, producing beards and heavier muscles. Testosterone does help promote sexual desire and the ability to get an erection. Though in men, the primary effect of lowering testosterone is to reduce sex drive rather than the ability to get an erection. In fact, testosterone replacement is clinically effective for sex drive only in men who are low in testosterone—it is not indicated for men complaining of erection problems and normal libido.

The process of the gradual decline in levels of testosterone in men is called andropause. This testosterone decline doesn't have the same impact and is not as rapid as the estrogen loss that women experience. In men ages forty to eighty the decrease in total serum testosterone is about 0.4 percent a year. The decline begins to increase after age sixty, but there is considerable individual variability and andropause is not noticeable in all men. Some men will remain sexually active into their eighties and nineties, although the frequency may be somewhat lower than when they were in their forties and fifties. The symptoms associated with andropause can include a lack of energy; fatigability or listlessness; diminished productivity and a disinclination to work; decreases in muscle, bone mass, libido, and appetite; poor concentration and memory; physical hypersensitivity; and increased irritability and sometimes depression.

If there is severely limited desire or persistent impotence or inability to ejaculate, have your physician check your blood and hormone levels, including serum testosterone, complete blood count (CBC), prostate specific antigen (PSA), and basic serum chemistries. If a low testosterone level is discovered, you may be a candidate for testosterone replacement, which can be in pill form, injections, implants, patches, or gels. The gel form, which absorbs through the skin, has become a popular means of treatment due to its ease in application and in the ability to adjust doses. You should begin to see some improvement in erections within a two-week period; however, desire may begin to increase sooner. Remember that increasing libido does not necessarily result in improved sexual performance or an improved relationship. Testosterone is just part of the story—not a panacea for all sexual or relational ills.

It is important to be under the care of a physician because there can be side effects such as water retention, an aggravation of hypertension, and an enlarging of the prostate. Certain conditions, such as prostate cancer, would contraindicate the use of testosterone replacement therapy. Keep your doctor informed regarding any effects of treatment, whether positive or negative.

Sexual Challenges in the Older Male

As a man ages, it is likely that he will notice some changes in his erections. These were noted earlier and are not considered to be impotence. Some men do experience erection difficulties that are more serious than the normal changes of aging and they may be caused by psychological factors (performance and stress issues, intimacy conflicts) or physical problems. Illnesses such as diabetes, vascular disease, urological or neurological conditions, and others can lead to impotence. Heavy drinkers and smokers may suffer damage to the blood vessels in the penis and this can lead to impotence as well, as can certain medications. Sometimes a combination of physical and psychological factors contribute to erection problems. In this case, an injection or a pill won't solve the problem.

The treatment for impotence will depend on what is causing it, whether physical, psychological or both. A number of treatments can be very helpful, discussed fully in Chapter 21, "Common Male Malfunctions." One of the most significant developments in the treatment of erectile dysfunction occurred in 1998 with the release of an oral impotence pill, sildenafil (Viagra). Viagra takes about fifty to sixty minutes after ingestion to be effective and works in the context of existing sexual desire, in that it does *not* restore libido. It is generally initiated with a 50 milligram tablet, and adjusted to 25 or 100 milligrams depending on adverse effects or efficacy. Viagra is contraindicated in a patient taking nitrates in any form, as it can result in a precipitous drop in blood pressure. No man should take Viagra or any other prescription medication that has not been prescribed specifically for him.

There are several other ways you can either prevent or lessen the effects of impotence, including adhering to a low-fat diet with regular exercise; eliminating smoking; expanding your definition of *sex* so that ejaculation is not the goal of lovemaking; having more frequent sexual contact; sharing more information and feelings with your spouse; and only taking the medications that you absolutely need.

Some men may struggle for years with premature ejaculation. As mentioned earlier, one benefit of aging is that the time leading up to ejaculation is often lengthened, allowing for more active thrusting. If premature ejaculation remains a problem, both older men as well as younger men respond to the use of the serotonin-based medications, such as paroxetine (Paxil) or clomipramine (Anafranil). These medications have as a side effect delayed ejaculation, which effectively treats this problem.

PHYSICAL PROBLEMS AND THEIR IMPACT ON SEXUAL BEHAVIOR

There are more creaks and groans from the body in general as you grow past your forties. Some specific illnesses like arthritis, ovarian and uterine problems, heart disease, bladder incontinence, prostatitis (inflammation of the prostate gland), some types of headaches, and lower back pain will become more common. Health changes will have an impact on your sexual performing and attitudes, but the loving couple will make choices to allow their lovemaking to continue.

Sexual Effects of Disease and Disability

Diseases with direct effects on sexual functioning include those associated with nerve damage such as diabetes mellitus, alcoholic neuropathy, and multiple sclerosis. Diabetic men have a greater chance of becoming impotent and in fact, impotence can be an early indication of the disease. Women with diabetes can experience vaginal dryness, a loss of sensation in the genitals, and are at greater risk for yeast and urinary tract infections. This disease can be managed by a rigorous adherence to dietary and medical instructions, which will minimize the sexual effects of the disease.

Any chronic disease that causes generalized pain can have an indirect effect on sexual function. Chronic pain is common in aging, and both the medication, as well as the inability to focus, can affect lovemaking. Other common problems include prostate enlargement and cancer, which may require the removal of the prostate. This can but does not necessarily produce impotence; more likely it may cause retrograde ejaculation, with the ejaculate going into the bladder during orgasm. This doesn't destroy sexual pleasure, but requires adjusting to different sensations. Peyronie's disease is an upward bowing of the penis, which may make erections and intercourse painful. Consult a urologist, and know that the condition may not preclude sex in other forms and in a majority of the cases can be corrected with surgery. After childbirth(s) the vagina can be stretched or torn, making it very loose and not as pleasurable for either partner. Plastic surgery can correct this problem.

A hysterectomy, other surgeries, or a heart attack will naturally take the focus off love-making for a while. Sometimes a hysterectomy or other surgeries, after physical healing, enliven making love, with the fear of pregnancy and monthly cycles gone or the pain decreased. But some diseases, like the threat of another heart attack, can dampen sexual desire and contact. The mate who had the heart attack is fearful of excitement, and the partner can be overprotective as well. This is a time for believing and following medical advice: fewer than 1 percent of heart attack fatalities occur during sex. Most heart attack patients are encouraged to resume sexual activity at the same time they begin other physical activities.

Medication Effects

Many times it may be the medication and not the disease or disability that causes the sexual problem. As we grow older, the likelihood is that we will be taking multiple medications. At midlife, medications are often prescribed to lower blood pressure, regulate heart conditions, treat depression, control ulcers, and treat a variety of aches, pains, colds, and allergies. Over two hundred commonly prescribed medications can influence sexual function or enjoyment. The most common sexual side effects include decreased libido, impotence or difficulty getting or maintaining an erection, loss of sensation in the genitals, increased vaginal dryness, or a difficulty with ejaculation in men or orgasm in women. (The sexual impact of specific medications is described further in Chapter 18, "Low Sexual Desire and Frequency.")

The Viagra Years: Blessing or Curse?

The advent of Viagra has undoubtedly had a major impact on the thirty million men in the United States with erectile dysfunction, and has been received with pleasure by many older couples, as partners have been able to experience revitalized sexual function. However, utilizing medical manipulation to enhance the performance of a man's penis will not heal a relationship that is not working.

The rapid return of sexual function in one partner will create problems if the other partner does not want to resume sexual relations. This can be true of a woman who may be secretly relieved her husband is impotent because she had adjusted to a life without sex, and avoiding sex was a fine way to avoid intimacy. Another woman may be willing to become sexually active again but finds her body uncooperative. She will need to slowly ease back into sex and her husband will need to appreciate and understand this adjustment. Viagra can also create a crisis for a man if his wife expects him to be able to return to normal function and he no longer has an "excuse" not to be sexually intimate. Remember that Viagra restores the capacity for an erection, not libido.

Some men will take their newly discovered erections and be prone to wander, to perhaps find more willing companions. There may be a flurry of affairs and divorces resulting from differing expectations and unmet needs. Viagra could force some couples to face relational problems they have long been ignoring. This may be quite troubling and result in more distance for some couples; but for others, Viagra may help strengthen their marriages by pushing them to resolve outstanding issues.

The impotence pill reminds us again that a healthy marriage and intimate lovemaking are about connection and not penetration. It's not about the penis, but about the person and the ability to relate intimately.

Sexual Problem Solving

One couple had multiple physical problems to deal with as they grew older. Unfortunately, a multiplicity of issues are common with aging. Arthritis ran in the wife's family, and even with her medication, it was very painful as she approached sixty. Joints ached, and some positions of intercourse that she had enjoyed were not possible anymore. Intercourse had also occasionally become painful with some vaginal soreness. The husband experienced lower back pain from a deteriorating disc, and tendonitis in his right elbow and shoulder. He was glad his heart and blood pressure were fine and that he suffered no prostate problems. His physician didn't think the back problems warranted surgery, but let him know there would be chronic pain on some days. He found it difficult to be sexual when the pain was there, and like his wife, he found that certain positions weren't comfortable.

They loved each other and had built a very mutually satisfying sex life that they refused to give up. Making love kept them smiling and connected in wonderful ways. No matter what the circumstances, they were determined to enjoy making love on a frequent basis for the rest of their lives.

Fortunately this couple had learned to really communicate, which helped them do effective problem solving. They were also creative, flexible, sensual, and passionate. In spite of the effects of aging, they still liked themselves, their bodies, sex, and each other. Here is the list of solutions they began to implement:

Heating pads and warm baths. Loosening arthritic joints and stiff backs before making love helped. Baths could also be quite sensual; shared, they became a part of loveplay. The couple came to associate relieving rubs with erotic arousal. Rubbing his back and arms often preceded fooling around and some fun sexual times. (She was careful to wash her hands before touching sensitive genital tissue after nearly sending him through the ceiling one time with Ben-Gay on her hands.)

Maximizing medication and heeding medical advice. There were windows of time when both felt better after taking pain medication or an arthritis treatment. During those times, they found it easier to focus and enjoy each other sexually. The pain medications the husband was taking seemed to decrease sexual interest, and his doctor changed the prescription on one and lowered the dosage on another. Both also got regular medical checkups and advice. They learned about their physical problems and what would or wouldn't hurt his back or her arthritis. The couple was surprised how much freedom their physician gave them medically, and he encouraged them to maintain an active love life.

New moves and selected positions. The husband found he could sit propped against the headboard of the bed with pillows and heating pad on his lower back and be comfortable. The wife could then sit between his legs with her back against him or lie back with her genital area in his lap. These positions allowed her to be pleasured with less wear on both of their bodies. They practiced the positions of intercourse that allowed them to lie down and stay less active, enjoying the "crosswise" arrangement and the ease of certain rear-entry positions. She missed the wife-on-top position, which had been a favorite, but her knees just wouldn't permit it anymore. She substituted a side-by-side position allowing her to have more active participation. The wife also found that, when her hands ached, oral stimulation was a good alternative. It pleasured him in fun ways and let her feel very sensual, too.

Lubrication. They made sure to have lubricants handy. When her arthritis was bothering her, she had more difficulty focusing on arousal and becoming lubricated. Thus they always augmented their lovemaking with artificial lubrication to take the burden off both of them. They bought extra pillows to prop up and get comfortable, and soft music helped set a soothing atmosphere.

Playing through the pain. This husband and wife had heard of athletes who said they would play through the pain, and they found that if they only made love when both felt good, it would seldom happen. (Note: Never play through the pain without being sure medically that you are not further damaging tissue.) The couple increased their communication and trusted each other when one expressed a desire to make love. At first, both had a difficult time tuning out the winces and grimaces of pain and not losing their arousal, but they got better at knowing when to adjust or even stop loveplay. Both were pleasantly surprised to find that sometimes making love and having orgasms actually diminished their pain.

Attitude readjustment. There were losses with aging and physical illnesses but so many gains, too. The couple learned to adapt and focus on the positive side. Part of grieving was crying over the loss of a favorite position but not allowing its absence to become an obsession. They enjoyed sex and intimacy and engaged in self-talk or sharing together when self-pity or obsessing began to creep in. They reveled in how much they were learning about sensuality and a deeper intimacy. Once she had to sternly lecture him when he thought he was losing his grip as the world's greatest lover, affirming for him that sex was much more than firmness of erections or vigorous thrusting.

RELATIONAL CHANGES WITH MATURITY

Have you had your midlife crisis? You may respond, "But I didn't know everyone had to have one," or "But I'm only forty-one, and that seems a little early to be into midlife." Actually, the phenomena of "midlife crises" occur throughout life. They might be better titled "identity" or "purpose in life" struggles, as all involve realizing goals and dreams and creating deeper intimacy. Areas that are usually included are sexuality, relationships, spirituality, career and life pursuits, and meaningful leisure distractions.

Sex after forty-five has to consider not only the physical changes but also the midlife relational changes that occur in the crucial years leading up to and including retirement. Middle age keeps getting pushed back, so we are not sure what middle age is anymore. For this chapter, a definition of midlife is not crucial because we are examining the sexual cycles of a couple's life from forty to eighty (or beyond), where much reevaluating goes on. During these years, we constantly reassess many parts of ourselves that have great impact on our sex lives: intimate companionship, sexual passion and variety, career development and retirement, and children in later stages of leaving the nest (notice we said, "stages of leaving the nest," because we don't think they ever leave completely).

Sex is different as we age and as marriages mature. That does not mean we give sex a lesser priority or lose our intimate passion. This section explores two aspects of relational changes that affect sex as we mature and grow older: (1) our environment and (2) our individual and relational needs.

CHANGING ENVIRONMENT AND RELATIONAL
AND INDIVIDUAL NEEDS

Children are stressors as they enter the teenage years and begin struggles for independence, then parents incur the expense of their children's college educations, and eventually, the nest is empty. This can have a positive and a negative impact on a couple's sex life. On the positive side, there is more time to get together with greater privacy and flexibility. The negative emotional stress is the feeling of loss, especially as children become adults and launch out on their own. Parents can lose a sense of purpose and, in their grieving, lose touch with each other.

All of these environmental factors take time and energy away from making love and focusing on the marital relationship. Sometimes parents get too much identity from their parental roles and have a difficult time readjusting to being best friends and lovers. The greater time together can be scary, but the excuses for lack of intimacy and infrequent sex have to be faced head-on. A couple will need to learn to expose impasses and not be afraid of confrontation and honest discussion. Unfortunately, all couples do not work hard at exposing impasses, resolving problems, and deepening companionship.

Midlife issues. The forties and fifties bring many career decisions to the forefront: Will my dreams ever be realized, and will I achieve the level of success that I had hoped for? This can bring on a full-fledged midlife crisis. You may have to grieve over some of your unachieved goals and change gears.

Midlife career changes and whole new career directions are common in today's marketplace. The wife may be back in the job market after full-time homemaking, and she faces many new decisions as she revs up a vocation she put on hold for the sake of mothering. The husband may be in the most productive and busiest time of his career—fighting for time to keep everything balanced and to enjoy making love.

All of this affects intimacy and a thriving sex life. The husband is entering a time when he has less sexual energy but a greater desire for intimate connecting. The wife may be entering a time of more sexual enthusiasm with greater independence and openness to explore and enjoy, or she may be experiencing the physical changes and emotional turmoil menopause can sometimes bring. As their bodies begin to age, their circumstances are a kaleidoscope of changes and challenges. Sex may be ignored and intimacy put on the back burner as the husband works through his challenges, and the wife works at varying jobs from launching children out on their own to balancing her own career.

There will be a search for individual identities in this time, with a need to learn to practice forgiving and the skills of grieving over losses. Young adult children complicate the picture. There can be some panic as you wonder if you might have missed the perfect mate and maybe it is now or never, because you do desire the deeper intimacy of midlife. But don't think that you know your mate perfectly or that there are no new horizons sexually to discover. You will want to revive mystery and plan sexual surprises, avoiding routines and not neglecting frequent and passionate lovemaking. It may even take getting out of town to overcome this. Be selfish sexually as well as nurturing as you individually put some pizzazz back into your love life.

Retirement issues. The fifties and sixties present even more changes as the transition into retirement is made over the coming years. Retirement can be structured differently for every couple. It may be going into early retirement and a new career or easing into more leisure time when one comes to mandatory retirement and there is nothing else to fill the vacuum. Both mates can get frustrated by the husband being underfoot for the first time in their lives.

Grandparenting can bring special meaning and enjoyment, but you may have to add into the equation a major illness and the recuperation time involved. This is also the time in life when you start dealing with the loss or needs of your aging parents, possibly calling for you to make difficult decisions or adjust your living situation.

Circumstances will hit the relationship with attending grief and losses. You may wonder if it is too late to establish a deeper level of intimacy in your marriage, but you do have tremendous opportunity for renewal. You are entering the years where the blessings and curses of the aging process become more apparent. Sex after fifty or sixty can become more exciting and intimate, and you can achieve a level of affirmation and togetherness as you celebrate this part of your relationship. Learn your limitations and flourish within them. Old dogs *can* learn new tricks—so be creative and experimental.

One couple had major adjusting to do when the husband was forced into early retirement at age fifty-two. It presented a financial crisis because there were still college bills to be paid for their last child, and the husband's field did not offer an immediate lateral shift. This was also tough because they were just adjusting to their last child's leaving the nest. The wife grieved more over her empty nest than she expected but launched into a part-time job that helped fill her need for personal identity and fulfillment. Her father also passed away after a struggle with cancer—an expected event, but it still left a hole in her life.

The husband became depressed, and the whole relationship suffered. But they rallied together. The wife grieved through her losses and started healing. She was able to get more hours at work, and he shifted into a lower-paying but personally gratifying job. They had to make major decisions a year later when an opportunity came up in his original field that would necessitate a move geographically. He turned it down, especially for his wife's sake. She enjoyed being near her daughters and liked what she was doing. Plus, they had already moved three times because of his job over the years, and both felt a deeper need for roots and stability. The couple had also purchased land in the country where they were going to build a cabin and get away from the rat race. Both found nature very therapeutic to their souls, and the cabin was a mutual goal for their sixties and seventies.

The couple valued their intimacy and worked to lessen the toll of the environment on their companionship. There were some lean sexual times during his depression and job fluctuations, but their marriage slowly changed—for the better—during these times. She became more independent and he less driven, and sex came back to its place of priority.

What did this couple need as they matured into the retirement years? He wanted and valued a deeper sense of sharing and connecting with her as he risked his feelings and was tender and playful. She desired this, too, but she also wanted an autonomous identity—to feel competent and in charge of herself. Her job helped create this feeling, and her greater sexual initiative was affirming. It was a time for reevaluating selves and the relationship. They needed healing and a grieving through to acceptance of the many losses they were experiencing.

Lovemaking became an important part of the healing. Neither minded living with ambiguity and uncertainty as much as they used to. They trusted their intimacy and found they could connect, separate, and reconnect more easily. In fact, sometimes the wife needed this process as she launched into her own career and endeavors. Both also wanted to know they were heading toward a stable retirement and that there were some things they could count on. Sex evolved into something very special in helping to meet these varied needs and staving off environmental pressures. This husband and wife entered into a very intimate time—a second, or maybe the third or fourth, honeymoon.

Later life losses. As a couple moves into their seventies and eighties they are well into retirement and facing the fact of losing each other eventually, as health deteriorates. It is a time when suffering can build character as you transcend yourself and let go of control. You may fight to establish new boundaries as you set up new ground rules concerning leisure routines and chores. Don't isolate, or become too codependent. Sexually, the older body will creak and groan, but don't let inertia set in. Continue to enjoy sexual closeness even if it doesn't frequently include intercourse—though it may. Fight for your privacy if you are living with your children, and enjoy the fruit of many years of bonding and sharing. Say nice things to each other, and hold each other close. You will start to fear losing the other person, and it will be okay to desperately clutch the other one near now and again. Sex can have a transcendent beauty in this time of life, admirable for a younger couple to emulate.

Connecting Versus Penetrating

As you lie with your mate and experience the intimacy of holding hands, caressing faces, hugging close, and stimulating sexual excitement, you are energized and affirmed. Making love is a safe haven where you can delight despite the environmental pressures. As you age, this becomes even more important, and your sex life is symbolic of your ability to still be in charge of your marriage and your destiny. But, the vast majority of older males continue to believe that all sexual expression must involve penile-vaginal penetration. Many of these same men may believe that the interpersonal relationship should have little influence on their ability to have an erection. These beliefs are recipes for sexual and relational disaster.

As we age, we can mature in our concepts of lovemaking. If sex is to be a celebration, we need to have a relationship to celebrate, and this is truer than ever as we grow older. If a couple develops their abilities to connect and communicate, and acquires many ways to achieve intimacy besides just sexual intercourse, they have a healthy repertoire to draw upon when disease or disability strikes. They have a much greater ability to successfully adapt to changes inherent in the aging process, because they have developed their understanding of making love.

Nurturing Each Other's Spirit

M. Scott Peck in his bestselling book *The Road Less Traveled* defined *love* as "the will to extend oneself for the purpose of nurturing one's own or another's spiritual growth."[2] This definition challenges us to put love into action and begs us to answer two questions if we are to be good "lovers." First, what is it that nurtures my own or my spouse's growth? Not just what arouses them or makes them temporarily feel good, but how can my nurturance make a difference in his or her life? The second question to consider is, what areas in my life or my spouse's life are in need of additional growth? My ability to communicate? My ability to resolve conflict? My unresolved issues with family or friends? My relationship with God? There may be many areas of potential growth and each of them will *enhance* my ability to legitimately love my spouse.

My ability to better nurture my spouse will manifest itself in the bedroom as we celebrate the effort we have put into our relationship. In aging, bodies do not respond with the same reflexive arousal as when younger but need the attention and nurturing of a partner in special ways. Older mates thus feel a greater sense of mutuality and power in their lovemaking. A husband may need his wife to stimulate his penis into an erection and help him reach a climax in ways he did not in earlier years. This can be very exciting and bonding to a wife as she enjoys being more aggressive and playful in her sexuality. Her husband involves and counts on her more, and she enjoys this form of nurturing. A man may acquire greater tenderness, sensitivity, and patience that make him a much more adept lover. Couples have fun feeling needed and engaging in mutual nurturing with a deeper sense of connection—the appreciation of being skilled and generous lovers.

Developing and Protecting Intimacy

Making love can become a healing agent, a special form of nurturing, a statement of our independent selves, deep and intimate communication, and a celebration of life. After forty-five, you especially need God's gift of sexuality to heal losses, reaffirm your sense of self and attractiveness, encourage playfulness, and express love. Not only is this deepening of intimacy important to bind wounds and protect the relationship, it is exciting to realize that it is much more likely to be achieved as you mature with your mate. Aging brings greater flexibility, knowledge, the ability to prolong pleasure, and a desire for deeper intimacy.

God desires us to mature and gain wisdom with age. Sex can become even more special after forty and fifty and eighty. Mature men and women are even better equipped—mentally and emotionally and physically—to bring their intimate companions and themselves greater pleasure. Your fulfilling partnership can achieve a level never before experienced, and your lovemaking can be an integral part of this whole process.

James K. Childerston, Ph.D., FICPP, MP, is a licensed psychologist in private practice and is board certified in Psychopharmacology and Medical Psychology. He teaches with the Psychopharmacological Institute and with the Institute for Sexual Wholeness. Jim is coauthor of Purity and Passion: Authentic Male Sexuality (Moody Press, 1994). *Jim can be reached at* jkc@nfis.com.

Carolyn Childerston, B.A., is the office manager for Childerston & Associates. She is completing her M.A. in Biblical Counseling at Trinity College and Seminary. Jim and Carolyn have five children and reside in Hagerstown, Maryland. Carolyn can be reached at cari@nfis.com.

CHAPTER TWENTY-ONE

Common Male Malfunctions

HERE'S THE BAD NEWS. Most men will struggle with four common dysfunctions, at various levels of complication, during the course of a marriage: blocked sexual desire, delayed (retarded) ejaculation (difficulty achieving an orgasm), premature ejaculation (climaxing too quickly), and impotence (erectile difficulties). A whole chapter (Chapter 18) has been devoted to the fourth common sexual problem—lack of desire. The good news is that medical and psychological solutions exist to help resolve these malfunctions.

One of my professors in sex-therapy training stated that a man's penis may be one of the most honest parts of his anatomy. This is so often true. The guilty, hurt, tired, depressed, or distracted man may be unable to focus his sexual attention, and his penis accurately reflects his mind, body, and emotions, with erections and climaxes more difficult to achieve. The man who is angry with his wife may use premature ejaculation to passively sabotage her pleasure and get back at her. The husband who empathizes with his mate's discomfort with sex may become impotent to take her off the hook.

Sexual responses and malfunctions can be very complex. This chapter can be a starting point as you press through to finding the help you need to resolve the problem.

BEGINNING THE TREATMENT OF SEXUAL DYSFUNCTION

Okay, men, so you've known something is wrong but were unsure you could admit it or where to go for help. We like to fix things on our own. Here are some of the beginning steps.

Understand the Complexity

Your sexual problem may very well be partly or primarily a physical or medical problem. This will require the assistance of a medical doctor who can diagnose and treat it. Many other factors may be contributing to your problems as well. Your relationship with your wife correlates with your sexual enjoyment. Husbands don't like to sleep with the enemy, or an angry or distant person. Her sexual responsiveness and problems affect your responsiveness. If she is having pain in intercourse, husbands don't want to hurt their mates and will back off or lose erections.

Are you exhausted, depressed, under stress, or tremendously focused on your job? All these impact your sexual performance. Some personality styles create a propensity for sexual dysfunction. The worrier who is sensitive to environmental stress and anxiety will be more prone to performance anxiety. Attention deficit and obsessive-compulsive disorders can contribute to thinking and behaviors that help prolong impotence or delayed ejaculation.

Chronic masturbation or sexual addiction can siphon off your sexual energy and create lack of desire, delayed or premature ejaculation, and an inability to truly be sexually intimate. Your sex therapy may need to include dealing with your addiction or ceasing masturbation. Overcoming sexual difficulties must address all areas that contribute to the dysfunction in order to be effective.

Seek Medical Intervention

In any sexual malfunction, ruling out and treating any physical problems is the place to start. Get a thorough physical to check things like blood pressure, low testosterone, thyroid, and prostate difficulties. For complications like ED (erectile difficulties) you may need to find a urologist who specializes in sexual problems. Medicine has grown in its ability to diagnose blood flow and nerve problems and to repair them with surgery.

Find Counseling

This may be a marriage therapist to help with relational problems that are interfering with your sex life. You may need a counselor with skill in sexual issues or a trained sex therapist to help diagnose and coach you through some of the self-help exercises developed later in this chapter.

DISEASES AND MEDICINE COMPLICATIONS

Start with the physical and then proceed to the psychological. If you are battling diabetes, working on your relationship with your wife will help, but you will need to understand the effects of the disease first. Conversely, just dealing with the medical and healing the physical will not put you in a place to want to make love to your wife.

Diseases and Sexual Dysfunction

Prostate enlargement and cancer can require the removal of the prostate. This can produce impotence, but because of improved surgical techniques it's not necessarily so. More likely it can cause retrograde ejaculation, with the ejaculation going into the bladder during orgasm. This doesn't destroy sexual pleasure; however, it may take some mental readjustment to allow a climax to feel as exciting again.

Cancer treatment with radiation and chemotherapy can affect sexual desire and functioning in various ways. Check with your physician whether the effects are short-term or must be adjusted to and worked around, as mates get back to sexual pleasure in different forms. Diabetes can also affect blood flow and create erectile difficulty.

Peyronie's disease is a bowing of the penis caused by trauma, which can make intercourse painful or impossible. Consult an expert; this condition runs a course of around eighteen months in which medicine can make a difference in the physical dysfunction in some men. After the trauma to the penis has run its course, surgery can be helpful for some men, to correct the damage and allow intercourse.

Side Effects of Medications

All medicines have side effects and many can affect sexual functioning. This can occur through direct sexual side effects as a result of the medication (impotence, delayed ejaculation, or lowered libido, for example) or indirectly through other side effects that impact one's mood or motivation for sex (for example, sedation, dizziness, nausea, headaches). (This is discussed more thoroughly in Chapter 18.) Check with your doctors regarding any use of antidepressants, antihypertensives for high blood pressure, and some ulcer medications. Sometimes adjusting the dosage, switching the drug, or adding another agent can help; or depending on the medication, a brief day "vacation" from the medication can help sexual functioning.

FOUR COMMON MALFUNCTIONS

It helps to understand some of the causes of the male malfunction as deeper changes are effected. In all of them, performance anxiety can play a continuingly greater role. The more the dysfunctions are reacted to, feared, and focused on, the more likely they are to occur. Both husband and wife have an important role in preventing this from happening. Sometimes rolling over and going to sleep without making a big deal of the malfunction is the most therapeutic response. You can enjoy making love again later.

These malfunctions will not always go away once the cause has been diagnosed and understood. They have become a pattern maintained by the anxiety. Psychological-change strategies are included to help you intervene in this destructive cycle.

LACK OF DESIRE AND FREQUENCY

Many myths exist about men, such as usually being horny and having instant erections. Actually, men are deeply affected by fatigue, relational conflict, and their strength (weakness) of being able to focus their energy on the task at hand. Work will sometimes take precedence over sex.

Don't feel you are less of a man or that something must be terribly wrong because you are the partner with low desire. You aren't operating in a vacuum and some good reasons are contributing to your lack of desire. Explore and find solutions to implement in your personal life and your lovemaking. Don't settle for sex every three or four months or simply to please your wife. God intended you to make love and be a lover. Don't cheat yourself or your wife. Chapter 18 has been devoted to this very complex sexual dysfunction.

DELAYED EJACULATION

Delayed, sometimes called retarded, ejaculation is less common than premature ejaculation and impotence. If we define this phenomenon as a complete inability to achieve an ejaculation, it is indeed rare. If we expand the definition to being unable to achieve a climax (or achieve a climax easily) through intercourse, it is less rare. A more accurate way to help us deal with this roadblock is to consider delayed ejaculation to be any time the husband cannot reach a climax as quickly as he desires. That is a more common occurrence.

Understanding Delayed Ejaculation

Some of the common causes of delayed ejaculation vary, depending on the situation. With one widower, it was a combination of guilt and a new mate, which mentally and emotionally interfered with his ability to climax in his partner's vagina. Another man experienced stress and anxiety about a variety of midlife experiences. His wife, with her own stressors, was not as active in the lovemaking process. All combined to lessen his sexual focus and arousal.

Other common reasons include letting sex lives become routine, and a husband's finding his wife and lovemaking less arousing. As less excitement is incited while making love, going over the edge into a climax happens less readily. Some husbands focus too much on the wife's pleasure and consequently neglect their own buildup of sexual tension and pleasure. In a similar manner, a wife may find herself not as aroused when she more exclusively focuses on playing with and stimulating her husband. It is difficult to keep a balance in focusing on both helping your mate and attending to your own feelings and arousal.

The husband sometimes finds the vagina too loose or too lubricated to give sufficient friction. If that is so, the wife can practice Kegel exercises and tighten the muscles of her vaginal opening. She may wish to consult a gynecologist or a cosmetic surgeon to tighten the vagina if Kegel exercises don't improve friction. But proceed with caution. It might not be the vagina at all but a lack of sexual arousal and focused concentration on the husband's part. The ability to focus on growing sexual arousal is a crucial part of great sex.

Sometimes emotional scars, family repression, or sexual guilt or intimidation interfere with a man's ability to experience pleasure with intercourse. Often the husband can climax with manual stimulation but through intercourse only with difficulty. Stopping masturbating and allowing the sensations of the penis in the vagina (very different from a hand) to grow erotically arousing may help. Perhaps he has been so indoctrinated about keeping himself pure and not getting girls pregnant that intercourse, even in marriage, seems wrong on an unconscious level. Maybe he viewed his mom as seductive, and as a boy, he shut down his sexual feelings; now he avoids active interaction with women. Maybe he struggles with homosexual feelings and needs to deal with this issue. He may have experienced an abusive sexual relationship with a woman and be fearful of rejection or inadequacy.

Medical Interventions in Delayed Ejaculation

Delayed ejaculation can be drug-induced. A common side effect of the SSRI (selective serotonin reuptake inhibitors) antidepressants, which increase serotonin levels like fluoxetine (Prozac), sertraline (Zoloft), and paroxetine (Paxil), is that they can delay and affect the ability to be orgasmic. You should attempt to have an open discussion with your doctor about the nature of the medications you are taking and the according risks of sexual dysfunction. Inform your physician of any side effects you may be experiencing, so that they may be specifically addressed at each visit and so that adjustments can be made. Non-drug-related methods should be introduced first in order to better minimize expense, additional side effects, and inconvenience. The following are guidelines to consider in attempting to manage medication-induced sexual dysfunction.

1. Wait for spontaneous remission of side effects. Side effects are often more severe in the initial weeks of treatment and later diminish. However, treatment-emergent sexual dysfunction tends to persist.

2. Decrease the medication to a lower dose. Sexual dysfunction is often dose related, so lowering the dose may be helpful, as long as it is not lowered below the therapeutic threshold.

3. Try partial or complete drug holidays. This will not work for all medications or in all medical conditions. However, for SSRI-induced sexual dysfunction, reducing or holding the medication for a weekend can reduce or eliminate the dysfunction during that time. This will not work for Fluoxetine (Prozac) because it is too long lasting for this to be effective.

4. Change to a different medication with fewer sexual side effects. For example, the antidepressants with the fewest effects on sexual function are Bupropion (Wellbutrin), Nefazadone (Serzone), Venlafaxine (Effexor), and Mirtazapine (Remeron). Be cautious in switching from Paroxetine or Fluoxetine to Nefazadone because of a significant drug interaction, which can create unpleasant physical side effects such as shortness of breath or interfere with the liver metabolizing other drugs, but is not fatal or seriously damaging to health.

5. Use a secondary agent to decrease sexual dysfunction. Adding an adjunctive agent may be possible in many cases, but concern should be given to the possibility of additional side effects or interaction possibilities. The following are possible adjunctive agents:

- a low dose of bupropion (Wellbutrin), 75 milligrams once or twice a day
- Yohimbine, 5.4 to 10.8 milligrams as needed before intercourse
- Viagra, with 50 to 75 percent response rates (this is contraindicated in those with cardiovascular disease or those taking nitrates)
- Cyproheptadine (Periactin), 4 to 12 milligrams one to two hours prior to intercourse
- Dopamine-stimulating drugs and psychostimulants: Amantadine (Symmetrel), 100 to 200 milligrams once a day, Lisuride, Bromocriptine (Parlodel), Dextroamphetamine (Dexedrine), and Methylphenidate (Ritalin) have all been used with varying success.
- Ginkgo biloba, 60 to 180 milligrams twice a day may be effective in vasoconstrictive sexual dysfunction. Side effects include gastrointestinal disturbances, headache, and general central nervous system activation.

A Change Program for Delayed Ejaculation

Emotional issues may emerge as you and your mate do the following behavioral work. Read the chapter on sexual communication and talk as you do these exercises. You and your mate can be healing agents for each other. Process the emotions and dispute the negative messages with positive affirmation statements. The husband may wish to repeat, "I have climaxed easily before; I know I can climax again," or "Intercourse feels so good, I will enjoy this experience for a while."

Focus on the journey. One man, struggling with delayed ejaculation, developed a fascinating metaphor from whitewater rafting. He saw sex as a great party in which there were fun and orgasms. He saw himself in a raft on a river heading for the party—some exciting rapids. No matter how hard he paddled, he always got stuck on snags, and he could never reach the rapids.

His wife had also gone through some of those feelings as she became orgasmic in the earlier days of their marriage. She had learned the hard way about loveplay and that curious paradox in sex: the goals you anxiously worry about and strive for are never achieved. The only way to reach most sexual destinations (for example, orgasm, increased desire, erections) is to forget about the goal and start enjoying the journey. She told her husband, "The party begins the minute we get into the raft and ease into the river. Forget about the rapids!"

The husband quickly identified with the idea of enjoying the journey. He and his wife loved to raft, and some of their most memorable trips had been floating down a river with no rapids above the Class Two category (rapids in Class Five are adventurous and usually take a guide). He remembered sunny Saturday afternoons with occasional lazy paddling to maintain their position in the river as they relaxed, ate, drank, and talked. One time they were on a mountain river while the mountain laurel and rhododendrons were in full bloom. On the same trip their guide had them all get out of the raft on a calm stretch and float. The water was so cold it took the breath away at first, but the beauty and adventure were among the most exciting memories of the trip.

The husband started hitting the rapids again as he began to enjoy the journey. Laughter, variety, spontaneity, and excitement returned. In a childlike fashion he began anticipating and expecting their lovemaking to have a lot of little thrills (Class Two rapids) and got truly excited about them. In awe and wonder he noticed sensual delights and unexpected pleasures. Rafting was fun once again.

Return to playfulness. Take a shower together and play at soaping each other up, and enjoy the relaxing feelings of the shower spray beating down on you. Gently towel each other dry as you nurture and care for each other. Now get your favorite snacks and beverages and have a nude picnic in your bed. Don't worry about sex, but try to tell some jokes and laugh together. Gently and sensually caress each other's body as a part of this picnicking. Playfully explore every inch of your mate's body, and come up with at least three new facts you did not know previously. Include a thorough and fun exploration of each other's genitals. Relax and be companions. Do not let this lead to making love or overt sexuality.

Practice genital pleasuring. Chapter 11 focuses on genital pleasuring. Turn to that chapter and practice the exercises on "Genital Exploration and Massage." This exercise is designed to decrease anxiety and increase warm playfulness and to allow sexual arousal without the goal of intercourse or climax. Don't let it lead into making love on the day you do it—let it be an end in itself and not a means to an end.

Focus on building pleasure and tension. An interesting paradox occurs with the idea of focusing. As discussed, focusing on an orgasm will have a negative effect and create performance anxiety. Creating orgasms requires the necessary stimulation and focusing in on personal pleasure and arousal. So, bad focus (performance) and good focus (pleasure and arousal) must both be addressed.

In these final exercises, you will limit orgasms to intercourse with the penis in the vagina. This allows sexual tension to build and pursues the goal of ejaculation within the vagina.

Exercise 1: The husband orchestrates making love to include the things that he finds stimulating. Both partners focus on building his sexual pleasure and tension. This can include oral and manual stimulation of the penis. Allow the sexual tension to build for ten to twenty minutes before beginning intercourse. Tease and play as mates—enjoy each other. The husband should zero in on aspects of his mate and lovemaking that he finds arousing and sexy. Get away from negative thinking and routines. The goal of this exercise is building sexual arousal and focusing on pleasure, not having orgasms or worrying about what isn't happening.

Exercise 2: This tension-building exercise is centered on intercourse. The husband again orchestrates and utilizes whatever position he finds most exciting to him—changing position if he desires. He begins with slow thrusting and concentrates on the feelings of the penis. He may fantasize about past sexy scenes together and focus on building sexual tension in the penis and genital area. He should allow himself to receive pleasure and enjoy it, forgetting about the goal of orgasm and concentrating on the sensations of thrusting. If the husband desires, the wife may take her middle finger and forefinger and, reaching down, grasp the base of the penis as it comes in and out of the vagina. He should thrust more rapidly for a minute, slow down, then repeat this several times. Before stopping this exercise, he should thrust vigorously for a couple of minutes and enjoy the feelings.

Bridging manual arousal into an orgasm with intercourse. Exercise 3: Begin with the husband once again orchestrating sexual arousal, and allow tension to build. This time manually or orally stimulate the penis to the point of ejaculation, then immediately insert it into the vagina and continue stimulation with thrusting. He may have some mishaps as he perfects knowing the point of ejaculation. The husband should keep trying, with succeeding sessions as needed. If he doesn't climax within a minute of insertion of the penis into the vagina, he should withdraw it and again stimulate the penis manually up to ejaculation and then bridge over into active thrusting in the vagina.

Stop after trying five times. You are trying to decrease performance anxiety, not increase it. You may need repeated sessions to break down inhibitions and anxieties. It can be a fun time of bonding lovemaking as you practice until you are able to break through the delayed ejaculation. Have fun and enjoy focusing on your pleasure and arousal.

3. PREMATURE EJACULATION

Wives feel cheated and both mates feel frustrated with premature ejaculation. Sometimes the husband is unpredictable and may last longer, only to relapse in the next lovemaking session. Couples often settle for this unsatisfactory condition, even though this malfunction can respond to treatment.

Understanding Premature Ejaculation

Premature ejaculation may happen because some men are born with a greater sensitivity to sensual and sexual stimulation, but it can also be a learned behavior. When adolescent boys are first experimenting with sexual feelings and behaviors, it is often something they are afraid of being caught doing. If a boy is in the bedroom or bathroom masturbating and wondering when someone is going to knock on the door, leisurely taking time is not an objective. Sex can become nonrelational, with a focus on attaining orgasms quickly. These habits can be carried into marriage and making love. Part of the change strategy for this dysfunction is ceasing masturbation and pairing arousal with making love.

Premature ejaculation can also be an outcome of emotional tensions. A husband may be anxious or feel pressured, which can interfere with his control—if he is worried about climaxing too quickly, it becomes a self-fulfilling prophecy. A man can also use ejaculating prematurely to passively get back at his partner as he expresses his anger and aggression. He may unconsciously say to himself: "I don't like to be controlled; I'll get her and come so quickly that she won't enjoy the experience."

Some wives are capable of having an orgasm with intercourse and prefer this method of stimulation. A problem occurs when she needs the husband to last eight to fifteen minutes and he begins to feel this pressure. Performance anxiety usually produces what a couple fears—climaxing prematurely. Sex researchers Masters and Johnson say that a man will often climax in under two minutes if actively thrusting. So we may not be dealing with premature ejaculation here, but a matching up of orgasmic desires.

Premature ejaculation may also occur by being too aroused and not knowing how to control the pace of lovemaking and the stimulation of the penis—stopping before the point of ejaculatory inevitability.

There are two stages to the male orgasm. The first stage includes contractions of the prostate, and the sphincter muscle closes off the bladder so the ejaculate goes out through the penis. The second stage is actual ejaculation. This includes muscle contractions along the urethra, seminal duct system, and penis, which expel the semen.

The first and second stages are only a few seconds, but with greater self-awareness, a man can anticipate it and feel a climax coming. Before this point, interventions must be made and the arousal interrupted. The pre-ejaculation and ejaculation stages are too late—with the completion of climax inevitable here. Once a man has passed over the point of ejaculatory inevitability, there is no returning; even a bucket of cold water won't stop it.

An important part of controlling premature ejaculation, then, is recognizing the bodily signs when getting close to climaxing, and backing off from active stimulation. The husband has to learn to stop and start and slow down as he regains control before passing the point of no return. Putting this arousal process on a scale of 1 to 10, with 10 being a climax, the key is knowing when you are approaching 7 and 8 and beginning to slow down. A 9 will usually be too far.

So how long must a husband last before he is not considered "premature"? Premature ejaculation can't really be defined in terms of time. It is better defined as the husband's not being able to control when he chooses to ejaculate. It is climaxing too quickly to mutually enjoy the experience of intercourse, and can vary from couple to couple. I remember more than one couple where the wife was complaining about premature ejaculation and when I asked what that meant to her, she said, "Oh, he can last only about ten minutes." Most wives would call her blessed. Certainly anything more than five to ten minutes should not be considered premature, though it may still be a problem to the wife who can and will want to climax through intercourse. An advantage of growing older is greater lasting power, with an ability to thrust longer.

Medical Intervention in Premature Ejaculation

The class of antidepressants referred to as SSRIs often affect sexual functioning. A common side effect is orgasmic difficulties with delaying or making climaxes more difficult to achieve. You feel like you are ready to ejaculate and yet you can't. A low dose of these drugs (for example, sertraline [Zoloft], paroxetine [Paxil], or citalopram [Celexa]) can increase the arousal time before ejaculation. Other antidepressants like clomipramine (Anafranil) can also have the similar sexual side effects of the SSRIs and can also be helpful with slowing down ejaculation.

It is sometimes difficult discerning what are legitimate effects of a drug and what is a placebo effect by creating confidence. Another issue with drug therapy is that though they can sometimes be effective, they do not deal with the psychological issues that helped create the problem. Psychotherapy along with drug therapy can often be more effective.

A Psychological Change Program for Premature Ejaculation

The following exercises are based on the stages of male orgasm and recognizing the point of inevitability. The Kegel exercises tighten the PC muscle in the genital area and around the prostate and help control ejaculatory inevitability. Remember the importance of being able to accurately recognize the physiological signs that you are approaching seven or eight on your ten-point scale.

Use Kegel exercises. The PC muscle in a man can be an invaluable aid for controlling arousal and helping to postpone ejaculation. It can be identified by starting to urinate and squeezing off the flow or, when standing, making the penis jump.

For one week, exercise the PC muscle by contracting it two times a day with ten repetitions per session. Contract the muscle while you count one thousand one, one thousand two, and then relax the muscle. Repeat this ten times and stop. Don't be macho and try to hold it tight longer or do thirty repetitions. You will grow sore and not accomplish any more.

During the second week, repeat the two sessions per day with ten repetitions. Hold the count for one thousand one, one thousand two, one thousand three, and then relax. This will help you identify the PC muscle and exercise it so it can more tightly grip the genital and prostate area. It will become a reflexive action that you can do easily and effectively.

Stop, contract PC, break, and start. Practice these stop-and-start exercises for three months. It takes time to break old habits and learn new skills. There should be no intercourse or orgasm during these three months, except while practicing this program, or the skills can be jeopardized. It will be helpful to block out two to three thirty-minute sessions per week. Wives, you can sabotage the whole process to your own detriment by not having the discipline to postpone your own pleasure while new skills are being learned. Granted, intercourse will not be as fun for you with starting and stopping, but the ultimate goal, better control, will be enjoyed by both of you.

Exercise 1: Start by manually stimulating the penis to the point of ejaculation and then stop and contract the PC muscle (tighten for the duration of one-thousand-one to one-thousand-three count). You may want to stop too soon rather than risk pushing close to the point of ejaculatory inevitability. Become aware of your physiological arousal, and start training yourself when to stop. Allow a brief minute or so interlude as sexual tension decreases after the PC tightening—take a break from any active stimulation and be close. (A younger man will need to take a longer break than an older man, to increase control.) Now repeat the process until you have practiced for fifteen to twenty minutes.

Here is a summary of this three-step technique for controlling ejaculation: (1) stop any movement, (2) contract the PC muscle, and (3) take a short break (a few seconds or more) from any stimulation of the penis as arousal decreases.

You can practice this exercise alone, but it is important to approximate real life with the sexual stimulation of your wife present. It also helps to have your mate aware of the skills you are learning and to participate with you. Your wife will profit from knowing that one extra pump or thrust may be too much. She is probably frustrated and needs to understand that you cannot, by sheer will, lengthen your staying power, but you can learn skills that will help. At the end of the session, allow your mate to bring you to an orgasm. Practice this exercise until you feel you are able to recognize your point of ejaculatory inevitability and can stop and decrease arousal. You should be able to comfortably stimulate the penis, with stopping and starting, for fifteen minutes without ejaculating.

Exercise 2: The next step is called the quiet vagina. Begin with active loveplay manually and orally, and if you approach ejaculation—stop, contract the PC muscle, and break to decrease arousal. After your mate and you are aroused sexually, enter her vagina but do not thrust. Just leave your penis in her quiet vagina. The wife is passive with no movements; she lies comfortably in a penis-in-vagina embrace. You will experience a special one-flesh closeness even though there isn't active stimulation. If this gets too exciting, withdraw the penis and use the stop-and-contract technique as needed.

After you are feeling less aroused sexually (a brief minute, or maybe two if you are younger), remove the penis and begin again with loveplay. Repeat the quiet vagina five or more times over a twenty- to thirty-minute period. You are slowly teaching yourself that you can be in the vagina without climaxing. Practice this skill until you can comfortably have the penis contained in the quiet vagina without ejaculating and until you are increasingly aware of your ability to keep from climaxing. Do not continue to orgasms with rapid thrusting at the end of these sessions. If you want release, do it manually so you don't interrupt your training of responding slower in the vagina.

Exercise 3: After initial loveplay and arousal, enter the vagina with slow and *shallow* thrusts (partial containment). The wife should remain more passive and allow you to enter about an inch and slowly move the penis in and out. If at any point in the thrusting you feel you are getting near to ejaculating, stop, contract, and go to the quiet vagina. If arousal is too high to remain in the vagina, withdraw completely as you stop and contract. Then go back to a quiet vagina until arousal decreases and you can begin the slow thrusting. Practice this until you feel able to control ejaculation during your thirty-minute lovemaking session. Again, don't ejaculate with thrusting but get relief manually as needed. You are learning new habits and working on orgasm control.

Exercise 4: After loveplay and arousal, practice slow and *deeper* thrusting (full containment). The wife again remains passive. Don't be surprised to discover that she finds this stimulation very arousing and exciting to her; this is a very stimulating way to enjoy intercourse. Use the stop-and-contract technique whenever you approach ejaculation as you maintain control during your thirty-minute session. At first it may be necessary to *completely withdraw* the penis and stop all stimulation and then begin again with the quiet vagina. Don't berate yourself when you slip up and climax. Neither partner should make this a federal offense, but laugh and know you will do better next time. You are learning together to maximize God's gift of sex. Even while building skills, lovemaking can be playful and intimate. Practice until you can accomplish this exercise comfortably and not ejaculate during intercourse.

Exercise 5: After loveplay, begin intercourse. This time practice varying slow with *rapid* thrusting. This is a crucial skill of the mature lover: intermittently varying rates and depths of thrusting. Intercourse thrusting might be charted like this: slow-deep, rapid-shallow, stop, rapid-deep, stop, rapid-deep, slow-shallow, slow-deeper, stop, rapid-shallow, and so on. As you approach an orgasm, the thrusting will become more vigorous and rapid. In this exercise, deliberately vary your rates of thrusting between rapid and slow. Whenever excitement builds toward ejaculation, stop immediately and practice your technique for decreasing sexual tension. Again as you progress, you may be able to use your stop-and-start technique without withdrawing. At the end of the session, choose when you want to ejaculate and enjoy it.

Practice for a lifetime. You have taken three months to practice new skills and to achieve your goals: being able to choose when you wish to ejaculate and enjoying prolonged intercourse. The stop-and-start technique with contracting the PC muscle is a skill you will need to incorporate into your lovemaking for the rest of your life. You will also be able to vary the rate of thrusting through intermittent stopping with the penis in the vagina and tightening the PC. You may discover that there will be periods in your lovemaking when you relapse and premature ejaculation comes back to haunt you. Take the time to go through the whole program again. You may be able to abbreviate it to a month this time. A great sex life takes some skills. Congratulations on learning some new ones.

4. IMPOTENCE

By the age of forty, around 90 percent of men have experienced one or more times of having difficulty getting or sustaining an erection. It still surprises most couples when it occurs, with an overreaction by both mates. This malfunction is prone to being made worse by anxiety and frustrated reactions.

Understanding Impotence

Erectile problems can be caused by physical or psychological problems, or by a combination of both. All men will have erections come and go during lovemaking as they focus in on their mates, but they should return easily with stimulation. A total lack of erections or a lack of firmness in the erection could point to physical problems. The process of aging makes erections more difficult to achieve without direct physical stimulation and they may slightly decrease in firmness. The presence of nighttime/morning erections or the ability to get erections in self-stimulation would point to psychological causes.

The most common psychological cause of impotence is performance anxiety. Getting sexually aroused and getting an erection depends on the autonomic nervous system. A man doesn't will an erection to occur—it happens as he is stimulated, physically and emotionally, into arousal. These reflexive nerve responses are short-circuited by anxiety. Psychological impotence is usually not the first time an erection does not occur. Impotence happens with the subsequent fear of not getting or of losing an erection.

It's Friday night and the husband is exhausted and has had too much to drink. He cannot get an erection. Saturday morning he fearfully tries to make love again. He, and sometimes his wife, are no longer present in enjoying lovemaking. They are mentally up on the bedpost as spectators, wondering if he will get an erection this time. This performance anxiety becomes the kiss of death.

Various forms of stress can also decrease your ability to focus on sexual feelings and become sufficiently stimulated. Environmental stressors can produce an inhibiting feeling such as *depression*, which is a common cause of sexual problems. You will want to discuss with your doctor whether it might be a factor in your life. *Grief* is another emotion that can be a real sexual depressant and create less desire and an inability to become aroused. *Relationships* also have an important impact on your sex life. It may be the depression and grief of your close relationships that are creating the loss and hurt. It is a myth that men are never affected by their emotions and always have a strong libido.

Other emotional and relational problems that many men face are anger, fear of rejection, rigid childhood sexual training, and guilt. *Anger* and other intense emotions efficiently sabotage great sex. Making love to someone you are fighting with and feeling hostile toward is often not possible. If you do not want intimacy or are afraid of it, your penis may be very honest and not react with arousal. Perhaps you fear rejection or pick up on your wife's signal that she does not want to be close or sex is not fun for her. This too can create erection problems. Perhaps you were raised in a rigid home where sex was viewed as wrong or dangerous, and this *squelched sexuality* spills over into your marital sex life. *Guilt* can be an excellent sabotaging emotion. Guilt about being impotent can compound the problem; you feel you're not being there sexually for your wife. You want to nurture her but just do not feel like it, physically or emotionally.

Just trying to make love, regardless of your physical and mental states, can also contribute to erection problems. Your wife may want to make love and experience some closeness. You may have had a particularly trying day at work and are exhausted. You hate to turn her down and you too desire to be close. But when you are unable to achieve an erection, the whole evening deteriorates further for you. Better skills at making love and connecting without having to have intercourse and erections, as well as healthy assertiveness, can help take care of some of these situations.

Certain physical problems can interfere with getting erections. The body mechanisms for achieving erection and sexual arousal are the endocrine system (hormones), the vascular system, and the nervous system. The hormones trigger desire, and the autonomic nervous system sends a signal causing the penis to engorge with blood and become erect. Diseases like diabetes, multiple sclerosis, and kidney problems can interfere with the nervous system and its functioning. Some surgeries like prostatectomy (removing the prostate) may destroy nerve paths. Radiation treatment can affect nerves and blood supply, creating leakage from the penis. The blood supply can also be disturbed by diabetes or arteriosclerosis.

Medical Interventions in Impotence

An insufficient level of the hormone testosterone can create lack of desire and difficulty functioning. Hormone deficiency can be checked with a simple blood test to assess one's testosterone level and also the luteinizing hormone (LH) levels. LH levels are necessary to determine whether a person may have pituitary or hypothalamus deficits or even testicular failure. Once this assessment is completed, the physician can determine whether testosterone replacement is appropriate or not. Remember that testosterone replacement is clinically effective for the improvement of desire or sex drive in hypotestosterone males. It is not particularly effective in restoring erections.

Drugs can also interfere with sexual functioning. They can depress or interrupt the nerve messages and affect the ability to get or retain an erection. The most common offender is alcohol. The more alcohol, the greater the negative effect on erectile functioning. Prescription medications, such as antihypertensives for high blood pressure or antidepressants, can also have an effect. Consult with your physician. Different medications have differing effects on the body chemistry of individuals. As discussed earlier, it may be possible to adjust the dose or change the medication to minimize the side effects. For more information about medication effects, refer to Chapter 18, which discusses low sexual desire and frequency.

The most common treatment for ED (erectile dysfunction) is sildenafil (Viagra or another PDE5—phosphoresterase 5—inhibitor) with a success rate of about 70 percent. It is taken orally an hour or so before lovemaking and helps the penis respond to stimulation. Viagra enhances the action of cyclic GMP, a chemical released in the production of nitric oxide in the nerve cells surrounding the penis, which has the effect of widening the blood vessels in the penis. Cyclic GMP inhibits the effect of PDE 5, an enzyme that is abundant in impotent men and blocks arousal. Viagra only works when there is sexual desire, so it won't work if you slip it in your husband's coffee. It is truly a "spirit is willing, but the flesh is weak" drug. An improved ability to perform, however, can create confidence and greater desire.

As with any medications, Viagra does not resolve the relational problems. I remember one client telling me, "I can get it up now, but I still don't want to have sex with her." I often encourage clients to try Viagra even when psychological impotence is the problem; it can give a confidence boost and be helpful in breaking the performance-anxiety cycle.

If Viagra (or equivalent) doesn't physiologically work, consult a urologist. Other drugs may be tried, administered orally or under the tongue, that deal with other parts of the body and central nervous system, like apomorphine or phentolamine. Sometimes chemical injections that can be self-administered (prostaglandin E, phentolomine, or papaverine) are other proven means of treating ED. Prostagladin E (Alprostadil) also comes in pellet form that can be inserted into the urethra, which then dissolves into the bloodstream. It is important to keep under a physician's care with drugs and their contraindications with some diseases. The injections should not be utilized in men with certain blood diseases like sickle cell anemia. If the erection does not subside after four to six hours—this is called priapism—seek medical help immediately or you may risk the possibility of permanent impotence.

There is also a vacuum pump that your physician can prescribe to pull blood into the penis, with a rubber ring to maintain the erection. It is interesting that some of the nuisance of self-injections or the vacuum pump make these methods more difficult for people to follow through on. Newer surgical techniques have been perfected to deal with blood flow and nerve damage. A urologist who specializes in sexual dysfunction can help diagnose whether these surgical interventions are feasible.

A physician can also help in sorting through the advisability of a penile prosthesis after truly determining that the impotence is indeed physiological and permanent. The most commonly used prosthesis is inflatable (a second is the semi-rigid rod) and inserted in the penis with a pump mechanism in the scrotum. Psychological counseling can help sort through both mates' feelings and sexual needs. Impotence does not prevent a man's having orgasms and ejaculation, and some couples adjust to the impossibility of having intercourse, emphasizing other aspects of making love to feel content and close. Others find that a prosthesis revolutionizes their sex lives.

A Change Program for Psychological Impotence

An important part of dealing with impotence is heading it off before it becomes a chronic dilemma. Couples can wisely and lovingly handle some of the psychological issues and prevent an occurrence of impotence from evolving into a recurrent problem. Couples must remember to minimize the erectile difficulty and not overreact. *The wife has an important role* in taking incidents of impotence in stride and not panicking. She can emphasize that impotence is normal with all men and can help both forget about trying to have sex immediately, waiting until another time when they are rested and able to focus on pleasure. Minimizing the incident is the best medicine. Caress, play, and enjoy each other as you take the focus off intercourse! This is not a commentary on your skill or attractiveness as a lover. Learn to initiate and refuse concerning your lovemaking so you don't attempt sex when you are truly not in the mood.

If the ability to get or sustain an erection is an ongoing problem, the following program can eliminate performance anxiety and increase sexual arousal. Please don't panic, and do some self-talk as you enjoy each other inside and outside the bedroom. Engage in a lot of physical touching and close companionship.

As impotence gets into its vicious cycle with failure increasing anxiety and leading to more failure, making love can come to be dreaded. This is just another chance for pain and disappointment, and eventually, you will avoid sex entirely. Making love must be reclaimed as a sensual, relaxing, erotic experience. An essential part of dealing with impotence is redirecting your energy to pleasuring and getting rid of performance anxiety.

Sensual touching. Do this sensual touching exercise without worrying about an erection. In fact, if the husband does get an erection, do not make use of it right now. Block out thirty minutes for this session, and relax with sensual feelings as each mate assumes the role of active toucher and passive touchee for fifteen minutes. Remember, this exercise is to distract from performance and get each of you re-involved in your sensual companionship. Do not engage in intercourse or other lovemaking on the day you do sensual touching.

The active toucher: Touch the passive partner in ways that feel good to you. This touching is oriented toward individual learning and experiencing—not mutually attending to the partner. Focus only on personal feelings and enjoyment of sensuality—there are no performance needs. The goal is selfishly enjoying touching the passive partner in ways that give personal pleasure.

Experiment with a variety of touches and strokes. Start with the touchee lying on the stomach and begin at the top of the head and slowly work your way down to the feet. Have the passive partner roll over and work from the feet to the head. It is best not to have any communication at this point but to revel in individual sensations. Exclude any touching of the breasts or genitals. If you are aware of areas of the body that your partner does not like to have touched, in love and respect stay away from these areas.

The passive touchee: Lie passively and allow the active partner to touch you. Often the touches that pleasure the active toucher also give stimulation and pleasure to the passive mate. You can increase self-awareness as you learn what areas and types of touching give you the greatest pleasure. Focus on and enjoy your feelings. You can ask for them and repeat them while making love at a different time. You are also learning about your lover—what kind of touching and stroking the other enjoys. When you are the active partner, don't confine your touching by this information or begin to attend to your partner's needs. Do your active touching for yourself.

Repeat this exercise two or three times a week for two weeks as you take the focus off intercourse and erections. Enjoy your mate's body and your sexual responses.

Genital pleasuring. Without fear and performance anxiety, the male and female genitals need to be comfortably and playfully stimulated into arousal. The husband needs to realize that it is normal for erections to come and go during lovemaking and that he can get them back—as well as maintain them—during intercourse. Sexual arousal is an involuntary response to loveplay and enjoying the mate as lover. The wife has to deal with her fears and fatigue as she involves herself in making love to her husband's penis for her pleasure and not just to make him respond. Sensual touching helps; so can nondemanding genital pleasuring. (It would be helpful to read Chapter 11, which describes genital pleasuring.)

Exercise 1: Assume a comfortable sitting position, facing each other, with the wife's legs overlapping the husband's and the penis accessible to her vulva. Using the penis as a wand, the wife takes the flaccid penis and brushes it over her vulval area as both receive erotic stimulation. This exercise does not depend on an erection. Let the husband, as she lies back, also use the penis to touch the clitoral area, labia, and mouth of the vagina. Both should relax and enjoy the sensual experience of the moment, delighting in the genital-to-genital sensations with no expectations. If the husband gets an erection, he should use it to stimulate the wife's external genital area. Don't engage in intercourse, but repeat this exercise at least twice a week for two weeks. The husband should refrain from orgasms during this time.

Exercise 2: Assume a comfortable position with genitals to genitals, and begin enjoying each other. If the husband experiences an erection, he should use it to stimulate the clitoral area. As the wife becomes aroused, he should gently place the penis at the mouth of the vagina and penetrate half an inch as he manually continues to stimulate the shaft of the penis. He is relaxing, then becoming comfortable with enjoying and maintaining an erection in the vagina, almost like the quiet vagina exercises for premature ejaculation. Now he should withdraw and reinsert the penis a little deeper; repeating this process as he enjoys the penis in the vagina without active thrusting. Do this two or three times a week for two weeks. Manually bring each other to an orgasm at the end of a session if desired.

Exercise 3: Start off with exercises 1 and 2 and engage in loveplay. As arousal builds, use a position of intercourse that feels great for both of you. Enjoy this process without demand as neither worries about erections, which may be lost and re-stimulated. If lost for the evening, don't keep trying but hug and hold and wait until the next time. The goal is not an orgasm but sensuously focusing on the experience of intercourse. Start with slow thrusts that are shallow and slowly penetrate deeper, enjoying the feel. Playfully begin varying the pace with more rapid thrusting. Enjoy this intermittent pattern of slow and rapid, shallow and deep. Come to an orgasm when you are ready.

For a month, combine the three exercises. Relax and be sensual; allow the desire and arousal to build. Keep your energy focused on sexual enjoyment as you allow your body and reflexive nervous system to do its erotic thing. God designed you to be a lover for your mate, if you will get out of your own way.

If trouble recurs with performance anxiety and loss of erection, don't panic. Simply back up to sensual touching and start the process over. Enjoy again the pleasure of touching and being close together as you redirect your emotional energy to making love.

Male malfunctions are not catastrophes—they can be worked through. Other skills can be helpful as you and your mate work through these issues. Learn to communicate effectively and work on expressing emotions. These skills are invaluable for problem solving. Creatively enjoy variety and cultivate the ability to be sensual and create ambiance. Above all, build a loving companionship that is full of playfulness, honesty, and erotic tension.

CHAPTER TWENTY-TWO

Common Female Difficulties

(WITH DEBRA L. TAYLOR, M.A.)

IN AN AMAZING WAY, God created humans a complex interaction of body, mind, emotions, and relationships. Women, unlike men, usually do not compartmentalize these various parts of themselves, but create an interactive whole. Their minds and hearts are probably their most important sex organs. Almost every sex therapy case with wives in our practice has involved some *combination* of emotional, relational, and medical problems. A physical problem (for example, pain with intercourse) will, over time, affect the way a woman feels about herself. These feelings then impact how she treats her partner and how she feels about her marriage, and may ultimately create a marital crisis. This crisis will make the original physical problem worse. It is nearly impossible for women to separate their sexuality from the context of their relationships and their total beings.

The complexity of a woman's sexuality has many facets. These interact to enhance or diminish her interest *in* sex and responsiveness *during* sex:

- health
- previous sexual experiences
- sexual abuse
- family sexual training (or lack of training)
- religious teaching and experiences
- medications
- feelings about her husband and her marriage
- the ages of her children

- energy level
- how she feels about her body and her appearance
- what she believes her husband feels about her body
- hormones

Mary came to see us because she and her husband of ten years had stopped having sex due to her intense vaginal pain. She was forty-five years old, worked full-time as a computer word processor, and had no children. She had taken birth control pills until her late thirties, when her husband had a vasectomy. Her menstrual cycles were irregular, and she had major mood swings until about ten months before coming to see us, when her periods had stopped. Mary was currently having mild hot flashes, but her mood was better. In addition to pain with intercourse, Mary complained of lack of sexual desire. She had tried artificial lubricants, but she still felt like she was being torn apart every time she and her husband attempted intercourse. Her inability to have intercourse and her lack of interest in sex were creating stress and frustration in her marriage.

Mary's mother died of uterine cancer in her early sixties, and Mary's sister had recently been diagnosed with breast cancer. Mary had decided that she would not take estrogen due to the risks associated with her family history of cancer. But she currently was exercising, eating carefully, and taking calcium supplements and other vitamins.

We referred Mary to an ob/gyn who specialized in vulvar pain. When she was examined, the doctor discovered severe genital atrophy. Her labia were thin, and insertion of a small speculum was difficult and extremely painful. She was obviously hormone deficient. Her bone density scan showed loss of bone mass and blood tests confirmed that she was menopausal. Her total testosterone was low and her free testosterone was negligible as well.

Because Mary was unwilling to take estrogen, her physician agreed to topical therapy and started her with estrogen cream daily to build up her vaginal walls. A 2 percent testosterone ointment was prescribed to be applied on the vulva and clitoris to help with desire. She also began taking a selective estrogen that would help prevent osteoporosis without activating estrogen receptors in her breasts or uterus.

Mary and her husband began sex therapy together, starting by increasing nonsexual touching and an agreement not to attempt intercourse. As her vagina became more stretchable, she began using a set of graduated dilators, inserting them daily. She continued using the dilators until she could comfortably insert the largest one with lots of lubrication. Her husband was very supportive and patient, and after four months, they were able to have intercourse. She reported still feeling tightness, but said it was becoming more and more comfortable. Because sex was no longer painful, she was actually looking forward to having intercourse with her husband.

Mary's case illustrates how a physical problem (menopause and hormonal deficiencies) can create a sexual problem (pain with intercourse), which causes more problems (lack of desire and marital stress).

SEXUAL PROBLEMS

Most women will encounter a variety of sexual challenges and difficulties over a lifetime. The most common sexual problems are desire difficulties, arousal difficulties, orgasm difficulties, sexual pain disorders, hormone problems, problems due to medications, blood flow problems, and exhaustion.

Desire Difficulties

If you are not interested in or receptive to sexual touching or having sexual intercourse and this is upsetting to you or is causing relationship problems, you may have a sexual desire problem. Problems with sexual desire can involve never feeling any sexual interest or receptivity, or when you have a lot less interest in sex than you used to. Desire disorders are the most common complaint reported in sexual surveys and the most common reason women seek out sex therapy. However, this sudden "epidemic" of low sexual desire may actually reflect our current cultural bias. Over the past two hundred years we have shifted from expecting "virtuous women" to *lack* all sexual desire to our society's current view that women *should* desire sex at least as *much* as (most) men do.

As this book is being written, researchers, doctors, sex therapists, and writers are working to better understand sexual desire. Pharmaceutical companies are investing vast amounts of money on research to "solve" sexual desire problems. Many current "experts" propose that the problem is not with women's sexual desire as much as the assumption that women's sexual desire and men's sexual desire are or should be the same. In fact, most women in long-term relationships are far more motivated sexually by a desire for intimacy and closeness rather than a desire for physical stimulation or orgasm. (Chapter 18 deals extensively with sexual desire problems.)

Arousal Difficulties

Difficulty with arousal before or during intercourse involves the inability to attain or maintain adequate genital lubrication, swelling, or another physical response such as nipple sensitivity, or sensitivity of the clitoris or labia. Arousal problems may result from emotional stress, such as depression or ongoing marital tension, a lack of sufficient stimulation, or a physical problem such as diminished blood flow to the vagina or clitoris.

Some newlyweds may never have explored their sexual feelings and simply stimulating the clitoral area will not immediately create arousal. These women may need to go through the exercises of Chapter 17 on becoming orgasmic, as they tune in to their sexual identity and feelings—learning the skills of sexual arousal.

Initially, women experiencing low or no arousal with vaginal dryness should try using commercial lubricants, vitamin E, or mineral oils when they engage in sex. Inadequate stimulation contributes to arousal disorders, especially in older women (see Chapter 20, "Sex After Forty-Five"), and may be helped by taking more time to touch each other and fondle, or using a vibrator to increase stimulation. Often women who develop arousal problems are thinking negative thoughts about themselves or their partners while making love. (Most women are not even aware they are doing this negative thinking until they are given the assignment to "listen" to themselves the next time they are sexually involved with their spouses.) Negative thinking *is* a turn-off.

Taking a warm bath before intercourse can help a woman to relax and also may increase arousal. Check your body and your mind for anxiety and distractions. Anxiety inhibits arousal, so exploring and learning anxiety-reduction techniques (deep breaths and making choices about what to focus on) can be helpful. Though not an easy task, arousal is dependent on keeping your body, mind, and heart truly present in your lovemaking.

Orgasm Difficulties

An orgasm is an intense sensation occurring at the peak of sexual arousal and followed by release of sexual tension. Physically, an orgasm is a series of rhythmic muscular contractions of the vagina and uterus accompanied by sharp increases in pulse rate, blood pressure, and breathing rate, and muscle contractions throughout the body.

Some women have never experienced an orgasm (see Chapter 17 for a more complete discussion of becoming more easily orgasmic); others become distressed because their orgasms are less intense than in the past, or delayed. Less intensity may be a natural product of aging; the most common cause of lack of orgasm is insufficient stimulation and arousal. The inability to be orgasmic can also be caused by emotional trauma, sexual abuse, hormone deficiency, and insufficient blood flow or damage to the pelvic nerves due to surgery. Some medications (see Chapter 21, under "Delayed Ejaculation") can slow down the orgasmic response and may need to be changed. Orgasm can also be inhibited by stored-up resentments against your husband.

Sexual Pain Disorders

There are three common types of sexual pain disorders: dyspareunia (pain with intercourse), vaginismus (involuntary muscle spasms of the lower third of the vagina, which interfere with or make it impossible to have intercourse), and vulvodynia (vulvar pain). Other causes of pain with sex include endometriosis and interstitial cystitis.

Dyspareunia. This involves recurrent or persistent genital pain associated with sexual intercourse. It can develop due to vaginal infections, thinning of the vaginal lining during menopause, bladder or urethral infection, pelvic inflammatory disease, endometriosis, some vaginal or vulvar surgical procedures, as well as various psychological issues or relationship problems.

Vulvodynia. This is a syndrome of unexplained vulvar pain, often causing limitation of daily activities, sexual dysfunction, and even physical disability. The vulva consists of the pad of fatty tissue at the base of your abdomen (mons pubis), the labia, the clitoris, and the opening of the vagina. The pain in the genital area can be burning, itching, stinging, or rawness, and may be constant or intermittent and is very sensitive to touch or contact. Because for some women the pain is especially intense in the vestibule (mouth) of the vagina, it is sometimes called vestibulitis. It can last for months or years, but can suddenly vanish.

Prior to the 1980s, vulvodynia was relatively unknown. Many doctors are still unfamiliar with vulvodynia, and patients are often misdiagnosed (and mistreated) or undiagnosed (and untreated). The pain is not always accompanied by visible signs, so many patients are told, "It's all in your head." It is important to be assertive if you or your wife is told this about pelvic pain. I often tell my clients, "No, it is not in your head, it is in your vulva, and it is painful. Find a doctor who will believe you, help you track down the cause of the pain, and help you alleviate the pain!" As more is learned about this syndrome, it is important for patients to work with a knowledgeable doctor, because the type of vulvodynia a patient has affects the treatment significantly.

Depending on the specific diagnosis, treatment may involve oral calcium citrate (Citracal); fluconazole (Diflucan); tricyclic antidepressants (Elavil, Tofranil); anticonvulsants (Tegretol and Neurontin); topical corticosteroids; dietary changes (a low oxalate diet—that is, avoiding beans, beer, beets, berries, celery, chard, chocolate, eggplant, some grapes, green peppers, peanuts, rutabagas, spinach, squash, and tofu); topical estradiol cream; intralesional interferon injection; topical testosterone; physical therapy with biofeedback; surgery (to remove the hypersensitive tissue of the vestibule and hymen); or laser therapy. Because vulvodynia tends to be chronic, attending a support group (www.vulvarpainfoundation.org and others) can be very helpful.

Vaginismus. This is the involuntary contraction of the muscles of the outer one-third of the vagina when penetration is attempted (or with the anticipation of penetration). The muscle spasms can occur only when attempting intercourse, or in some women the spasms also occur during a pelvic exam or when trying to insert a tampon. Vaginismus often develops as a response to painful penetration; it can also be due to past abuse or sexual phobias. (However, the cause is not always clear. We have treated several women who had no known history of sexual abuse or trauma, no especially repressive sexual upbringing, and no explanation for why they experienced this condition.)

Treatment of vaginismus involves progressive muscle relaxation and insertion of gradually larger dilators (or similar objects such as tampons or fingers) into the vagina. Successful treatment requires the woman, and later in treatment the couple, to spend time daily in this relaxation and insertion process. (Treatment for vaginismus has a very high success rate and will be detailed at the end of this chapter.)

Two other pain disorders that affect women's sexuality should also be noted:

Interstitial cystitis. This is a chronic inflammatory condition of the bladder that causes urinary urgency, frequency (sometimes up to fifty times per day), and burning, often accompanied by lower abdominal, vaginal, and rectal pain. The causes are unknown. Interstitial cystitis can be a debilitating disease, often found with sexual dysfunction, particularly vaginal, labial, and pelvic pain as well as arousal and orgasm problems. Approximately 700,000 Americans have IC, and 90 percent are women.

Endometriosis. This occurs when the endometrium (the lining of the uterus that grows during each menstrual cycle and is sloughed off in menstruation) grows in a place other than the uterus. This can happen in the ovaries, fallopian tubes, rectum, bladder, vagina, vulva, cervix, or lymph glands. The most common symptom of endometriosis is very painful periods with excessive bleeding that last an unusually long time. Endometriosis is serious and should be treated by a doctor; it can lead to sterility if left untreated. In some cases hormone therapy or medications can regulate it; in other cases laparoscopic surgery is used to remove the endometrial tissue.

Hormone Problems

Estrogen, progesterone, and testosterone influence women from the time they are developing as fetuses to the time they die. Fetal development, puberty, the ongoing menstrual cycle, pregnancy, postpartum physical and emotional reactions, breast-feeding, perimenopause, and menopause—all of these experiences are shaped by hormones.

Although medical researchers have advanced our knowledge dramatically in the area of hormones, we still have much to learn. For instance, there are still debates regarding hormone replacement therapy and currently a great deal of research is being done on supplemental testosterone in women.

It is normal for a woman to experience loss of desire in the months after giving birth. Some newer research indicates that a percentage of women experience loss of sexual interest for years after the birth of a child. These women, when tested, have almost no testosterone in their systems. Why? Medical science doesn't know yet. It may be an adrenal failure or ovarian problem, or initially, it may be because oxytocin (released when women breast-feed) suppresses testosterone, and without testosterone women have little or no sexual desire.

When a woman breast-feeds, she produces high levels of prolactin. Prolactin stimulates milk production, but it also inhibits ovulation, lowers estrogen levels, and decreases sexual desire. Lowered estrogen over a period of months causes the vaginal lining to become thin and dry (as it does during menopause); therefore, intercourse hurts. We cannot stress enough: when sex is painful, emotionally or physically, DO NOT "PLAY THROUGH THE PAIN." Get help! Painful sex does not get better by ignoring it or trying to play through it. Often, it further traumatizes and creates more sexual difficulties.

Over 80 percent of the two thousand Christian women surveyed in the National Study on the Sexuality of Christian Women (NSSCW—published in *Secrets of Eve*) reported that PMS (premenstrual syndrome) affected their sexual desire. Over 80 percent of these women also said they experienced increased marital conflict during those three to fourteen days prior to the beginning of their periods. With the most common symptoms of PMS being anger, anxiety, edginess, bloating, breast tenderness, clumsiness, depression, difficulty concentrating, emotional volatility, fatigue, headaches, and insomnia, it's not hard to understand why many women experience a drop in sexual desire or sexual responsiveness during this time of the month!

During menopause, most women experience sexual changes due to hormonal shifts. (They also tend to experience a worsening of their PMS symptoms.) Because the ovaries are gradually shutting down, there is less and less estrogen. Vaginal secretions (lubrication) diminish, less blood flows to the vagina (so there is less engorgement of the tissues during arousal), and sometimes nerve apathy develops, leading to numbness. Muscle tone in the vagina declines, and the muscles don't contract as easily (or not at all). Up to 40 percent of menopausal women develop dyspareunia if they do not use some type of estrogen replacement. Though not the total answer, artificial lubrication is a necessity.

Problems with Medications

Throughout this book we have highlighted problems that medications can cause, so we will only briefly discuss medications in this chapter (see Chapter 18 for more information). However, it is imperative that patients keep in mind that *all* medications have side effects, and most have sexual side effects. Often these side effects are not well known or understood, especially with a medication that is relatively new. Also, many doctors are not comfortable talking with their patients about the possible sexual side effects of the drugs they prescribe.

Many drugs have both a direct effect on the brain and central nervous system (CNS) and a local effect on the genitals. Sometimes a drug's action on the brain or CNS may produce contradictory effects on the body, sex organs, and arousal. For example, birth control pills may balance out a woman's hormones but may also decrease testosterone levels and therefore negatively affect sexual desire. Some women find birth control pills increase vaginal lubrication, but others find a decrease in lubrication, more yeast infections, and pain with intercourse. Remember, too, that most medical research in the past was done on males and then (maybe) *applied* to females. There is so much we don't know yet about our sexual physiology and how medications specifically affect women.

Antihypertensives (blood pressure–lowering medications) often cause sexual dysfunction in men, and we hypothesize that they may cause difficulty with arousal and orgasm in women. Recently calcium channel blockers (such as Procardia and Cardizem) have become more popular, partially because they have less effect on sexual functioning.

Antidepressants are well-known culprits in sexual dysfunction (but then, so is depression!). Nearly half of the patients who take the tricyclic antidepressant Anafranil (clomipramine) experience delayed orgasm. The newer SSRI antidepressants Prozac (fluoxetine) and Zoloft (sertraline) cause delayed orgasm or an inability to reach orgasm in as many as 60 percent of the patients who take them. Paxil (paroxetine, also an SSRI) can cause loss of sexual desire.

Sedatives (such as Xanax and Valium) are prescribed to treat anxiety, but they also frequently cause loss of arousal or sexual desire. Antiseizure drugs (such as Dilantin and Tegretol) cause sexual problems and perhaps low sexual desire. Antiulcer drugs (like Tagamet) are highly effective in treating ulcers or serious heartburn and may affect arousal in women (it is known to cause impotence in some men). Antihistamines, such as over-the-counter cold and allergy medications, dry women up—both in their nasal passages and in their vaginas, causing decreased lubrication.

So what do we do if we need to take any of these medications? Patients need to become better informed. Ask your doctor and your pharmacist questions about potential side effects. Be brave—ask about possible sexual side effects! Keep a journal of your reactions, particularly possible sexual changes, when you begin to take any medication. Especially with the busyness of our lives, it can be difficult to remember when a problem began, and whether or not it seemed to coincide with a change in medication. This is especially true when you consider that some effects only show up as a medication reaches its "therapeutic dose" in your body— sometimes as much as six weeks after you begin to take it!

Ask your doctor (and pharmacist) what alternatives there may be for a medication prescribed for you—is there a similar medication that has fewer sexual side effects, or even a sex-positive effect (such as the antidepressant Welbutrin [bupropion] instead of Prozac)?

Blood Flow Problems

Arousal, engorgement, and lubrication are affected by low blood flow to the pelvis. The most common causes of low blood flow are coronary heart disease, high blood pressure, high cholesterol, and smoking.

More than half of all women in the U.S. over sixty-five have high blood pressure. It is the most common chronic illness in the United States. High blood pressure is the abnormal increased pressure of blood flowing in the arteries as they feed our organs and tissues. In most people the cause is unknown. Factors that contribute to high blood pressure are a high-fat diet, being overweight, a lack of exercise, and heredity. It is well known that high blood pressure is one of the chief causes of male erectile dysfunction. We hypothesize that women also experience damage to the blood vessels due to high blood pressure, making them more susceptible to the buildup of fatty deposits (plaque) along the inside walls of the arteries, and therefore more prone to coronary heart disease. High blood pressure in women probably causes decreased pelvic and genital blood flow, and contributes to decreased sexual arousal, decreased vaginal lubrication, and pain.

Exhaustion

It is important to understand how crucial a woman's energy level is to her sexual health. Many men can be dead-tired and still be interested in having sex with their wives; most women report that feeling tired wipes out sexual desire, and for some, the ability to experience physical arousal and orgasm.

The average woman barely gets six and a half hours of sleep most nights. "So, what's the big deal?" you may ask. Almost all human beings need eight or more hours of sleep per night for optimal functioning. Sleep research shows that blood supply to our muscles increases during deep sleep, allowing the body to recover from the physical stresses of the day. Chronic sleep loss may speed some aspects of aging, can alter hormone levels, and can affect the body's ability to burn carbohydrates. Disruption in certain types of sleep lowers the pain threshold in women with fibromyalgia, arthritis, and headaches. Sleep deprivation causes crankiness and forgetfulness. Obviously an energized lover and fun lovemaking correlate to sleep and being rested.

While most surveys report that the most common sexual difficulty of women is lack of desire, one of the surprising findings of the NSSCW was that the most common difficulty reported by these two thousand women was "difficulty finding the energy for sex." Comments from the participants underscore this struggle, such as "I just don't have the energy to be bothered with sex. This may only be temporary, but right now I don't even care if it is or it isn't"; and "Since having children, ages 3, 4, and 6, I find it hard to summon the desire and energy for sex. I sometimes wonder if this is normal. After kids all day the last thing I want is more physical contact (sex) at night. When we first married, I wanted sex more than my husband—now it is reversed, and he's frustrated and feels the withdrawal of my love and support. Help! Will this change?"

This comment about small children is representative of many of the written comments we received from mothers. Over half of the women with children living at home, especially small children, had greater difficulty finding the energy for sex. As our culture speeds up, dictating to families that they become busier and busier, this problem with exhaustion will only get worse. Apparently, this busyness and tiredness is affecting not just women, but men as well: "We both don't have the energy to be troubled about sex. We both work at full-time jobs and come home exhausted every evening. On weekends, church and our kids consume all our free time. Sunday evenings we can hardly make it to bed and often fall asleep exhausted in front of the TV. Will we ever escape this frenzied cycle?"

The answer to that question is no. Not without some serious communication, review of priorities, major lifestyle changes, and then the discipline to follow through on those decisions.

TREATING PAINFUL INTERCOURSE

Prior to visiting your gynecologist, think through some of the facts surrounding your pain and identify its onset: Did it begin after a painful honeymoon (or first intercourse) experience? Or after childbirth? Or a surgery?

Think about your attitudes surrounding sexuality. Did your parents talk with you about sex? Was your upbringing open and communicative or restrictive? Has sex always seemed wrong, dirty, or intimidating? Was there sexual abuse or painful (emotionally or physically) sexual experiences?

How do you feel about pregnancy? Do you want to have children (or possibly, more children), or are you afraid of becoming pregnant?

Have you ever had a vaginal infection? A sexually transmitted disease (STD)? Have you had sex with more than one partner, and if so, were you tested for sexually transmitted diseases? Women, especially, often contract an STD but have no symptoms.

When and where does the pain occur during lovemaking? What is its intensity? (Think in terms of a continuum: mild, to somewhat painful, to painful, to extremely painful, to excruciating.) Does the pain begin as you experience arousal, or is it as the penis enters the vagina? Is it with all types of thrusting, or only with deep or rapid thrusting? Does the pain increase with orgasm? Does it remain after intercourse?

After thinking through these questions, tell your physician details about the pain. Careful medical diagnosis and treatment are necessary for treatment to be successful. Sometimes your general practitioner can provide this care, but it may take the specialized attention of a dermatologist, gynecologist, or surgeon. In selecting a physician, be a good consumer. The following are fair demands:

- To be treated with respect
- To have a nurse present
- To be properly gowned or draped
- To have adequate time taken for the exam and for questions to be answered
- To have questions answered in language you understand and each problem carefully

explained. Explanation should be given as to the diagnosis and prognosis. If any procedures are recommended or medications prescribed, these should be explained and possible side effects described.

- To know the exact cost of each medical or surgical procedure, its probability of success, and a general idea of the recuperation time and physical discomfort during and after the procedure
- To have questions answered regarding the physician's experience in treating your condition, and the number of surgeries of this type that the physician has performed. This may also include inquiring into her or his training in this area.

Try to develop a supportive relationship with your doctor. Be *persistent* in finding the cause of your pain and the proper treatment for it. Exercise your right to change doctors to get the best care you can.

Although most of the physical causes of pain will need a physician's attention, you can make some interventions on your own. If you are fairly certain you have a yeast infection, some medications can be purchased over-the-counter. If you have used a new lubricant or spermicide and develop irritation or pain, try changing to another brand.

Commonsense Interventions

Keep on hand plenty of artificial lubricant, which is sold in most pharmacies and even in grocery stores, in a gel or a more liquid form. You can also use natural oils, from coconut or almond to olive oil. These are edible, don't interfere with oral stimulation of the genitals, and also may be appealing for scent or consistency. Vegetable oils (corn or safflower) work fine if you have forgotten to purchase another type. The advantage of artificial lubricants is that they are often water soluble and easier for the vagina to self-cleanse. Use lubricants generously when the vagina is irritated or there is anxiety. It is amazing how much pain can be prevented by using common sense!

Gentle and *slow* are crucial words in overcoming painful intercourse. Creating a safe and tender atmosphere is important in dealing with stress and tension. Unwind together. Work on relaxing and being playful. Allow the wife to set the pace, with plenty of time for loveplay and arousal before attempting intercourse. Try using a position (such as wife on top) that lets her control penetration and depth. Take your time and enjoy the process. Be imaginative in creating ambiance.

Stop when there is pain! Shift your position. Stop thrusting, or stop deep thrusting. Prop a small pillow underneath the hips or lower back, use more lubrication, or go back to loving, playful caressing. Relax again. Use your creativity, but *never* ignore the discomfort. Continuing with painful intercourse and hoping it will just go away almost always increases the problem.

If no immediate intervention helps, stop making love and just hold each other, or bring each other to orgasm in other ways until the problem can be checked out medically.

Use birth control wisely and increase precautions if the possibility of pregnancy is a source of anxiety during intercourse. The husband may need to get a vasectomy, or the wife may need to consider tubal ligation. Discuss together how you might handle an unexpected pregnancy.

Both partners may need to utilize greater care and take responsibility for birth control. Some couples have conflict about the type of birth control they use, or resent that only one is responsible for it. Talk together on how to make birth control a more unified decision. Be honest. *Never* lie to your partner by "forgetting" to take your birth control pill. Carry your birth control with you; if it is important to you not to become pregnant, don't take chances. Sexual passion can be wonderfully strong, but you are never "out of control." Pregnancy doesn't "just happen"!

Psychological Interventions

If you were raised in an environment where sex was never discussed or was considered "bad" or "dirty," undertake a personal education program. Reading a book like this one and doing the exercises with your mate will be very helpful. Communicating about sex and developing a comfortable language will assist you in becoming more at ease with sexuality as well. Tune in to your self-talk, your fears and inhibitions about sex. On your own, examine your beliefs about your sexuality and the "meaning" you have developed about sex. Do you know how God feels about sex? Do you feel as He does? (That is, that He created sex as a wedding gift for you, to be used throughout your married life for unity, for connection, for fun, for comfort . . . you get the idea.) Do you need to commit to constructing a new "meaning" for sex in your life?

A loving, empathetic partner can be a marvelous sounding board, or you may need to talk with a same-gender friend who will truly listen to you in a way your spouse cannot. Talking can help you get beyond embarrassment. There is no question or topic too silly or taboo to discuss and resolve.

Spouses who employ their creativity and work together to increase their enjoyment of sex don't always need professional intervention or a sex therapist. Increase your enjoyment of your senses; learn to tease and to play together. Read passages aloud from this book, or from the Song of Solomon (in a modern translation) to desensitize yourself and to become more sexually open. Enjoy the exercises recommended in this book: take showers together, become comfortable with nakedness, have picnics in bed, plan sexual surprises, and get into sensual massage. Let making love and enjoying your bodies permeate your relationship.

Survivors of sexual abuse often need specific therapy to help them deal with unresolved feelings and reactions that impede sexual pleasure. Professional counseling may also be needed to deal with the guilt of a sex-negative religious background or to resolve premarital or honeymoon experiences. Extramarital affairs can be crippling and need an experienced marriage counselor.

Never feel inferior if you cannot work out problems on your own. Maturity allows us to reach out for the help and wisdom we need. God created persons with different gifts and gives individuals the intelligence, skills, and abilities to help us. Don't settle for living with the pain—physically or emotionally.

Desensitization Exercise for Painful Intercourse

A couple experiencing painful intercourse becomes sensitized to pain and begins to expect it. With the following exercises, you are going to stop associating pain and fear with intercourse. It is possible to address the physical causes and the emotional causes of painful intercourse, but to still have your body and mind react automatically with anxiety to the idea of lovemaking. You need to desensitize your mind and body—to change their expectation from pain to pleasure.

Schedule at least thirty minutes for each of the following steps. Each step may need to be broken into a series of practice sessions. Repeat each step twice or as many times as needed. Allow these three exercises to stretch out over two or three weeks. Do not try to rush this process. You may need to take a week or a month prior to beginning the exercises to hug nude, caress, and enjoy loveplay to become comfortable and relaxed together.

Step 1. Engage in loveplay that is relaxing and fun for ten to twenty minutes, allowing emotional bonding and sexual arousal to take place. Liberally apply lubricant to the opening of the vagina and the head of the penis. Choose a position in which the woman can touch and guide the penis as she brushes the penis over the inner lips, lightly touching it to the opening of the vagina without penetration. (This may be as much desensitization as is possible in the first session. If so, stop. Proceed to the next part of this exercise in the next session.) Under the wife's direction, touch the head of the penis to the opening of the vagina, then let the head of the penis enter the vagina an inch; stop, gently leaving the penis there for several minutes. Remove and apply more lubrication. Now slowly penetrate two inches. Repeat this procedure to three and four inches, knowing it may take several sessions to reach this point. Apply more lubrication and insert until the penis is fully contained in the vagina. Leave it there until the erection begins to ebb. If there is pain at any point, stop. Touch and enjoy each other's bodies again for several minutes, then proceed with the exercise, or wait until the next session. Do not start any thrusting with this experience. Manually stimulate each other to orgasm at the end of the session, if you want to.

Step 2. Repeat the slow containment of the penis from step 1. Again, apply plenty of lubrication and proceed slowly and gently. When the penis is fully contained, remove and apply more lubrication. Now start with shallow penetration, and slowly thrust ten or fifteen times to a depth of an inch or so. Remove the penis and apply more lubrication; thrust slowly at a depth of two inches. Remove and apply more lubrication if needed; softly thrust with full penetration. Use as many practice sessions as you need to accomplish this step. If there is any pain, *stop*, touch and caress each other, then go back to thrusting at a more shallow depth. Do not attempt to ejaculate with intercourse; instead bring each other to climax manually or orally.

Step 3. Enjoy loveplay and apply lubrication as you begin with gentle penetration and slow thrusting in the outer two inches of the vagina ten to fifteen times. Remove the penis and lubricate as you thrust halfway ten to fifteen times—then fully penetrate and slowly thrust. Now try more rapid thrusting at a shallow depth. Remove the penis, lubricate, and enjoy thrusting deeper, being careful not to cause any pain. If there is pain, try to shift positions or thrust more shallowly or more gently. If the husband is having trouble refraining from ejaculation, stop and allow his arousal to subside, then continue. Allow the husband to reach orgasm, and manually bring the wife to orgasm if she has not climaxed.

You get the idea of desensitizing. You are gradually, carefully having intercourse with adequate arousal and lubrication. If there is pain, stop or shift as you make sure this experience is relaxed, pain-free, and unpressured. Take as many practice sessions as you need to accomplish all three steps comfortably. You will find that reaching a goal (for example, the head of the penis in the vagina) does not automatically ensure you can start at that point in your next session or that you can proceed further. Growth can be slow, and you may have to reach a goal several times before the desensitization is permanent.

Overcoming Vaginismus

The following program will help overcome vaginismus. The wife should do the first two exercises alone; the husband should be included for the last two exercises.

Exercise 1. Take a warm bath, and adjust the bedroom temperature so it is comfortable to be naked. Lock the door to assure your privacy. Take a finger and lubricate it well; place it at the mouth of the vagina. Allow any emotional or physical tension to subside. (With each step, take a few deep breaths and let them out slowly through your mouth. Relax and expel the tension through the exhaled breath.) Gently insert the end of the finger, just slightly penetrating, and leave it there as you breathe and relax. Do not remove the finger for five minutes or more as you become used to an object being in the vagina. Now insert your finger to the first knuckle and again leave the finger there; relax. If the vaginal muscles start to spasm, stop and slowly breathe as you relax. (Note: for some women an inanimate object like a tampon, syringe cap, or some type of dilator is less threatening than an animate finger; varying sizes of candles can be purchased inexpensively and utilized with condoms over them—then proceed to fingers.)

To get a greater feeling of control, practice deliberately tightening the PC muscle on your finger as in the Kegel exercises. (See Chapter 17, "Women Becoming More Easily Orgasmic," for explanation.) Repeat this part of the exercise two more times, inserting the finger more deeply into the vagina, stopping each time to breathe deeply; do the Kegels and become more acclimated to an object being in the vagina. Repeat this exercise daily or several times per week over the coming weeks.

Exercise 2. Take a bath and get comfortable. Start with one finger deeply penetrated into the vagina (always use plenty of lubrication). Hold the finger in place and relax with deep, slow breaths. Wiggle the finger inside the vagina, relaxing and acclimating to the different sensation. Now slowly insert two fingers to the first knuckle. Stop for five or more minutes; allow yourself to relax, and acclimate to the new feelings. Insert the fingers farther; relax. Move the two fingers, breathing deeply and relaxing.

Exercise 3. The husband now becomes a part of this process. He must listen to the wife's instructions, with encouragement and patience. Relax together and touch each other's bodies in pleasurable ways. Lubricate the husband's fingers (make sure the fingernails and cuticles are clipped—place a condom over finger if needed); begin with one finger, inserting it slowly. Hold the husband's finger in the wife's vagina for five minutes; relax. Follow the procedure in exercises 1 and 2, but use the husband's finger instead of the wife's. Once he can insert two fingers comfortably, he should move the fingers gently inside the vagina, with the wife relaxing, until this is comfortable. It may take weeks or even months to accomplish this exercise.

Exercise 4. Now you are ready to begin becoming comfortable with the feel of the penis. Do this by going through the exercises in the preceding section on desensitizing.

It may take two months to slowly work through these exercises, even after you have done preliminary months of therapy and sexual growth. It may take you longer—that is *fine*. If there is pain or anxiety at any point along the way, be prepared to go back to caressing, holding each other, and sensual touching, then continue with the exercises.

Remember, *never* try to tolerate pain in lovemaking and intercourse. Pain needs to be explored medically and resolved through treatment or therapy. If you are already trapped in the vicious cycle of anxiety, fear, tension, or pain, work out the emotional and physical parts of the problem first. Then slowly move through the desensitizing exercises. If you get stuck, seek out therapy. You are not alone, and pleasurable sexual intercourse can be yours to enjoy. Don't give up! Persist!

CHAPTER TWENTY-THREE

Making Love When You Have a Disability

DISABILITIES GREATLY IMPACT many couples' lives and relationships. Lovemaking may be a part of the fallout, but a good sex life can still be created. A committed, loving relationship factors in as the most important part of making love, and this can actually deepen with the interdependence of struggling through a disability. The mind is the key sexual organ and it can help you build new sexual sensations, attitudes, and techniques.

The frustrating news for the person or couple with a disability is the same for any couple facing new challenges in their marriage (children, aging): you will have to work to learn additional skills, build more erotic fantasy, and tailor your own warm, unique, and exciting lovemaking together.

This first section explores five needed skills to enhance lovemaking. The second section considers temporary disabilities, the nondisabled spouse, the effect of medications, preparation for lovemaking, and pregnancy. Section three lists practical suggestions for increasing sexual enjoyment, and the final section looks more specifically at three categories of disabilities: birth defects, accidents and injuries, and illnesses.

FIVE NECESSARY SKILLS

Every person with chronic pain, muscular dystrophy, or cancer has not faced the same journey. Disabilities and varying levels of severity present different challenges in roles and attitudes of males or females. But there is much commonality in working through a disability to a fulfilling sex life. Certain skills make a difference if learned and employed consistently. This section discusses five of them.

1. Creating a Positive Sexual Self-Image

Everyone struggles at times with body image and the comfortable enjoyment of masculinity or femininity. This can be especially true of a disability, but please don't let this label and color you as a lover. You don't have a big "D" on your chest. You have a special personality and the ability to play and be very sexy and romantic. It is an exciting phenomenon that we have the ability to become what we think we are. Our attitudes and beliefs about ourselves are crucial. (It may help to read Chapter 16 on body image and feeling sexy.)

Two men can have gone through a similar set of experiences and be in wheelchairs. One likes himself and thinks he is an interesting and attractive man. He comes across that way and is appealing to the opposite sex. The other man is insecure and angry. He does not think he is special or sexy. He also comes across that way. Being sexy has to do with an attitude and not the way the body looks.

Granted, the disabled person faces unique challenges. You may have to be in a more dependent role than you desire. Mobility and autonomy may be limited, with someone helping to attend to your bodily functions or your spouse assuming a more active physical role in making love. Unless you expand your concept of masculinity or femininity, you may constantly be threatened.

Develop your masculine or feminine soul with the character traits of a great lover: the ability to be playful, honest, gently loving and nurturing, forgiving, and self-disciplined. These characteristics are essential for becoming an accomplished sexual partner and truly sexy, whether disabled or nondisabled. Real masculinity or femininity is based on being a creation in God's image and goes way beyond body parts or disabilities.

Sex is also much more than intercourse, certain physical activities, or the ability to have an orgasm. You can kiss and have stimulating arousal strapped into a hospital bed. Persons who have paraplegia, a hearing impairment, a visual handicap, or a similar disability can be intensely sensual and develop differing senses in ways that others don't. Making love is a marvelous personal and relationship quality that doesn't have to be lost through physical problems. Challenge your attitudes and develop your tremendous potential in new and creative ways. Do some self-talk as you work through to liking yourself and being gently confident in ways that draw others to you.

2. Communicating

If you want to live as a comfortable friend and lover, learn to communicate with your spouse about the loss of personal control and many other emotionally loaded topics. Certain disabilities require you to rely on others when dealing with bodily wastes, handling menstrual cycles, or choosing when to pass gas is often taken out of your hands and made a public matter.

Talk to your mate, become excellent sounding boards for each other, and learn how to dialogue. (See Chapter 8 on communication-skill building for a more developed discussion of these principles.) In dialogue, one partner keeps quiet and carefully listens while the other partner assertively expresses needs and feelings. The one who stays quiet focuses on the message being communicated—trying to walk in the other's shoes. The listener detaches from his or her personal feelings or the need for a rebuttal—trying to clarify and really understand the message. The speaker puts the message into assertive, responsible, and courteous "I" language ("I feel hurt when you don't initiate making love to me, and I wonder if I'm still attractive to you") and not blaming "you" language ("You don't ever make love anymore—you must hate me").

A great listener is sure he or she has objectively contained personal opinions and has focused on and understood the message; the listener will then make an empathy statement before giving a rebuttal. (An empathy statement is only about twenty seconds and tells your mate that you are acknowledging his or her reality—you are not saying that your mate is right, but you are giving a little summary that conveys you understand and acknowledge the other's perception of things.)

You will often hear some of the same feelings, needs, and struggles over and over. Remain an active listener as you help your mate work through grief and other issues to a better sense of resolution. Express and process your feelings; you are having to deal with some very tough and private issues, which may be laden with anger, despondency, excitement, sadness, helplessness, and hope. Understand and work through these feelings to a deeper sense of intimacy.

Take the time and energy to talk about the structure of your sex life. You are into a new and challenging era that will take creative problem solving. Provide courage and romantic creativity for each other as you find different ways to make love. Talk through possible ways to adapt moves, and brainstorm on solutions to overcome the disabilities. You will find good communication invaluable as you determine not to lose God's wonderful gift of sexuality within your intimate companionship.

3. Expanding Your Senses and Knowledge of Sexuality

We all have a body and mind that God created to enjoy pleasure, but we use only about one-third of their full sensual capacity. Individuals and couples need to more fully allow their bodies to take in sensual pleasure—which so easily spills over into their sexual lives. Look more carefully and take in colors, textures, and the visual joy around you. Go to a decorated mall or a botanical garden and revel in the sights. Stop and listen, with your eyes closed, to the world around you. Surround yourself with music, or go to a stock car race and hear and feel the power permeating the air. Eat more slowly as you notice the tastes and smells. Visit coffee shops or bakeries, buy some potpourri, eat spicy, ethnic foods, or enjoy a new perfume. Go through your house and touch the objects with your mind focused on your fingertips. Enjoy smooth and rough, cold and hot, soft and hard, oily and dry.

We are still learning how the brain takes in and stores information. It is exciting how one sense can be disabled and another will expand. The person who is blind develops a keener sense of hearing and touch; the person who is paralyzed from the waist down takes on greater sensuality with chest, neck, and face. A part of this is the concept of phantom feelings or the power of the mind. The person with an amputated arm may still feel itches and pain on occasion. In a similar way, the person with no sensation in the genital area can experience a phantom orgasm within the sexual cycle as excitement builds. Different sexual behaviors and parts of the body can take on new meaning—creating a sense of warm closeness or exciting arousal.

All lovers have to continually work at staying out of routines and expanding their sexual behaviors and mental store of erotic images. Mates with disabilities need to expand their sensuality and modify behaviors as their lovemaking grows in its arousal and joy. Become more creative, sensual, and varied. Your lovemaking can surpass the meaning, variety, and enjoyment of the nondisabled couple, who take so much for granted.

4. Choosing Optimal Times

Understanding medications and using medical advice. Medications can help you feel more like making love. The person with arthritis or other types of disability might want to have sex when the medication is having maximum effect. Likewise, the person on dialysis will feel better right after the treatment, before the toxins have begun to build up again—this can be a much better time to enjoy sex. Creatively discuss and work through your special situation with your mate as you both increase your ability to make love meaningfully.

Medications can also have a negative effect, creating less desire for sex or reduced ability to perform. You must learn to minimize the negative side effects of some medications (for example, antidepressants, painkillers, blood thinners, and blood pressure treatments). At times medications can be changed to a different brand that has fewer physical side effects on you. With some medications, making love right before taking them will lessen their effects, or perhaps it is possible to periodically reduce the dosage or take a brief drug "vacation." Consult with your physician about skipping one day of medication in order to make love.

Ask specific sexual questions of your medical doctor about what is permitted physically and what is not. Ask for and find pamphlets on your particular disability. Be an informed lover and determine what physical sensations and types of sexual activity are possible as you maximize lovemaking.

Planning that enhances romance. You will enjoy sex more when you are rested, relaxed, and able to focus on your sensual feelings. You will have to consider more than just medications. For the person with spinal cord injury or with spina bifida, it will be necessary to plan around urination and catheterization. For the person with paraplegia or quadriplegia, if your mate helps you dilate the rectum for bowel movements, wait several hours and allow that to be separate from being lovers and making love. Like any couple with a dynamic marriage and sex life, you will have to use your creativity and common sense to create timing and energy for lovemaking.

Prioritize may become a theme word. The energy to do what you used to do probably won't be there. Face those important difficult questions: What can I let go of? What do I want to save energy for today? Quality lovemaking will depend on your planning.

5. Grieving

Elisabeth Kubler-Ross and other psychological researchers have demonstrated that people go through various stages and feelings when they are grieving a loss. You and your partner may have experienced multiple losses: the marriage as it was, autonomy, dreams and expectations, sexual self-image, and mutual health—to name a few. The one-flesh companionship has been shaken up in many ways, and the sexual part may be most obvious.

The first reactions in grieving are usually shock and denial. You can't believe this is happening to you. Then come anger, bargaining, and depression as the reality settles in. The anger may be at God or at any available target. You may bargain with God and ask God to take away the disability with the promise that you will make drastic changes. Withdrawal into isolation may occur as the issues are worked through. Eventually, the disability is accepted and equilibrium returns. However, life has a way of triggering the losses over and over again, so flashbacks into the grieving process are likely.

Sometimes Christians get stuck in the grieving process as they engage in self-pity or hope for God to miraculously cure them. There is no way around this grief. The point is to work your way through it to acceptance and healing and new alternatives. If you repress the tears and anger, they will come back to haunt you later. The nondisabled mate will have to find the time and space to grieve, too—you cannot stay strong for your partner throughout the whole process.

Build a solid support network that you can lean on. Christ designed the church to fulfill this role of being a healer. Allow your loving brothers and sisters to take you up in their arms and hold you while you angrily yell at God and uncontrollably give in to your tears over the injustice that you are experiencing. With sin in the world, bad things happen to good people, and that is what God gave us the grieving process for—to slowly work our way through the pain and hurt of life's unfairness until we heal.

IMPORTANT AREAS TO CONSIDER

Most couples will experience temporary disabilities and the side effects of medication, especially as they grow older. Both partners have necessary roles in taking the initiative for remaining sexual and encouraging needed adaptations.

Temporary Disabilities

Most couples will encounter some physical disability during the course of their marriages. Some of them—a complicated pregnancy, pneumonia, broken bones, yeast infections, a heart attack, or surgery—are temporary in nature. But unless you make the necessary adjustments in your lovemaking, these temporary conditions can completely shut down your sex life to the detriment of your marriage and intimacy. Temporary disabilities can create long-term effects in the love life of a couple.

Much of this chapter, which is primarily addressed to persons with permanent disabilities, will also apply to those of you with temporary disabilities—as you creatively enjoy different but satisfying lovemaking sessions. You may have to adapt and focus on sexual activities other than vigorous intercourse and the pursuit of orgasms as you learn to caress and hold each other and be close emotionally and physically. I remember cracked ribs and intense pain when I stupidly placed a ladder on wet leaves and fell ten feet. Sex became a lot more gentle.

Don't assume that you must forgo sex for the duration of the temporary disability. Talk to your physician and learn about your physical condition, whether it is high blood pressure, a hysterectomy, broken ribs, or poison ivy. Don't be embarrassed to ask specifically about making love; plan on being as sexually active as you can—despite the temporary disability.

Overcoming Dual Disabilities

Sometimes both partners will have disabilities. In this case, there will be a need for extra creativity and a willingness to reach out practically for help from people outside the marriage. Each should avoid prejudice against the other's disability. It is unfortunate but true that sometimes a disabled mate can have more difficulty dealing with a partner's disability than a nondisabled mate. With maturity and wisdom, each can be an even more empathetic source of encouragement and motivation for the other than a nondisabled mate. (Much of what is written in this chapter applies to a marriage with dual disabilities.)

The Nondisabled Partner

The feelings of the nondisabled partner will range all over the map, much as those of the partner with the disability, from despair to optimism (sometimes false optimism over a possible cure), from anger and discouragement to joy and pleasure. Sometimes it may be difficult to switch from the role of nursing or helping your mate with the disability to being a passionate lover.

As the nondisabled partner, you will probably have to assume a more active physical (not emotional) role sensually. You may have been asked to do things, like dealing with bowel or bladder accidents or perhaps trying types of oral stimulation, that you might have found unpleasant in the past. New behaviors will be required as you pleasure your mate. As lovers, learning new and effective lovemaking techniques is seldom comfortable or smooth, whether you are disabled or not. It may be helpful to talk to a therapist or a physical occupation counselor regarding any problems. But whatever you do, don't treat your partner as fragile. You need to process your feelings, too, as you work through to practical solutions in your lovemaking.

Stay creative and pray for extra strength. Your stamina and hope will be essential commodities, especially if your mate is adjusting to a recent disability and is reeling from the blows to self-image. Create an effective support network for both of you as you affirm your sexual partnership. Marital trauma and even divorce can occur because of lack of knowledge. Remember that because you wish your spouse felt better or the fact that he or she seems to look better doesn't matter. Keep seeking out information and courageously facing reality because your mate may have a disability that doesn't always show (Lupus, MS).

Medication

Many sexual problems caused by medications are often caused not by the disability but by the medication required because of the disability—or perhaps by the medication required to deal with the depression caused by the reaction to the disability. You cannot just stop taking the medication, but you should be aware of possible sexual side effects. Check with your pharmacist or physician so that you can be informed of any negative effects of particular medications; each one reacts differently with various body chemistries, and a given medication may not negatively affect you.

Common sexual problems are loss of or decreased sexual desire, impotence in the male or inadequate lubrication in the female, less physical sensation in the genital area, more difficulty in achieving or decreased intensity in orgasm, delay or pain in ejaculating, and priapism (a sustained erection to the point of being painful). Some common drugs that have side effects are certain tranquilizers, antidepressants, hypertension medications, blood thinners, stomach and digestive treatments, and chemotherapy. (Read the body busters in Chapter 18 to gain more knowledge.)

Sometimes one medication can be exchanged for another that will have fewer side effects on a given individual. There may be a period of time before taking the medication that is more conducive for making love, or the possibility of taking a drug vacation. Creating atmosphere and being rested can increase libido as well, and increased stimulation time can offset lack of genital response. Also, the male can still have an orgasm and ejaculate without an erection. Like other challenges to a great sex life, problems caused by medications must be met with knowledge and creative alternatives.

Preparation for Sex

The couple with a disability will have more things to remember in getting ready to make love. Like other couples, you will have to plan things like birth control and artificial lubrication. It is wise to have towels and other cleanup needs handy for those inevitable accidents that will occur. You will also have to sort through timing and use optimum minutes or hours that can enhance lovemaking.

Don't neglect having a water-soluble lubricant available (and use it liberally with continual application because it will dry out). Some brands like Wet or Astroglide seem to last longer than K-Y Jelly. Most water-soluble lubricants are glycerin based and cause a reaction in some people; using vegetable or natural oils may be an acceptable alternative. Women with spinal cord injuries or diabetes will have nerve or circulatory problems that prevent natural lubrication. These women can be more susceptible to vaginal and urinary tract infections that cause subsequent problems with intercourse. Stress, grief, pain, and other aspects of a disability can also prevent adequate lubrication.

Take care of bladder and bowel needs prior to making love, especially if intercourse is involved. Often in today's medicine, if there is an indwelling Foley catheter, intercourse may be inadvisable as a result. If a condom catheter is being used, it can be removed immediately prior to intercourse. In the case of spina bifida and some other disabilities in which intermittent catheterization may be needed, it is important for females to catheterize and empty the bladder both before and immediately after intercourse. This step can help prevent cystitis and other infections.

Bowel needs can often be taken care of well in advance of making love. Sometimes it may not be possible to remove an ostomy bag, but you can drape a towel over it if you prefer. Don't forget as you prepare to make love that sexiness originates in the mind. Create a mood and revel in your sexual power and attractiveness as you look forward to making love with your mate.

Pregnancy

A disability generally does not affect fertility—but with some it does. Certain spinal cord injuries in men or some chemotherapy may nullify the possibility of creating children. Some illnesses such as breast cancer or those requiring medications that could affect the baby may render it inadvisable to become pregnant. It is also necessary to be careful with birth control and guard against an unwanted pregnancy. Sometimes the disabled person can have an adverse physical sensitivity and reaction to latex condoms or antispermicidal chemicals, so you must exercise caution.

Practical considerations of whether or not to have children must be faced with the mind and not the heart. With the disability, will there be a way to adequately provide for a child's care? If it is a life-threatening illness, is it fair to bring into the world a child who is likely to be raised by a single parent? Can you as mother-to-be go off certain medications without serious emotional or physical threats to your health? Is there a high risk to the child that the disability will be genetically passed on? This is actually a very low probability—but could you raise a disabled child?

The woman with spina bifida or a spinal cord injury is capable of conceiving and carrying a child through pregnancy. But she must monitor medications and health concerns and kidney and bladder functions and avoid infections. Having damaged nerves doesn't mean that tissue and organs are not functioning healthily. Thus a woman with a spinal cord injury may not be able to feel the beginning of labor pains, but a monitoring device can be utilized to signal when they occur.

The male with disabilities may not be able to father a child because of lack of ejaculation or infertility caused by fever or testicle damage. With a lack of erection (for example, from diabetes), an ejaculation can sometimes occur, and artificial insemination allows the semen to be placed in the wife's vagina at the mouth of the cervix or within the uterus. There is also a technique called electroejaculation in which the doctor takes the semen out of the body by electric stimulation. With spinal cord injuries, benign prostate hypertrophy, and prostate surgeries, occasionally retrograde ejaculation occurs: the semen goes back into the bladder instead of out through the penis. It is sometimes possible to separate fertile sperm from the urine and use them in artificial insemination.

If you want a child, carefully think through what childbearing and child rearing would mean. Explore the possibility of fertility and take advantage of modern medicine.

PRACTICAL SUGGESTIONS

Making love as a couple with disabilities will necessitate creativity and knowledge. Here are some further words of advice and points to think through and discuss.

Love Through the Pain

Sometimes your mate may want to make love despite feeling some physical pain. Learn to enjoy together times that may be less than optimal. With careful communication, you can be sensitive to your mate's needs and know when to engage and when to stop. You may have to do more of the stimulation, but it can still be mutually enjoyable. Sometimes your disabled mate may want only to be held or lovingly caressed, which still gives opportunity for closeness. At other times your disabled partner may wish to nurture you but not become fully involved. Learn to recognize those special times when it is important to make love as you play through the pain and discomfort.

Creatively take steps to minimize the pain with strategically propped pillows or taking pain medication right before lovemaking. One friend told how much neck support and pillows that supported elbows and knees assisted. She never thought of assembling props as a part of lovemaking before her disability. Learn new positions of intercourse that decrease stress on joints or muscles; the nondisabled partner can take the more active lead as both of you stay practically creative.

Acquire Adaptive Creativity

Sex will be different, but don't assume that there is a different set of lovemaking techniques for disabled couples. Much of what is discussed in this book—especially the ideas of utilizing your imagination and learning new ways to be sensual—applies across the board to lovers. If you are more recently disabled, don't abandon all that you used to do. It might take some creativity and adaptation, but you may still enjoy these exciting or warmly connecting techniques. Don't accept a label and think you are incapable of "normal" sex—whatever that is. Like any couple, enjoy your sensuality and cultivate a wide repertoire of exciting behaviors.

Develop Expectations and Humor Concerning Accidents

You will pass gas sometimes while making love, or you may have a bladder accident. But then, so do couples without a disability. Expecting and preparing for accidents helps prevent you from overreacting when they do occur. Making love demands that you keep a sense of humor because the unusual and funny will happen often. Frustration can reign, or you can laugh and allow the intimacy to go on unbroken. Great sex is built on being playful companions; take the mishaps and mistakes in stride.

THREE CATEGORIES OF DISABILITIES

Most disabilities can be listed under three broad categories:

1. *Birth defects:* spina bifida, cystic fibrosis, cerebral palsy, mental disabilities, sensory deficits (blindness, deafness)

2. *Accidents and injuries:* chronic pain, spinal cord injuries, traumatic brain injury, loss of limb or mobility, sensory loss (sight, hearing)

3. *Illnesses:* cancer (breast, prostate, uterine, testicular, and so on), endometriosis, heart attack, stroke, arthritis, depression, diabetes, chronic fatigue syndrome, lupus, fibromyalgia, muscular dystrophy (genetic but often doesn't appear until adulthood), and multiple sclerosis.

Gather information about your specific disability. There are videos, pamphlets, and associations dealing with many of these disabilities, such as spina bifida, cancer, deafness, endometriosis, depression, and spinal cord injuries. Following is a sampling of disabilities within each category and the possibilities of warm, connecting lovemaking.

1. Birth Defects

Being born with a birth defect does not make a person less sexual. Most people have sexual feelings and at puberty will undergo normal development into adult sexuality. (Note: Some birth defects do affect the reproductive organs and prevent normal development.) These disabilities do create special social and sexual challenges.

Children with birth defects or chronic illnesses are often not allowed to develop a sense of modesty as nondisabled children do. The genital area is not treated as private but is a part of caregiving, with bladder and bowel care and medical exams. Developing a comfortable understanding of nudity and privacy and the personal nature of genitals and sexuality may require special tutoring and values education.

Children with spina bifida often go through puberty early. And many individuals with spina bifida do not have any sensations in the genital area. During intercourse, a woman with spina bifida has to take special care with lubrication, which does not occur even with sexual arousal. Her damaged nerves may not signal her body to react normally with vasocongestion (blood rushing to the genital area, which then becomes swollen, with lubrication sweating through the vaginal walls as a part of this sexual excitement phase of arousal). Without artificial lubrication every three minutes or so, it is easy for the skin to break down. With tender tissue, twenty seconds of dry rubbing could create an abrasion.

She also may be prone to cystitis and urinary tract infections, so care should be taken to empty the bladder both before and after intercourse. (A primary cause of cystitis and infection is *E. coli* bacteria, which reside in the colon.) She should also be cautious to prevent any contact of waste material with the vagina. A woman with spina bifida may not be orgasmic, but she can be a sensitive, sensual lover who enjoys her sexual feelings and the interaction with her husband.

The person with mental disability, whether by birth or by illness or injury, faces a unique set of challenges. Sexually the individual will often mature normally and possess normal sexual drive and desire. However, the social skills and ability to live self-sufficiently may be seriously impaired, perhaps denying real independence even in marriage. The disability may also have set this person up for sexual victimization. All these issues must worked through to establish a marriage and lovemaking that are meaningful and healthy. Caregivers will have to be sensitive to the person's need for privacy and as much independence as possible, and will have to teach them sexual skills, boundaries, and values. Mentally disabled couples do work through to good marriages and sex lives—again, with creativity, healing, skill building, and helpful caregivers.

Whether spina bifida, cerebral palsy, blindness, or mental disability, the individual will have to work on overcoming developmental deficits by developing social skills and building a healthy self-concept. The individual will need friends and family who can see the whole person, not just the disability. Many of the other parts of this book will apply and can be helpful.

Gender identity, a good sexual self-image, and sexual feelings will be affected by the disability. Some sensations (maybe even genital feelings and orgasms), sexual techniques, and some experiences may be impossible. Creative adaptability will be crucial as the individual and couple become sensual in a variety of possible ways. The blind person, for example, may find different types of intercourse or touch exciting, over the sighted person who may want more visual stimulation.

2. Accidents and Injuries

Chronic pain hits the young and old. It may be an old sports injury, back problems, a knee or hip replacement, severe arthritis, or nerve damage from a mastectomy or other cancer surgery. Sex may be the farthest thing from a person's mind when the pain is intense. For some, making love or an orgasm may intensify the pain, but for others it can be a relief and distraction. Unfortunately some pain medications can negatively affect sexual desire and may need to be adjusted if possible.

Athletes often play through their pain. Some pain is an indication of injury (female pain in intercourse) and should not be played through, as it risks incurring further injury. With many types of chronic pain, however, if you wait until it feels okay, you will never make love. Some things help: increase your communication and trust each other when one expresses a desire to make love. You may have a difficult time tuning out the winces and grimaces of pain and not losing arousal. With practice at hitting the optimal times and knowing better when to adjust or even stop loveplay, sexual frequency increases. Often the mate without the pain needs to initiate and encourage with pillows and props and some seduction.

Though a spinal cord injury is not the most common disability, it does bring about changes in a couple's sex life in a more dramatic way than some of the other disabilities. There are four parts to the backbone, and the spinal cord (the nerves) runs through the center of it. Usually, there is a loss of sensation and movement from the point of injury on down if it is a complete lesion (severing of the spinal cord nerves). There are seven cervical vertebrae in the neck, and an injury to these bones with a complete lesion can cause quadriplegia (paralysis from the neck down). If the injury occurred in the lower, thoracic vertebrae (there are twelve of them), it can cause paraplegia, with paralysis below the site of the injury. Below the thoracic vertebrae there are five lumbar vertebrae and one sacral bone (tailbone) at the lowest part of the back.

Females with spinal cord injuries will not be able to self-lubricate, and a male spinal cord injury affects erections. There are two types of erections: psychogenic and reflexogenic. Psychogenic erections occur as a result of the mind thinking about something sexual and conveying arousal to the genital area through the nerves. Injuries in the thoracic and cervical parts of the spinal column often prevent men from experiencing psychogenic erections.

Reflexogenic erections result from direct stimulation of the penis or are perhaps caused by a full bladder or bowel. About 90 percent of men with higher spinal cord injuries are able to get reflexogenic erections though there is still no sensation in the penis. The problem is that these erections do not always occur when making love, or don't last long enough. Manual or oral stimulation can help, and a technique called "stuffing," in which the wife assumes the on-top position of intercourse to push the flaccid penis into her vagina, sometimes creates an erection.

Ejaculation is often impaired in most complete spinal cord injuries. This does not mean that the husband is unable to experience the pleasure of sexual arousal and the plateau phase, as well as the enjoyment of resolution after making love. Even though the actual nerve sensations do not occur, a person may be able to experience some of the old sensations of an orgasm in their mind with what is called a phantom orgasm.

Our minds are marvelous tools to create sensations and experiences even without the body reactions. Individuals with spinal cord injuries often find that nipples and neck and chin can become particularly sensitive to touch and sexual arousal even through to triggering phantom orgasms. Couples can also become more sensual with fingers and mouth.

Other types of injuries, in addition to that of the spinal cord, can affect the ability to enjoy making love. Loss of a limb or of one of the senses may have much more of an impact than anticipated—you might not have realized how much you depend on hearing your mate's groaning, heavy breathing, and talking for pacing the lovemaking or becoming aroused. You will have to use new senses and develop a new style. The loss of a limb may eliminate certain positions and methods of stimulation, demanding adaptation and change.

Traumatic brain injuries don't as often affect sexual arousal and behaviors (sometimes they can *increase* sexual desire and tuning in to sexual cues). The impact here is on the relationship, with less impulse control and angry outbursts that damage loving feelings and respect. Things may improve as time goes by, but psychotherapy or marriage counseling may be necessary to heal the relational damage or to teach anger management and impulse control. The medications required to treat emotional and physical impairment may have a negative effect on sexual desire and physical ability to experience arousal. Work with your physician to regulate medications as best as possible, to limit their negative side effects on lovemaking.

Injuries generally do not curb sexual desire and the ability to become sexually aroused and make love. Certain behaviors and physical responses may not be possible, and you will have to develop new sensations and techniques. Both partners will have to take time to adjust to the changes as both reestablish sexiness and the ability to comfortably make love; communicate and work through the feelings.

3. Illnesses

Because of nerve and vascular damage, a man with diabetes may have problems getting and maintaining adequate erections for intercourse. To minimize psychological anxiety, he and his wife may go to other activities in their lovemaking and not make erections and intercourse the be-all and end-all.

They may monitor blood-sugar levels and lessen fatigue as they choose optimal times for lovemaking. If the man's testosterone levels are at normal, hormone replacement may not help with erections or desire. But oral medication such as Viagra or an equivalent may improve blood flow. Or, injections into the penis of papaverine or prostaglandin may increase blood flow and cause erections firm enough to permit intercourse. However, the positive effects of the injections may lessen over time as the nerves and blood flow in the genital area become worse.

Some couples have found vacuum pumps helpful in creating erections. A vacuum pump placed over the penis creates a vacuum pressure that draws blood into the penis, creating an erection. A tension ring is then placed at the base of the penis to maintain the erection during intercourse.

If impotence becomes permanent, a penile prosthesis may be a possible solution. A semi-rigid rod or a mechanical pump is surgically placed within the two corpora cavernosa of the penis. With the semi-rigid rod of coated wire, the penis stays firm and is kept down with special underwear. The hydraulic-pump method is a fluid pump surgically placed in the scrotum with two inflatable cylinders placed in the two corpora cavernosa of the penis. The erection is achieved by pumping a bulb in the scrotum, which fills the two cylinders and can then be released when desired.

Diabetes does not have to diminish the man's sexual desire and the enjoyment of his wife's body and femininity. He can refuse to let illness dampen the closeness with his wife as a lover and sexual companion. They can work together to make good choices as they discuss the next part of their journey through impotence and disability.

Lupus, chronic fatigue, and fibromyalgia hit at the heart of a sex life: energy. It is also confusing to have a disease that can still be puzzling even to the medical community. How do you fight back? Daily fatigue wins out so often with its accompanying lack of motivation and desire for most things, including lovemaking. Watchwords will have to become *plan, prioritize, delegate,* and *pace.* You will have to choose what gets done and what is struck off the to-do list. Sex forces these kinds of choices too. Adapt to a workable pace and save up energy for the times it is needed. Intimacy is still necessary and possible. Keep disciplined and make "tough" choices.

With aging come increased chances of heart problems, arthritis, and other illnesses that can affect the sex life of a couple with permanent disabilities. Become a student of the illness and find ways to minimize its detrimental effects on your sex life; seek reliable medical advice and ask questions until you receive answers. Above all, stay creative and romantic as you remain sensual lovers. It can be wise to keep caregiving separate from your lovemaking and sexual enjoyment of each other. With illnesses, always keep an eye on effective timing.

Cancer can have particularly devastating consequences on making love. A wife's mastectomy, for example, can affect both partners. A beneficial approach is to learn about cancer, the surgery, the healing process, and the possible impact of the cancer and treatment on sexuality. Just facing the possibility of death—with the ensuing panic, grief, and depression—affects sexuality. The body-image dragon rears its ugly head with surgeries, especially with a mastectomy. An attitude restructuring may need to precede the discovery of new and exciting ways of arousal and sexual enjoyment.

Cancer surgery and treatment can also sometimes damage nerves, which leads to lack of erections or lubrication. New surgical techniques have resulted in fewer problems with prostatectomies (surgery on the prostate) and hysterectomies (surgery on the uterus and perhaps ovaries) with more damage still in female surgeries. Sometimes radiation and chemotherapy may affect sexual desire or physical arousal and lubrication over a period of months, until nerves and tissue can be regenerated.

Even a man dying of prostate cancer may evolve into a sensual lover. Despite his impotence, the love for his wife and their intimacy may reach a depth they never knew existed. Sometimes he may be too tired to make love, and he may just want to be held. But when they do make love, there may be a tenderness, a sensuality, and a passionate connecting that were never in their sexual relationship before. Their senses may be finely tuned to pick up touches, sights, and smells. And each may gently caress the other's face and back, allowing passion and connection to build, totally focusing on the moment of being together.

Being disabled, injured, or suffering illness can all be times of discovery about making love and building a better sexual relationship. Unbelievably, couples often become more in love and sexually intimate. Timing, taking initiative, following medical advice, and separating the roles of caregiver and loving partner are all important considerations. Creatively seek solutions to new obstacles as you patiently and proactively talk for hours. Lean on others for hope and encouragement and help. Don't give in but pester professionals for better answers. God will bless you on this journey you didn't ask for but are courageously willing to undertake.

CHAPTER TWENTY-FOUR

Survivors of Sexual Abuse

FRIGHTENING AND TRAGIC STATISTICS confront us. Recent surveys estimate that one out of three girls experiences a sexually traumatizing incident by the time she is seventeen—and boys are abused at almost the same rate. Confused couples experience revictimization in their lovemaking over and over again by the unhealed wounds from the past abuse. Mates therefore play an important role in helping their partners reclaim a comfortable sexuality and enjoy, perhaps for the first time, the ability to relate intimately and truly make love.

DEFINING *SEXUAL ABUSE*

Is sexual abuse only fondling of the genitals? Does it have to include penetration of the vagina or masturbation of the penis? No! Some of the worst cases of sexual abuse involve no physical touching at all. One young boy came home every day to find his mother in a see-through gown, and at night he would hear her with her lovers. The sexual confusion and abuse deeply traumatized him. One girl had the door taken off the bathroom and a window cut into the door of her bedroom. She had no privacy. Her stepfather constantly observed her while she dressed and bathed. Needless to say, the experience severely damaged her emotional and sexual development.

Sexual abuse involves any behavior, attitude, or verbal response that hinders normal sexual development, bringing distortion and inhibition to personal sexuality and married lovemaking. Your grandfather may have leered at you and made suggestive remarks. Mom and Dad may have refused to create an intimate relationship with each other and made you the little man or woman in the family. An adult secretly or overtly observing a child undressing or going to the bathroom, intentionally disrobing or exposing genitals, sleeping with a child, or rubbing the genitals against the child or masturbating in the child's presence; or siblings, cousins, or neighborhood children engaging in traumatizing sex play—all of these are clear examples of sexual abuse. More subtly, a form of sexual distortion occurs when the family refuses to talk about sex and makes it sinful or scary. This attitude definitely gets in the way of normal sexual development.

Having said all this, parents need not run scared or create unnecessary guilt. Some behaviors are not abusive, like washing children until they can wash themselves or cleaning the genital area when changing a diaper. Children need to be hugged and held with open demonstrations of physical affection, especially when they become teenagers. Sexual tension and awkwardness will naturally occur as parents and children become aware of each other as sexual beings, either before or at puberty. Respecting appropriate boundaries, privacy, and private parts naturally resolve these issues.

The bottom line is that sexually abusive situations have an entirely different atmosphere. Sexuality becomes confusing, and boundaries and relationships are blurred. The perpetrator is getting personal sexual gratification in inappropriate ways.

EFFECTS OF SEXUAL ABUSE ON THE SURVIVOR

In a healthy family, members have a right to privacy and state assertively that they don't like behaviors that feel invasive or hurtful. Family members respect and validate one another's feelings and set consistent boundaries of what is appropriate and what is harmful. Without creating and understanding limits, people can hurt each other and demand too much or too little of each other.

In situations where sexual abuse occurs, the boundaries are unclear and confusing. A person is just developing a sense of the self and his or her relationship with others from infancy through the teen years. This is when the rules are set for defining expectations and guidelines for sexuality and sexual relating, as well as for relationships in general.

These rules and sexual limits are distorted for the abuse victim. Even with milder abuse, a child knows something is wrong but feels powerless, out of control, and helpless to stop the abusive behavior. This becomes a strong influence in the whole personality makeup. The person often dreads being out of control in adult life and rigidly tries to keep everything tidy and running smoothly, but a terrible bind inevitably occurs. The abuse survivor values healthy control of his of her life but doesn't have the skills to set the boundaries that help maintain control of life's events. This can result in the person's being victimized over and over again.

Confusion haunts the personal and sexual relationships of abuse survivors. How relationships should function and how the boundaries are set eludes them. Lack of knowledge in how to express their needs, and even asking if they deserve to have their needs met, creates uncertainty. Discomfort and skill deficits with feelings abound. Because no one was there to validate their hurt and angry feelings, they begin to not trust themselves or their own feelings. Confusion and shame also creep in because the abuse may have created a sense of attention and connection that feels good but is difficult to keep separate from the trauma of the abuse.

Feelings of shame loom so large in the survivor's reality. They often think that they should have been able to prevent or stop the abuse, that somehow they are responsible. It must be strongly emphasized that *a child is never responsible for sexual abuse.* One adult, in looking back on his own abuse, wished he could have assertively said to his uncle, "Uncle John, you are not keeping proper sexual boundaries and are engaging in this activity purely for your own sexual gratification. I am not going to participate in these behaviors. I am going to report you to the proper authorities, and I strongly suggest you get some professional help." He laughed as he realized the impossibility of a nine-year-old child behaving so maturely. He still felt somehow to blame.

Masculinity and femininity, and sex and sexuality, are profoundly affected by abusive experiences. Abuse victims are usually sexualized earlier than God intended and in situations far removed from the loving relational experience He designed. Sex becomes associated with fear, pain, and control. The positive feelings of love, joy, and pleasure are absent or distorted. As persons try to alter these experiences and enjoy making love in the present marital companionship, flashbacks are triggered, and these people get stuck in past distortions over and over, as healing slowly takes place.

MATES AS PARTNERS IN HEALING

You and every other mate bring into marriage a whole backpack of garbage accrued in the years before you met each other. Because of the presence of evil and imperfection in this world, people hurt each other, and no one is exempt from these scars. That's the bad news. Now here's the good news. For every bad and hurtful relationship, there can be an opposite healing relationship full of love and truth. The fact is that wounds experienced in destructive relationships demand a positive healing relationship to regenerate wholeness.

How the Survivor Can Help the Partner

Both the partner and the marriage of the abuse survivor become victims of the abuse. Having your "survivor" mate turned off by sex or avoiding physical affection feels very personal. The partner can know the cause and be sensitive to the abuse issues, but personal needs and feelings still exist for the nonabused mate. The non-survivor partner may long for sex and desire to be close to his or her spouse without being pushed away because it's a bad day or week and the flashbacks have returned.

It's easy to start doubting one's attractiveness and sexual appeal. Am I lovable? Is something wrong with my technique and ability as a lover? Sexual appeal and ability have little to do with what is going on, and both mates need to remind each other that the abuse is dampening sexuality. The male partner may experience difficulty with erections, and both partners may suffer a loss of sexual desire. Grow adept at laying the responsibility at the feet of the abuse. The abuse is the bogeyman both of you are fighting *together*.

The excitement of making love diminishes when it seems full of confusion and, at times, painful flashbacks for the survivor. The nonabused partner sometimes wonders if both might be better served by eliminating sex from the marriage. This idea, of course, causes shock waves of anxiety for both—wondering whether either could remain in a sexless marriage. These and many other feelings haunt the marriage and have to be worked through. The partner, too, has to deal with grief as he or she wishes that the mate had not been abused and that the marriage did not have to cope with these devastating aftershocks. The partner comes to feel as helpless toward the abuse as the survivor does and has to work through to hope and healing also.

Partners can become furious at the perpetrator. Sometimes it seems that the survivor gets all the attention and the healing takes precedence over all else. The partner knows that until the sexual abuse is worked through, lovemaking will never flourish. But it can seem very one-sided. The partner gets lonely, too, and may have personal scars and unique types of woundedness. Feelings are stirred up both ways, and it is important that you encourage the partner to get help and create a support network as well; the abuse survivor has his or her plate full and cannot always be available for support. The partner must build those solid same-sex friendships and maybe join a support group. He or she will grow impatient or hurt in destructive ways without this help, and the survivor's growth will be impeded.

So how can a survivor help his or her partner?

1. Build and validate an understanding of the partner's position—feelings, needs, and reality. Your partner's reality and way of looking at life is probably very different from your own. Communicate empathetically as you walk in his or her shoes, and encourage your partner to deal with feelings in positive ways.

2. Keep affirming the commitment to your marriage and love for your partner. Even though sex may be difficult, maintain physical affection. Sensual caressing, with sex off-limits, can be very affirming.

3. Remind your partner that difficulty with sex stems from the abuse and has nothing to do with the partner's attractiveness or ability as a lover. Reaffirm your commitment to working at the sexual part of the relationship and your determination that you, too, want your lovemaking to flourish. Remind your partner that you think you are married to a sexually attractive lover.

4. Recognize and appreciate the efforts of your partner in promoting healing. Express thanks for loving you with respect and patience. (There will be relapses and impatience, but affirm your mate's helpful behaviors.) Encourage your partner to seek support with friendships, groups, and counseling.

5. Answer questions and try to be assertive in helping your partner understand what is comfortable and uncomfortable and what triggers flashbacks. Don't overreact to or take too personally your partner's frustration and anger and grieving. Both of you must continually affirm the difficulty of the healing process and your deep appreciation in tackling it together. Reassure each other of your intent to work through this to resolution and a great sex life with God's help.

How the Partner Can Help the Survivor

Sexual abuse destroys so much of the joy and freedom in life and relationships. Survivors appreciate mates who will take the time to try to understand their reality in a loving and patient way—to get into the reality of the wounded child and perceive how tough it was. Your mate needs your empathy in comprehending what abuse is all about.

The survivor needs to be reassured that abuse will never have to be endured again, and must be empowered to positively take charge of his or her life and sexuality. The survivor has the right to say no and set sexual limits. Remember, proper boundaries did not exist in the life of the survivor, or the ability to take charge of life and express likes and dislikes in the abusive situation. Healing depends on the survivor's ability to learn these skills. You, as partner, can encourage and model healthy independence and setting limits with safe, protective boundaries.

You can assume a crucial role in empowering the survivor and breaking the vicious cycle of revictimization. You can also help your mate to recognize potentially dangerous situations, assertively set limits, and confront as needed. These skills will be affirming and increase your mate's self-esteem. Make clear that the survivor deserves good things, and support your partner in accepting God's verdict that everyone is created worthwhile and special. Compliment and build up the survivor's strengths and abilities as you increase healthy self-awareness and self-directedness.

Empower the survivor as both of you keep placing the blame and responsibility for the abuse on the perpetrator. Your assistance will be invaluable as your mate grows beyond the disabling shame and guilt. Logically, the abuse will trouble you, and you will wish the survivor could have stopped the traumatizing behaviors sooner. Be careful not to imply that your mate could have done something about it, that somehow your mate chose to stay in the abusive situation. Your mate was a victim who did not choose to be victimized. He or she needs your support in distancing from the abuse and reclaiming the power to control life in a healthy way.

In a similar way, you need to work through any thoughts or feelings that the survivor is "damaged goods." Get beyond yourself. What happened to the survivor was not sex; it was violence and pain. Your mate needs your acceptance—not judgment or further victimization. You, as partner, did not ask for this burden of the abuse, and it creates many troubling side effects. Your mate did not ask for it, either. Cruel and vicious damage has been perpetrated, and the survivor's personhood and sexuality need hope and healing.

Be gentle and empathetic. Resist placing any sexual pressure, especially when he or she is going through the most traumatic part of healing and the flashbacks are terrible. They will avoid sex, and that is about all you can think of, like being in the desert without water. This too shall pass! Let your mate know that your companionship is much more than the sexual part of it. Learn to touch and hold apart from sex, and make love with your clothes on. Your mate's life and sexuality are not irreparably damaged. It is a shame that both of you are having to pick up the pieces, but both will be closer and more committed for having walked the journey together. Jesus is using you "to heal the brokenhearted, to proclaim liberty to the captives" (Luke 4:18 NKJV). It is a role that only you as partner can accomplish.

RECLAIMING SEXUALITY

The many facets of working through sexual abuse demand time and focused energy, but hope can break through. This section considers some of the significant issues, from finding a therapist to breaking the conspiracy of silence about the abuse to reclaiming sexuality. Many before you have worked their way through to peace, freedom, and healing, so courageously persist.

The journey differs for everyone. Many survivors have repressed their feelings for many years. Then perhaps in their late thirties, the feelings and flashbacks start to emerge, and life can become unmanageable. Sometimes the birth of a child, or a child reaching the age of their own abuse, triggers reactions and memories. Others find their marital sexuality seriously hampered, and they are nudged into working on the causes. Memories of the abuse can begin to surface that may or may not be already in the conscious mind. Repeated nightmares or flashbacks can begin as well.

Regardless of how the abuse surfaces or gets in the way, there comes a time when it is important to seek healing. Please don't put it off. It is scary even to consider confronting the memories with their pain and terror. Unfortunately, no shortcut exists for resolving sexual abuse; you must wade through the memories and resolve the pain and fears. Reading books or sharing with your mate or a friend is helpful, but working through the feelings and memories will most likely require the assistance of a professional therapist. Unlike other problems, the complexity of the issues usually prevents self-help.

Finding Professional Counseling

A professional therapist has been trained in psychological counseling and has special expertise in working with sexual abuse survivors. This counseling may come in several different forms. Working through the memories will probably take some individual work in a one-on-one office setting. Therapy groups help survivors work through their traumas together, and a group can provide support and also be effective for bringing memories to the surface and promoting healing. Sometimes more concentrated therapeutic time is needed to work through intense grief and pain—especially if the emotions cause the person to have self-destructive thoughts. This may require a stay in a hospital that specializes in working with survivors.

Recent rape victims need specialized care. In larger cities there are crisis centers where you can get immediate help and involvement in support groups. As with sexual abuse, the effects will not just go away. The feelings can be repressed, but they will likely come back to haunt you and your marriage. You are not "damaged goods," and there is healing! If you cannot go to a crisis center, seek out therapy that can help you and your mate resolve the feelings of anger, helplessness, fear, shame, and pain.

One reason abuse survivors do not get help is that they are not sure where to go to find professional therapy. Use the yellow pages wisely. It may mean driving to a larger city to find a professional with the needed expertise, but more professionals are receiving training in this area. Look under psychology and counseling centers or marriage and family therapists in the directory, then make some calls. Any therapist should be willing to give five minutes of time to answer questions.

In interviewing and selecting a therapist, consider these points:

1. Has the person had specialized training in working with sexual abuse survivors? Has the person been supervised by someone skilled in this area?

2. How many cases of sexual abuse has the person worked with, and is the therapist currently seeing any other abuse survivors?

3. Is the therapist familiar with helping a survivor work through repressed and confused memories of abuse?

You may be able to find a therapist recommended by a professional counseling agency. A pastor or a friend may know of someone to recommend as well. That is better than starting cold, but the phone interview is still a good idea.

After you have started therapy, be aware of several issues. Every therapist has a different personality and style, and you may get matched up with someone who doesn't fit well. Be a good consumer and find another therapist. Sometimes female survivors cannot get beyond the maleness of a therapist despite a gentle and sensitive manner. They need to find a female counselor who can work more effectively with them.

Therapists who work with abuse survivors need to be able to set healthy boundaries. By "boundaries," I mean the healthy definitions and limits of any good relationship. I am a father, grandfather, friend, mate, and therapist, and each of these relationships has things I will and won't allow, to protect that special relationship. Obviously, if there are any sexual advances, find another therapist. Lack of boundaries will probably be more subtle, like keeping the role of therapist versus friend clear for you, or maybe even starting and ending counseling sessions on time. Talk to the therapist if any boundary issues come up and you feel uncomfortable. Never tolerate your therapist's implication that the abuse was your fault—find another therapist if this happens. Your therapist should be able to accept and appreciate that some of your symptoms (anger, avoidance) are coping habits that have helped you survive. They will have to be worked through and replaced slowly.

This will be one of the most important relationships of your life. Choose the person carefully and then commit to the process. It won't be easy; the pain and confusion *usually get much worse before they get better*. It is exciting to slowly see the pain leaving and yourself empowered to enjoy life in an assertive and whole way. The only way to get through to healing is to put your boots on, with your therapist walking with you, and wade through the muck to the other side. You can do it!

Resolving Dissociation and Feelings

Dissociation is taking your sexual abuse and distancing yourself from it in your mind. This is an important mechanism you used to survive as a child. Abuse memories can be cataloged under the acrostic of BASK. It stands for Behaviors, Affect, Senses, and Knowledge. With dissociation, memories of the abuse are often taken apart and stored under each category. There may be behavioral memories (being pinned down, gagging); affective, or feelings, memories (feeling trapped, depressed, terrified); sensual memories (smelling a cologne, experiencing a certain look, hearing a sound, feeling chafed or sore); or stored knowledge (someone saying "just relax" like the abuser, or remembering the time of year when it happened).

With some survivors, there is fairly accurate conscious knowledge of the abuse, even though they may never have talked about it with anyone. With most, there is dissociation, and the events have been stored away and are not remembered or are very fuzzy and minimized in the mind. This is not unusual because often the mind was turned off during the abuse and the event was stored in bits and pieces.

The goal in therapy is reassociating the memories and empowering the survivor to let go and move on. The behaviors and feelings and sensed data and knowledge of the event are all brought back together and experienced. It is a painful process to go back and acknowledge what happened and know that the abuse need never happen again. You are remembering so that you can let go of the pain and effects of abuse.

The survivor doesn't have to remember every incident—some of the horror will be kept safely stored—to experience healing. But the "adult you" has to go back and re-associate with the wounded child or teenager and acknowledge and heal some of the pain—reassuring the wounded inner parts that the abuse is over and they can now be protected.

Forgiveness is not an instantaneous process unless you are God; He can instantly remove our sins "as far as the east is from the west" (Ps. 103:12 NKJV). With humans in relationships, we remember and hate and feel intense anger that certain deeds have been perpetrated on us and that our rights have been violated. Over time we slowly let go. Forgiveness is not condoning what the abuser has done or even choosing to ever see that person. It is a personal process that does not depend on the person who has hurt you. One woman who was kidnapped and raped was asked how she could forgive her rapist. She replied that he had stolen seven hours of her life and that was all he was getting. Forgiveness leaves the abuser to God's "day of vengeance" and frees your emotional energy for better uses than revenge, painful memories, and consuming hatred.

The Christian can appropriate God's love and power to do some of this inner healing. It is a *process* that lets Christ's healing presence into your pain. As you remember and reassociate the memories, you may want to work through them in healing prayer with a wise friend or counselor. One way to do this is to imagine walking back through your life and the traumatizing events with Jesus. Incident by incident you can pray and allow Him to put His healing touch on your hurts with compassionate understanding and restorative empowering.

Your Christian counselor can affirm this healing process by praying with you. After you have completed this inner process, it can be helpful to imagine Jesus gently holding you as one of His precious lambs, weeping with you that you have been wounded so badly, while His loving presence brings further comfort and grace to help you let go.

You may have to work through the hurt and anger over the idea that Jesus did not stop the abuse. It is a sinful, broken world, and evil deeds are perpetrated on innocent people. God did not create people to be robots but to have free will, so we can make true choices—unfortunately they are not always loving choices. Precious person, I want so much for you to know deeply that God does love you and He is appalled at what happened to you. Actually God buffered more than you know, and while the abuse was going on He was creating people in your future to help you heal. He shaped my life and writing hopefully to be one of those "angels," like your mate, to bring healing.

The primary feelings that you will have to understand and resolve are anger, pain, fear, and shame. The anger may have been repressed and never allowed to surface against the abuser or caretakers who failed to protect. There is special rage that occurs when you feel helpless and can do nothing about helping yourself. The hurt child was trapped and subjected to injury against his or her will without any recourse; you suffered both physical and emotional pain that you probably dissociated from. The pain has to be faced and lived through again, only this time you are *remembering in order to let go and be healed.*

The many fears must be confronted and better understood. The mind can then restructure the fears and make them manageable. It helps to go back and realize your reality as a little child—you can give that child reassurance that that was the past, and now there is more power and knowledge to prevent the same thing from ever happening again. There can also be mental reevaluation and restructuring of the shame. You can place responsibility squarely back on the perpetrator of the abuse, and the timid, shame-ridden attitudes can be challenged and overcome. The abuser's brainwashing should be brought out in the open and shown for what it is.

Breaking the Conspiracy of Silence and Confronting the Abuser

Sharing your story with your spouse will be therapeutic. Remember, though, that your spouse's reality will be quite different from yours. You may need some patience as you try to convey the feelings and reality of the wounded child. A professional therapist is helpful because of the ability to empathize and understand more easily.

You will have to decide how you choose to break the silence and secrecy. Deciding whether to confront the abuser and other people connected to you during the abuse will be very difficult. They may be deceased, or you may have no continued contact, so the work will have to be done by you alone. Be sure to prepare before you choose to confront.

The danger is in being revictimized or having greatly disappointed expectations if the confrontation is not carefully thought through and planned. Think through why you want to confront and what the consequences of the confrontation will be for you. Are you willing to risk losing relationships and contact with family? Do you have a good support system? Can you take a negative reaction, denial, or no response without being victimized all over again?

This concern needs to be strategic as you promote healing. If you don't confront people because you are full of shame or want to protect them, your reluctance needs further work in therapy. If there is legitimate fear of reprisal or no hope of anything but denial, don't confront and be revictimized. Perhaps you want no contact whatsoever, and you have dealt with your personal traumas and victimization in therapy. Thus a confrontation may serve no purpose. Think through this step with a wise counselor and make focused choices.

Healing and Reclaiming Sexuality

Wendy Maltz, in her book *The Sexual Healing Journey,* talks about the five false ideas most abuse survivors have in their attitudes about sex:

1. "Sex is uncontrollable." Sexual energy is wild and impulsive and cannot be controlled or contained. If it is unleashed, it probably can't be stopped and the desire is never satisfied. The perpetrator says he will stop but never does. Sex makes people irresponsible and divorced from everyday reality.

2. "Sex is hurtful." Sexual feelings and behaviors are emotionally and physically painful. Sex is full of betrayal and is really just using someone and can include hostility and rage. Physical penetration and rubbing caused torn skin and genital irritations.

3. "Sex is a commodity." Sexuality is an object or skill to use and is divorced from caring or relating. It is something to manipulate and bargain with, as sex is exchanged for attention, love, and power. Sex is performance-oriented and disconnected from emotion.

4. "Sex is secretive." Sexual behaviors are more exciting when sneaky or forbidden. Sex is shameful and should never be talked about with others. Sex is covert and furtive—never natural, or open to discussion, or possessing a comfortable knowledge, with a healthy sense of privacy and mutuality.

5. "Sex has no moral boundaries." Sex has no right or wrong with limits but is whatever feels good to the other person. It is a game with winners and losers. There is no respect, trust, fairness, consequence, or virtue.

Challenge with words and actions that sex is a commodity and tied into earning love and commitment. Be assertive as you make sex natural and a conscious decision with the ability to say no whenever needed. Reaffirm your Christian beliefs that making love is a mutual experience and based on a loving, intimate companionship.

Male abuse survivors sometimes struggle with same-sex fantasies and an arousal by penises. That is a consequence of their abuse and not necessarily homosexuality. They can work through it with reconditioning and arousal centered on the mate. Male and female survivors sometimes find pain arousing sexually or have erotic dreams about the abuse. That, too, is a product of the abusive conditioning. They did not invite the abuse, and the reflexive arousal does not make them seductive, masochistic, or wanting sex with the abuser.

Prone to guilt and shame, the survivor may try to work things through without talking about them, thus sabotaging efforts to change attitudes and become comfortable with new behaviors. Don't keep secrets. Talk about these emotionally loaded topics with someone who is safe. Love and acceptance can be so healing. You may wish to unload some of this on a therapist and not just your mate, but it is important to get things out into the open without self-condemnation. Change attitudes that say it must be something you did or asked for. Change can be encouraged by saying aloud or writing down affirmation statements of truth: "I was a victim"; "I deserve love and affection."

With male and female survivors, a reconditioning process is a vital part of the journey. So much of sexual arousal, or pain, is built on conditioning. Sex in abuse is associated with the false beliefs of its being uncontrollable, hurtful, and secretive. Mates can begin a new set of conditioning as they pair sexual feelings and behaviors with fun, loving, respectful experiences. This slowly starts to make a real difference.

The pain, fear, and shame are often reflexive reactions and have to be continually challenged with healthy self-talk and healthy behaviors. Flashbacks occur unbidden and can be very disruptive. In the midst of lovemaking, you may panic in a certain position or sexual movement. Something your mate says or does may trigger old fears or pain.

Don't discount your feelings and reactions. Sort through your memories of the abuse, and try to find triggers from the past, even if you have to stop your lovemaking awhile. It will help your feelings seem more manageable. Take a deep breath and slowly let it out as you calm your autonomic physiological response. You might say, "I am safe, and no one is trying to hurt me now." As you control your physical response, you will feel safer and more in control. Ground yourself in the present. Look around the room and notice, perhaps even touch, at least five things that are completely different from the abusive situation. Let your partner assist you in getting firmly back into the present. Tune in to your adult self and remind yourself that you now have more power and control. Above all, choose a new response or behavior as you alter the old reality and continue healing, even in the middle of lovemaking.

Change to a different sexual behavior, like engaging in intercourse rather than stimulating the clitoris. Find a way to alter the behavior a little and make it more acceptable as you try not to duplicate the past. One couple learned that it helped if the husband was already in the bed and the survivor chose to join him—rather than feeling her perpetrator was hovering over the bed and coming to her. Another couple took two years to slowly reclaim the breasts as erotic, and not body parts that triggered abusive flashbacks. Intercourse and other behaviors were fine—so they started there and he slowly started touching her sides, tummy, and around the breasts as they paired up safety and erotic pleasure with touch. Finally it was okay to actually touch the breasts.

Engage in a lot of pleasurable touching and holding before stimulation of the genitals. Again, try to understand what triggers the negative reactions and work through the feelings. Immediately do something positive with your partner that can change your present reaction. All of this may take only a minute or two, but it puts you back in control.

It is not fair that anyone has to suffer sexual abuse. You are to be congratulated because you are a survivor. You indeed are on a healing journey, and God will bless your efforts. Stay courageous, and know that you can work through to the intimate lovemaking you so deeply desire.

CHAPTER TWENTY-FIVE

Dealing with Infertility

(WITH WILLIAM CUTRER, M.D.)

ONE OUT OF SIX COUPLES has problems with infertility, according to recent estimates. That's huge! The desire for children is so natural and yet becomes very painful when it is unfulfilled. Infertility takes a tremendous toll emotionally on both the individuals and the marriage. The estimated 50 percent divorce rate for couples struggling with infertility perhaps is not surprising in that two of the top causes of marital breakups are involved—sex and money.

Despite efforts to minimize the influence, infertility and the attempts to overcome it will have a definite negative effect on a couple's intimate companionship and sex life. One research study showed that over half of the couples struggling with infertility experience definite changes in their love lives:

- Fifty-six percent of couples report a decrease in frequency of intercourse after diagnosis of infertility.
- Both women (59 percent) and men (42 percent) report a decrease in satisfaction with sex. Women (49 percent) also say they feel less comfortable with their sexuality.[1]

Couples often feel procreation is their God-given right and that children will be a natural outcome of lovemaking whenever they choose to begin a family. But that is not so for many marriages, and a season of turmoil begins with many difficult choices. This chapter will hopefully increase understanding, give helpful suggestions, and most important, encourage couples to come through this crisis still in love and spiritually enriched.

COMMON MISCONCEPTIONS ABOUT INFERTILITY

You as a couple have probably struggled with some of these statements or heard them from a friend. People in the lives of the infertile couple don't mean to be so insensitive and hurtful, but they often are.

It's just stress. Relax and hang in there; you'll get pregnant soon. This is well-meant advice, but infertility is not usually due to stress or emotional issues. In close to 90 percent of couples who seek medical help, there is a diagnosable physical problem. (The problem may still be medical in the final 10 percent but, like ten years ago with certain immune problems, it just can't be diagnosed yet. This 10 percent can struggle with never knowing why they cannot conceive.) It is also true that getting pregnant once does not ensure that you will get pregnant easily the next time. Fortunately, with improved techniques, medical help is effective, and more than half of the couples seeking treatment achieve successful outcomes.

Perhaps it is not God's will that you have a child, or maybe there is sin in your life that God is trying to remove. God has a will for each person's life, but infertility is usually a physical problem. It may have nothing to do with God's will about potential parenting. That is, like the disciple's question of who sinned and our Lord's response that this wasn't the point, it may simply be a chance for God to be glorified and His children to grow. God may use infertility to shape us into the person He wants, like other painful occurrences in our lives. It may possibly be a by-product of a sin issue, like an STD that created the infertility, but one still shouldn't "blame the victim" as we help him or her find forgiveness and healing.

It must be him/her. Nothing like this has ever happened in our family. Actually, most assume it's the female. If the guy is able to attain an erection and ejaculate, the reasoning goes, he's probably okay. The truth is that infertility problems are fairly evenly divided in causation, with roughly one-third the male and one-third the female and one-third a joint problem. Infertility usually isn't hereditary.

Wait until you adopt a baby. I bet you'll get pregnant then. Everyone has a story of this occurrence and is happy to hear it. Studies have shown that only 5 percent of couples spontaneously overcome their infertility and conceive after adopting—and 5 percent who quit treatment and *don't* adopt conceive as well. This misconception has the harmful, implicit suggestion that adoption is a cure for infertility rather than adoption being considered in its own right as a thoughtful decision and process.

Fertility tests are terrible. I hope we survive. Fertility testing for some can be painful or intrusive, though many husbands and wives find the process fascinating as they gain new knowledge and seek to overcome the problem. The pain, frustration, and stress often are caused not by the medical treatment but by miscarriages, continued disappointments, financial pressures, and fatigue. Infertility ranks on the stress scales right up there with the death of a loved one and cancer.

It's only a miscarriage. Miscarriages are often part of the infertility process, as they are for any couple attempting conception. Most medical studies estimate miscarriage rates between 20 and 30 percent, but the loss is not diminished because they are common or because the child is not brought to full term. Grieving must take place and the choice made about whether to continue with treatment. Every child has eternal value, even if he or she only survives a few days or weeks in the womb. We need to grieve with each other and our friends suffering miscarriages. As the Twila Paris song so beautifully reminds, any God-given life is "a visitor from heaven, if only for awhile."

I have no control over the medical treatment process. You are the consumer. You have the right to be informed about the treatment process and make choices about the costs: physically, emotionally, and financially. Educate yourself and never be afraid to ask questions or be a part of the decision making.

Infertility can mean some great sex while trying to conceive. For some couples, especially those women who struggle with sexual inhibitions and desire, trying to get pregnant can give motivation, enjoyment, and relaxing control. Unfortunately, sex on demand is not much fun, and infertility usually has a negative impact on making love instead of providing opportunity for more fun. The stress may aggravate already existing marital and sexual problems.

I must pursue this goal strongly. There is no price too great to pay to have a child of my own. During the process, before you finally give up, you will have to take a recess from your efforts now and again to regroup. Neither of you will want to give up, but one or perhaps both of you will come to a time when you want to stop the fertility process. You will have decreased motivation for the struggle, you will feel you have done all you can, and you will want to get life back to normal. There is a price in terms of health, financial security, and your marriage that is too dear. For some (not all), the joy of being adoptive parents may start taking precedence over having a natural child.

Maybe you should adopt and give a needy child a Christian home. The adoption process averages one to two years of waiting for an infant and approximately $15,000 to $30,000 in fees to an adoption agency. Those who are persistent still find it possible to adopt the healthy baby of their dreams, but it is not an easy road and not for everyone.

I will never get beyond the tragedy that I cannot have children. God will help you grieve and work through your anger and loss. Don't hold it in. Cry and share your tears with the Lord and another person. Lean on a support group such as RESOLVE (see the contact information at end of chapter). Your toughest job may be taking your unborn children with your precious dreams and placing them in Jesus' arms—leaving them there, forever, with Him. I (Doug) am crying as I write these words because I know what a painful experience that will be. The grief and loss will still be triggered again and again, but there is healing, and God fills the empty places with many special things.

ACKNOWLEDGING THE PROBLEM

After waiting and worrying about birth control, when the time is right to conceive mates experience increased freedom, and enjoy the extra sex, and anticipate becoming pregnant. You are letting the idea of being parents settle on both of you, sharing your dreams about what your child will be like and how the three of you will create a family unit. You wonder if you should be more systematic in tracking the most fertile time, but you don't think you need to bother; yet you make love more frequently when ovulation is most likely occurring. It's a good time in your life.

There Might Be a Problem

You may not be sure exactly when it starts nagging at you that something may be wrong. You know nothing is happening, and it has been months that you have been trying to get pregnant. It isn't panic or severe anxiety, but you probably need to do something. This starts your journey into the emotional, intrusive, hopeful, frustrating, and educational world of infertility. Your lives will never be the same. At first, it isn't too disconcerting, and there is still hope that nothing major is wrong. This is a time of becoming more structured with doctor's visits, checking ovulation, and the beginning of intercourse on demand.

The process begins with the wife having a basic pelvic exam. If no abnormalities are noticed, the time of the wife's ovulation begins to take on a relationship-shaping significance. LH ovulation predictor kits (purchased in drug stores to detect the surge in the luteinizing hormone [LH], which precedes ovulation by about twenty-four hours), a transvaginal sonogram, and perhaps BBT (Basal Body Temperature) charts will help to pinpoint the time of ovulation and fertility. It is recommended that you have intercourse right before and right after ovulation on alternate nights, to cover the fertile time. At other times of the month, you can be as spontaneous and carefree as you desire with making love—but at ovulation, planning is a necessity.

There Is a Problem

It will not take many months of focusing sex on conception, rather than making love, before sexual frequency and enjoyment diminish. As one woman at a RESOLVE support group meeting said: "I'm tired of sex when I don't feel like it and ending up looking like a stupid question mark afterward." She was referring to the recommendation of keeping her legs in the air after intercourse so the sperm will pool around the cervix and swim into the uterus. Unfortunately, medically she was going through unneeded contortions. Actually, elevating the hips is what is called for; just a pillow underneath with the legs prone is more comfortable.

Sex on demand can be demoralizing, and as the months go by, you will be forced to acknowledge that there indeed is a problem. Cutting through the denial takes time, and you may wonder, *Why us?* Further tests will be undertaken to pinpoint what is needed for further medical intervention.

TESTS AND SEEKING ANSWERS

This time of testing can feel very invasive, both physically and emotionally. It isn't just the tests. Emotionally, you want so much to have a child, and everywhere you turn you are reminded of your childlessness. You encounter babies in malls; you walk by the nursery at church; your family asks you when you will be having children. All these circumstances make it even tougher on you—with a broad spectrum of emotions from sadness to anger to hurt to fear.

Hormonal Testing

The endocrine system affects fertility and conception in many ways. God created a beautifully complex physical system to create life. The hormones and endocrine system help signal when the uterus should begin building up endometrial tissue in preparation for the fertilized egg. The ovaries are marvelously complicated; the hormones help eggs to be matured and released (the process termed *ovulation*) into the fallopian tubes on a monthly basis. Approximately half of female infertility is related to a problem with ovulation or the endocrine system.

Your physician may observe for egg maturation in the wife's ovaries with a vaginal ultrasound, and she may be given a fertility drug to help regulate or stimulate ovulation. Unfortunately, a possible side effect is the development of cysts. *Cyst* merely means a fluid-filled sac. Every normal egg develops in a tiny cyst called a follicle, but occasionally other types of cysts may develop and persist, interfering with the normal ovulatory process. In certain cases, these physical complications may need to be addressed medically.

Your gynecologist will generally start by doing a hormonal workup, and often begin the treatment with a drug like Clomid to help regulate ovulation. It's important to note that an early referral to a fertility specialist and/or reproductive endocrinologist is very important if your ob–gyn doesn't have a personal interest and training in infertility treatment.

The hormones thyroid, prolactin, estrogen, progesterone, and the androgens should be checked early (all through blood tests)—many successful therapies come from this source. Many physicians have vaginal sonograms in their offices to assist in evaluating and treating ovulation issues.

Sperm Count

Usually during the first medical tests, the husband's sperm sample is evaluated for the amount and healthiness of his sperm. In a "normal" ejaculate there are more than 40 million sperm per cc. Both the concentration of sperm as well as total count are evaluated. With counts below 10 million (10 million per cc)—along with other parameters such as the sperm being alive and motile—there is a significant problem.

Sometimes the husband gives a sperm sample at the doctor's office, or he may be able to take one in later. It is definitely not an ego-boosting or intimacy-enhancing process to walk in with jar in hand or to be required to give a specimen on demand. Infertility may come to seem like a maze in which you constantly bump into obstructions. Frustration and, sometimes, humiliation seem to be ever-present parts of the process. The movie *She's Having a Baby* may be interesting to watch as you empathize and laugh with another couple giving sperm samples and utilizing optimal times. A sense of humor and allowing God and your physician to give you perspective really help.

The husband may be afraid, before the results are known, that he is sterile. Such fears are normal. Both spouses should talk through what this would mean. It may affect the husband's sense of masculinity and have to be worked through by both. The wife can help him feel secure in his maleness.

You may decide that if the husband is sterile, you will begin adoption procedures. You may consider using a sperm donor. Many Christian couples reject the use of artificial insemination by donor. Infertility is full of ethical and personal issues that couples have to work through for themselves. The husband may fear his emotional reaction if his wife were carrying someone else's child. Some couples feel that the husband's sterility is God's closing the door on natural children for them. Both partners have to struggle before God and their consciences about when they believe He is saying enough is enough, and that He has another path laid out.

There are further tests and medical interventions for the couple whose problem is a low sperm count. A problem with hormone levels or sperm motility may respond to intervention with drugs. Sometimes having surgery on a varicocele (dilated blood vessels similar to varicose veins) in the scrotum or unblocking the ducts that carry the sperm is helpful. Semen can be processed to separate sperm from harmful antibodies, or the physician may prepare the sperm for direct insemination into the uterus, bypassing the cervix.

Hysterosalpingogram

The hysterosalpingogram and some of the other medical procedures are fascinating in their sophisticated biology, but the wife may find this exam very intrusive or even painful. In the hysterosalpingogram, radiopaque dye is injected slowly into the uterus. As the uterus fills up, there can be cramping (for a small percentage of women it is quite intense). The dye spills over into the fallopian tubes and out the ends of them if there is no obstruction. A fluoroscope and X rays are used to chart the flow of the dye as the test determines whether the tubes are open. Sometimes even this is inconclusive, as they can be open and "leak" the dye while still being quite abnormal.

Some women go through this test with no discomfort or reaction. With others, it can be among the most uncomfortable exams that they will experience. The husband can be Psalm 18:2 for his wife (a rock, a fortress, a shield, a stronghold) with strong emotional and physical support during this journey. Infertility will force a couple to depend on each other. Feeling helpless and uncertain creates deep discomfort, and at times you will wonder if the process is worth the toll it is taking on the relationship and the body.

As the tests progress, you may be disappointed again and again as nothing wrong is discovered or perhaps medical interventions prove futile. You may sometimes feel like you are going down a path with no clear map, in a foggy state of limbo, trying to reach a goal that is perhaps impossible. It is important to formulate a careful game plan with your doctor and deal with the worst-case scenario and the subsequent steps to pursue. You may begin to wonder, *Where is God in this process and what is He doing?*

Your faith will be challenged throughout the infertility process. Wonderful Scriptures can give hope and sustenance:

> Have you not known?
> Have you not heard?
> The everlasting God, the LORD,
> The Creator of the ends of the earth,
> Neither faints nor is weary.
> His understanding is unsearchable.
> He gives power to the weak,
> And to those who have no might He increases strength. (Isa. 40:28–29 NKJV)

But unfortunately, reading them is easier than incorporating them into life. Trusting and resting in the Lord come with a struggle, as you are continually driven back to relying on His strength. Sometimes you must see God's provision in the caring demonstrated through Christian friends. It is important to work through God's teaching on fertility.

There are interesting stories in Scripture, like Hannah, who is trying to conceive and so devastated she couldn't even eat. Her loving husband Elkanah gave helpful—perhaps more of a male "fix-it" mentality than empathetic—advice. He encouraged her, "Am I not better to you than ten sons?" (1 Sam. 1:8 NKJV). Somehow his support encourages her and she started eating again.

The Post-Coital Test

A sex life can be traumatized when genitals and making love cease to be for pleasure and bonding and instead are examined and utilized as a means of reaching the goal of pregnancy. This is certainly true of the post-coital exam. The couple have intercourse on the expected day of ovulation, no matter what the mood. Sexual arousal for both mates may take much longer than usual, and an erection more difficult to stimulate. Some couples cannot comply with the sex on demand, and the test has to be rescheduled. After intercourse, the couple go to the doctor's office so the wife can be given a pelvic exam.

Some wives find this test especially embarrassing and intrusive as mucous is taken from the cervix. For others, this test is still a learning experience or just part of the process of trying to unlock the mystery of infertility. The mucous is examined because it has certain consistency that changes with ovulation. A successful test shows the mucous to be more fluid with a sufficient quantity of sperm actively swimming in it. This exam can also check for sperm antibodies by checking for immobile or dead sperm.

Sex may disappear except around the time of ovulation. You may have temporarily lost the emotional bonding and sexual excitement of making love. There may be some release of sexual tension, but all in all, sex has become engulfed in the process of becoming pregnant. The post-coital exam may contribute to and symbolize this unfortunate fact.

Artificial Insemination

Your doctor may suggest artificial insemination. This procedure certainly won't nurture your sex life but again is part of the process that you are hopeful will make a difference. At the time of ovulation, the husband provides sperm and the physician inserts the sperm with a syringe at the mouth of the wife's cervix. This increases the chance of sperm swimming up into the uterus and to the fallopian tubes. But this procedure can get expensive, as it may need to be repeated for several months. Oftentimes the doctor will recommend intrauterine insemination, which, following sperm preparation, involves injecting the sperm through the cervix and directly into the uterus. Because only 10 percent of sperm make it into the uterus with normal intercourse, this technique, in effect, increases the number of sperm closer to the area where fertilization occurs: the fallopian tube.

Laparoscopy

On the advice of your gynecologist, you may decide to have a laparoscopy. A small incision is made near the navel after the abdominal cavity is inflated with carbon dioxide. The laparoscope is inserted to allow the physician to observe internal organs and especially to check for endometriosis. Endometriosis is a puzzling disease affecting women in their reproductive years. The endometrium is the tissue that lines the inside of the uterus and builds up and then is shed each month at a woman's menstrual cycle. In endometriosis, tissue like the endometrium develops in areas outside the uterus, adhering to the ovaries, fallopian tubes, and other areas of the pelvic cavity.

Endometriosis can be very painful and cause infertility. If it is present, a surgeon can remove the tissue and clear the ovaries and tubal area using laser or electrocautery. Some of the scarring and other damage may be irreversible.

MISCARRIAGES AND OTHER INFERTILITY ISSUES

At some point, the wife may discover she is pregnant. She takes a home pregnancy test, then confirms the pregnancy with the gynecologist.

It is fun as both of you tell all your friends and family who have been praying for you. You wonder how a child will change your lifestyle, and you are so happy. In your joy, the turmoil of the infertility process up to this point now becomes blurred. A baby is coming, and that makes up for everything. You are going to be parents! God has blessed you, and it is an accomplished fact.

Working Through Grief and Feelings

Then one day a couple of weeks later, you think something might be wrong with the pregnancy but don't want to face it. Some bleeding and discomfort occur—surely it's not *that*. Deep down, you know what is happening but can't accept it.

Eventually, though, you are physically faced with the fact that you have lost the baby. Both of you will be affected emotionally. No matter the stage of gestation, you have lost a life and will need to grieve. Both of you may find friends invaluable—particularly those who have been through infertility struggles. Miscarriages are common in fertile and infertile couples, but the fertility struggles may make the disappointment and grief even stronger.

Don't be shocked at the intense roller coaster of feelings that will need to be worked through, including anger at God that He has allowed your hope and happiness to be destroyed. You may wonder exactly what He was doing. Express this anger to Him; He can handle your strong emotions. Acknowledge the intense feelings of loss and the need to mourn the death of your child, along with all of your dreams and expectations for that life.

It may be especially rough or apparent to the wife, who carried the baby; yet the husband can grieve just as intensely. Husband and wife often grieve differently, and in nonparallel paths, but both must deal with loss. It is difficult to be there for each other in supportive ways, but both need to talk and be heard and to be held and comforted. Grieving is tough.

Some general observations on feelings may be helpful at this point in the discussion. During various times on your journey through infertility (maybe more apparent after a miscarriage), you will experience a range of emotions. The feelings of grief are denial, anger, depression, and a desire to withdraw and lick your wounds. Try to express these feelings and not let them build into deep resentment and depression. Support groups, and hopefully friends, can be empathetic sounding boards. Your intimate companionship will suffer under the onslaught of all these feelings, but work at maintaining communication. Mates have a special role in understanding and healing.

Infertility can be a great saboteur of a fun, playful, intimate, passionate sex life. Sexual arousal depends on your reflexive (autonomic) nervous system. Certain feelings short-circuit the arousal that normally occurs when spouses playfully enjoy each other's body, stimulate erogenous zones, and try to passionately connect. The main saboteurs of sexual enjoyment are anger, anxiety, depression, guilt, and grief. The couple struggling with infertility can experience these emotions weekly if not daily. Again, keep communicating and creating companionship, as you maintain perspective.

Dealing with Friends and Family

You told so many friends and family members about the pregnancy. You now have to repeat your story of the miscarriage, feeling somehow embarrassed and hurt and at a loss for words. Some people come through with flying colors as they express sympathy and say they are there for you in any way that would be helpful. Others feel a need to try to fix things or give helpful advice: "You can try again"; or "Maybe God didn't want you to be parents right now." Such advice doesn't help.

All who struggle with infertility have had to work through careless comments, advice, and very personal questions. Families can sometimes be more difficult than friends and acquaintances. You struggle with not isolating and try to be open to your church support group, family, and friends. You may want to withdraw and crawl into a corner, but together you can work at not doing this. Experience the healing that comes with support and talking things through with others.

You may sense that people are uncomfortable and do not know what to say about a miscarriage and infertility in general. Sometimes you just have to shrug off comments, and other times you can seek to educate and express your feelings.

Infertility and even miscarriages are difficult for people to talk about because they involve sex. You can be open about many topics, but in the Christian church and society in general, sex is still not openly discussed. Most infertile couples encounter this problem of having a "socially unacceptable" issue, much like those who have a hysterectomy (female problems) or a varicocele fixed (male problems). Embarrassment prevents people from discussing sexual topics and supporting one another at times when it is needed the most—certainly true with infertility.

Regarding infertility and miscarriages, think ahead and plan some responses so you can comfortably manage conversations and questions. You may want to develop three levels of responses to personal tragedy or struggles. The first level of response is for those who are superficially curious and whose questions and comments sometimes come unexpectedly. "When are you going to start a family?" or "My sister had a miscarriage once." A level-one response is polite but discourages further conversation until you wish to talk: "We're working on it," or "Thanks for your concern, but I don't feel like talking about it right now."

A level-two response is more open and self-disclosing for friends and family who are interested but not wanting or able to be deeply involved: "I am really hurting right now and would appreciate your prayers," or "It's so confusing; if you have the time, I would be willing to sit down and share more about what is happening."

A level-three response is for supportive friends and family you grieve with and count on for help. They want to know what is going on and will make sincere statements offering assistance. It is a more complete self-disclosure with tears and angry outbursts. You may sometimes have to make clearer what you want from them. You might have to say, "I need you just to sit and listen and hold my hand. You can't make it better, but thanks for being here."

It is helpful to think through how your family members choose to deal with problems and perhaps to do some reeducating. They may be judgmental or quick to give advice, or maybe they are silent and never talk about anything personal. The silence may be worse than the quick response. It is worth making attempts to change these patterns and include them in level-three responses. Because they are family does not mean you will always get the support that you wish from them. However, with encouragement and coaching, they may come through in ways that surprise you. Give them material to read, and keep them informed.

You may feel you are letting the family down, especially parents who desire grandchildren. Sometimes when you are wrapped up in your own grief, you may miss how others grieve over your loss. Take the time to talk.

Coping with Holidays and Constant Reminders

Holidays and traditional family times are tough, especially days like Mother's Day and Father's Day. It seems like there is a national day in which everyone gets together and celebrates your loss. You may cry and not want to go to church. Thanksgiving and Christmas can be even more painful reminders of family togetherness.

You don't want to go through another Christmas without a child of your own. You dread family get-togethers and anything that forces you to deal once again with your childlessness. You hate going through busy shopping malls and seeing all the seemingly happy families. Holiday and vacation times can be the pits.

Use common sense as you cope with holidays. Plan special events that minimize the focus on infertility and fill difficult times. Create your own traditions, and enjoy each other as a couple. Allow yourself to feel a little depressed as you reach out for support. Celebrate your faith, and enjoy music. Practice strategic avoidance as you choose not to participate in activities you know will be especially painful.

Sadly, infertile couples may experience more than one miscarriage. In this case, in a later pregnancy you are cautiously optimistic and do not tell everyone. But you cannot help having renewed hope and some anticipation. Could a baby truly be coming into your lives? Unfortunately, only weeks later the same cycle is repeated with another miscarriage. Grieving on top of grieving, along with continued efforts at becoming pregnant, can make life a blur at times. You may grow fearful of getting pregnant and going through another loss all over again. Sex may shut down completely. It isn't making love anymore but risking pregnancy, which can result in another miscarriage and more pain. The prolonged effort takes a toll on all areas of life.

FURTHER OPTIONS

Your gynecologist may complete the initial round of testing and treatment, then recommend a fertility specialist. (This depends on the level of expertise of the physician in infertility and the relationship of the patient to the physician.) A fertility specialist is usually a physician with training in obstetrics and gynecology who has added a subspecialty in reproductive endocrinology (the hormonal system) and infertility. The national organization RESOLVE (see contact information at end of chapter) keeps a list and will make referrals in a given geographic area.

Be an informed and well-educated consumer. Demand straight answers and quality care from the professionals you consult about infertility problems. If you are going through the journey of trying to conceive, please be proactive. Read, go to RESOLVE meetings, talk with those who have been through the process, and ask questions. Here are reasonable expectations in working through the infertility process and in dealing with your doctor(s):

1. Attend sessions as a couple, and both of you speak with the doctor. As a part of this process, make sure the management of both male (a urologist may need to be involved) and female aspects of infertility is coordinated.
2. Insist that questions be answered in language you can understand and that each procedure be explained before it is done.
3. Develop a supportive relationship with your doctor, but retain the right to change doctors to get the type of care you desire. Go with your hunches and find a doctor and staff with whom you are comfortable.
4. Know precisely what every procedure will cost financially, its probability of success, and a general idea of the toll in physical discomfort and danger to health.
5. Reserve the right to know when the price has become too high—physically, financially, and emotionally—and to stop without guilt or pressure to continue.

In Vitro Fertilization

The whole process of infertility, especially in vitro, can become very expensive. Unfortunately, health insurance does not cover a lot of infertility testing and medical interventions. Many couples cannot afford in vitro fertilization (IVF), with its price tag of $10,000 to $20,000 per cycle. There is also no guarantee for in vitro, though success rates have improved with increased technology and greater medical knowledge. Some claim as high as 40 percent, with success rates much higher if the woman is younger. After thirty-five to thirty-eight and older the rates drop dramatically. Some couples endanger their future financial security and completely deplete their savings as they struggle to overcome infertility. Be wise stewards of your money, bodies, and companionship.

As with using a sperm donor, there are ethical issues involved with trying in vitro fertilization; many view the fertilized egg as life. We (Dr. Bill wrote this bioethical summary) believe that unique, individual human life begins when the sperm penetrates the egg and the chromosomes align and activate. This would be the "fertilization event" whether it takes place in the body or in vitro (in "glass"—the petri dish). Thus, each one-celled human, in our view, is made in the image of God and is worthy of dignity and respect.

In the IVF procedure many eggs may be fertilized. The physician prefers implanting three or at most four in the uterus to ensure that one will develop. If high-order multiple birth results, some doctors recommend selective abortions to try to improve the chances of the remaining embryos. Your physician will work with you and can implant only two or three of the healthiest fertilized eggs. You may also not want unused fertilized eggs to be discarded without consideration, and they can be kept frozen. However, consider developing a plan for any "extra" embryos, as they represent life in its earliest form. You can have them implanted at a later time, or donate them to another couple willing to attempt pregnancy with your embryos.

The infertility process continually forces you to make personal and ethical choices. You are being forced to make interventions in a natural process gone awry. You are also trying to contain the strain on your bodies and your relationship.

In addition to in vitro fertilization, there are micromanipulative techniques that a fertility specialist can attempt. Two of these are GIFT (Gamete Intrafallopian Transfer) and ZIFT (Zygote Intrafallopian Transfer). These "high-tech" reproductive technologies are even more expensive. (Further information and explanation can be found in the book *When Empty Arms Become a Heavy Burden*—see the end of this chapter for more details.)

At this point, you may feel tremendous discouragement. Your life and marriage remain infertile and childless. Sometimes one of you will be depressed and the other will not know why. It might be the anniversary of a miscarriage or something that occurred during the day. You may begin feeling that you have done all you can. You still do not have any final answers. You may stop going to the specialists regularly.

You may continue to lash out at God and wonder, as more disappointments occur, "Is He still loving and in charge?" He often continues to demonstrate it through His caring people, but at times it's hard to see. Like your sex life, your spiritual life will take some special attention during the infertility process. Allow God and your supportive encouragers to be there for you as you deepen your faith through suffering—and resist growing deeply bitter.

LETTING GO

After a third miscarriage, one couple learned that there might be an antibody causing the miscarriages. The unfortunate thing was that the way to prevent the antibody from operating was for the wife to take steroids during the entire course of her next pregnancy. There was no guarantee concerning what damage this might do to her body.

That was it for her; enough energy and effort had been expended. Her body had been invaded for the last time, and she was through subjecting herself to further procedures and drugs. It was time to finally accept that she would never have the joy of carrying a child to term and giving birth. There was much grieving, but she was slowly looking forward to adoption and parenting. The importance of her own pregnancy was diminishing, but the need to parent was increasing.

Her husband was still not sure if indeed they had sought enough information and answers. He wasn't quite ready to give up, and still wanted a biological child and was angry with his wife for completely giving up. Her husband wasn't willing to accept and let go of his desire for a natural child. It took a major confrontation for it to finally sink in that she had indeed had all she could take! Even then his denial wasn't instantaneously dissolved. But it became increasingly clear that it was time to move on, and he became willing to check into adoption. (Obviously, all couples will not choose this option.)

When you decide to stop infertility treatments, a special kind of loss and grieving takes place in an ongoing manner that not everyone can understand. Part of the reason you may experience difficulty letting go is not knowing if you are truly infertile. Even if you do know, infertility seems a less concrete loss. Rather than actually losing a child, it is the more nebulous crying over never being a biological parent—nebulous, but very real and traumatizing.

It is not unusual for couples to experience great loss in frequency of sex and to develop problems like temporary impotence. For some couples, a vacation and time spent making love revive the old passion. Others may need to do specific sex therapy to resolve issues that have developed or that the infertility has brought to the surface.

ADOPTION

Some couples, after going through the grueling process of infertility, decide to live child-free. Reasons vary for not pursuing adoption: too old, too exhausted for yet another process, or unable to adjust to not having their own biological child. The decision not to adopt can be a wise decision that a couple must pray through and decide between themselves and the Lord.

For those who decide to adopt, they begin another long and complex process, including finding the right agency to list with. (Many books list adoption resources.)

All agencies differ in their requirements of prospective parents and the way in which the adopted child is delivered to them. Certain state regulations must be complied with as well. Couples feel like things are so out of their control during the infertility testing that they desire to be more in control of the adoption process. Unfortunately, this is not easily achieved.

Like many couples, you may be happy that one aspect of your relationship has returned to normal during the adoption process—your sex life. Intercourse once again is for connecting and is not regulated by ovulation. You are able to make love with all its God-intended excitement and intimate bonding, and you are becoming one flesh and not simply trying to get pregnant. It is great!

The Final Steps

During the final waiting period for a child, you are still grieving, and pangs will be triggered as you see a family together. One father, who has adopted children who are four and six years old, stated that the scars of the infertility process never completely go away. He and his wife have emotional reactions, but they have become less frequent and less painful.

One woman who recently adopted a child said she had to resolve three issues before she was ready to welcome the new child into her life. First, could she let go of fertility and accept that she would never have a biological child? She might never know why medically, but the issue needed to be resolved as forever finished for her. Second, could she take her unborn children (perhaps going to a place that is special and holy) and, with the necessary grieving, leave them forever in Jesus' hands? Third, was she able and ready to get excited about someone else's child becoming her own?

May God bless you if this is the path you choose to take. Adoption has wonderful rewards, and you quickly discover that the children are indeed your own—perhaps even more special because of this added process.

STEPS FOR SURVIVAL AND HEALING IN INFERTILITY

Here is a summary of some of the key points of this chapter:

1. Build and use freely a loving, nonjudgmental support network.
2. Express your feelings and carefully work through them.
3. Find someone, perhaps through the RESOLVE network, who has been through infertility and can be there for you. You will find a special camaraderie and kinship among the couples you start sharing with, and you won't feel so alone. The RESOLVE national office is at

1310 Broadway, Somerville, Massachusetts 02144. They can be contacted at their hotline (888-623-0744) or via e-mail at info@resolve.org; or for further information, see their Web site: www.resolve.org.

4. Be an educated and assertive consumer as you wisely find your way through the maze of infertility. Work with your physicians to formulate an overall game plan and the worst-case scenario so that you do not feel so helpless at each point of failure.

5. Realize your sex life will be affected. Try to keep as much privacy and loving tenderness as possible apart from ovulation. Take vacations and practice other parts of this book to sustain variety and playfulness.

6. Keep as balanced as possible, and resist letting infertility rule your whole life.

7. Choose to allow infertility to draw you together, not tear you apart. Communicate daily; continue loving and nurturing gestures; get away together as companions and ban infertility as a topic while away; make love as separate from infertility; enjoy times with other committed couples.

8. Keep close to the Lord. Be angry, cry, laugh, and allow Him to be there. He gently promises, "Come to me, all you who are weary and burdened, and I will give you rest" (Matt. 11:28 NIV).

Note: This chapter is only meant to be introductory. If you desire further information, take the time to read the more thorough development of a theology of infertility in *When Empty Arms Become a Heavy Burden* by William Cutrer and Sandra Glahn (Broadman and Holman, 1997)

William R. Cutrer, M.D., is a licensed ob/gyn who specialized in the treatment of infertility for fifteen years. He holds a graduate degree from Dallas Theological Seminary and currently is the Gheens Professor of Christian Ministry at the Southern Baptist Seminary in Louisville, Kentucky, where he teaches Sexuality, Marriage Enrichment, and Christian Counseling. He resides in Louisville with his wife, Jane, and is the author or coauthor of several books: When Empty Arms Become a Heavy Burden: Encouragement for Couples Facing Infertility *(Broadman & Holman, 1997),* Sexual Intimacy in Marriage *(Kregel, 2001),* Sexuality and Reproductive Technologies *(Kregel, 1998), and several fiction medical thrillers, including* Lethal Harvest *(a Christian Booksellers Association best-seller, Kregel, 2000),* Deadly Cure *(Kregel, 2001), and* False Positive *(Waterbrook, 2002).*

CHAPTER TWENTY-SIX

God's Sexual Emergency Room

REMEMBER EDEN FOR A MOMENT, and the supercouple Adam and Eve. They were the only mates ever who were truly naked, physically and emotionally, and never had a trace of shame or self-consciousness. Sex and marriage were at a pinnacle. They romped, played, and relaxed in God's presence. But in one moment, Adam and Eve destroyed it. They sinned and the world forever changed.

With cosmic creativity and design second to none, the Almighty jumped in and said, "I'll have to cover your private parts because you won't be able to handle naked as well now. I will rescue My gift of sexuality. I will deal with sin and invent skills to redeem your ruptured relationships."

So now when we're broken and hurting, especially sexually, we can come to God's emergency room. Our sexual breakdowns may be an affair, selfishness, skill deficit, neglect of lovemaking, or fetishes and addiction. This ER is equipped with the healing instruments for rectifying our distorted situations and helping us get back into God's love and light and wisdom. We must gain skill in using these every day, as we heal our relationships and regain integrity.

CONFRONTATION AND INTERVENTIONS

The apostle Paul told Timothy that he should learn to "correct, rebuke and encourage—with great patience and careful instruction" (2 Tim. 4:2 NIV). Paul knew that living in this fallen world would require us to hold each other accountable for growing and not becoming trapped by Satan's deceitfulness. Sexual sins especially appeal to the fleshly desires and are exciting. I appreciate Hebrews 3:13 (NKJV), which encourages us to look out for our fellow Christian brothers and sisters: "But exhort one another daily . . . lest any of you be hardened through the deceitfulness of sin."

We need to take on the qualities of Christ who "is able to deal gently with those who are ignorant and are going astray" (Heb. 5:2 NIV). We all know that there is a lot of sin and stupidity in this present broken world. Christians are not exempt from marital difficulties, broken sexuality, poor boundaries, or real skill deficits. But we can help keep each other conforming to God's guidelines.

A hurting, motivated wife came to me for counseling and said she had practiced submission, hoping to help her husband make some needed changes. I replied that submission would create an atmosphere in which change could take place, but that submission was not God's tool for accomplishing change. Confrontation was that needed skill. She needed to assertively confront but her husband, not angrily, but rather with "great patience and careful instruction" (2 Tim. 4:3 NIV). She felt she had already told him, but I encouraged telling him ten different times and in ten different ways as a part of patient instruction.

In confrontation, it also helps to sandwich the correction with encouragement. "Thanks for getting the door fixed"; "I really need you to call your mother and straighten out Thanksgiving"; "I do appreciate the help with the kids last night." Sandwiching rebukes helps create less defensiveness and the confrontation produces change.

We also have to care enough to confront. I think one of the reasons Jesus did not let the religious rulers throw stones at the woman taken in adultery, in addition to their not deserving to throw stones, is because they did not love her enough to stone her. We have to truly have someone's best interest at heart in order for confrontation to be effective.

Christ taught that when someone offends you, you should confront the issue first with just the two of you and see if you can resolve it. But if the person persists in denial, get some witnesses to corroborate what you are saying and hopefully to break through (Matt. 18:15–16). Today, with addictions, we call this situation an "intervention." Concerned friends and family assemble several people who know and love the individual and have witnessed his sinful shortcoming. Together you confront and shine the spotlight of truth on attitudes and actions while offering alternatives for changing the destructive behaviors.

Confrontation gets better with practice, but it's never fun or easy. God needs us to be that type of friend who cares enough to wisely confront.

Time Out: Whom do you need to confront? When? How?

CONFESSION

James wrote, "Confess your trespasses to one another, and pray for one another, that you may be healed" (5:16 NKJV). Elsewhere Scripture teaches, "He who covers his sins will not prosper, but whoever confesses and forsakes them will have mercy" (Prov. 28:13 NKJV).

Confession is crucial to healing intimate relationships that have been damaged by sinful behaviors.

The Process of Confession

Confession includes two important aspects:

1. Confession brings secrets to the light of day so we drain them of their power. Satan loves to operate in secrecy and darkness. Several years ago I remember having trouble keeping my thought life disciplined concerning a certain woman who would occasionally cross my path. There was no inappropriate interaction, but I did not like the way she could ring my sexual chimes without even trying! I finally told a friend of mine about her—the way I had coached others to confess their secret struggles. How interesting that the next time I saw this woman the sexual pull was gone.

Satan is the master of darkness, and the secrets we keep will fester and gain power. If we bring them to the light of day, God gives us perspective. I see this so often with extramarital affairs that have become so strong and damaging. They lose so much of their power when confessed.

2. Confession also allows God and a caring person to see our ugliness and still love us. We can begin to let go of guilt and shame as we separate sin from sinner. We find out we are not impostors but redeemable sinners when a person knows all of our ugly secrets and *still* loves us. This is a critical concept: we are called by God as confessors to help the transgressor know he or she is redeemable. I like the Twila Paris song about Christ and the line that describes Him as a confessor with "tender eyes that choose to forgive and never despise." He judged sin but was never judgmental of the sinner as He lovingly encouraged change.

An important part of this discipline is seeking out appropriate confessors, groups, and accountability buddies. It's usually not healthy to make our wives our only accountability partners or our primary confessors. Men need a same-sex friend to listen, hear confession, confront, encourage, and hold their feet to the fire.

Time Out: Stop right now and confess a secret sin. Tell a friend today.

REPENTANCE

Repentance is a frequent topic in the New Testament: "I hold this against you: You have forsaken your first love. Remember the height from which you have fallen! Repent and do the things you did at first" (Rev. 2:4–5 NIV); "Godly sorrow produces repentance leading to salvation, not to be regretted" (2 Cor. 7:10 NKJV). Repentance demonstrates we recognize and accept responsibility for destructive thoughts and actions as we choose to make necessary changes. Repentance means giving feet to our remorse and making a 180-degree turn in the other direction. It was amusing when one of my friends got his math mixed up and said repentance was a 360-degree turn. I thought, *"Wow, headed back in the same direction; how easy repentance is!"*

Wives so often say to me that their husbands get very sorry and make changes. The problem is that they usually only last about two months and then they relapse into old attitudes and behaviors. Godly character change that results in sexual integrity is a process with many ongoing choices that will continue over a lifetime. We must follow through on repentance and seek out all the destructive thinking and behaviors that are damaging our marriage and sex life and change them. Lovers can recapture their first love and move on to an intimacy they have never experienced before.

An important part of repentance is putting ourselves back into God's way of thinking and acting. This is so crucial sexually. Remember the basic theology that God created sex primarily for intimate connection. He wants each of us to seek out our own Adam or Eve and become married, covenant companions. He wants each of us to be soul virgins. Virginity is not merely the state of our bodies but the place of our souls in being committed only to our Adam and Eve in this present marriage (or future marriage, for singles). My wife Cathy and I are soul virgins to each other. Repentance is submitting to God's sexual economy and reconforming to His will and way.

Ultimately this is what godly sorrow, guilt, and our consciences are all about. They drive us to repentance and needed change so we get back into God's way of thinking. This way, we don't miss out on His best. Part of getting to the emergency room and experiencing the needed changing is our allowing the Holy Spirit to convict and guide. False guilt is a black cloud of unforgiveness, legalism, and crippling shame. Healthy, convicting guilt helps to flag mistakes and points out when we have violated our godly values. Good guilt motivates us to repent, confess, grieve, and get our act together (2 Cor. 7:10–11). This type of godly sorrow is critical to repentance and to keeping our sexuality on the straight and narrow.

Unfortunately deep, lasting change and repentance are difficult to follow through on. Here are some tips: paint yourself into a corner by telling others of your plans for change; find a same-sex accountability friend to assist you, but be very honest in the questions you want the other to ask you; build your relationship with God—He wants to pour His love, wisdom, and some godly sorrow into your life; keep consistent for six months to a year and it will start to become a habit. Making changes and then *continuing* to make changes is the only way that a great marriage and love life can be built and flourish.

Time Out: You know one very important thing you have procrastinated in changing that would help your marriage and your sex life. What is blocking the change? What two things could you do today that would start the change and repentance?

GRIEVING

"Blessed are those who mourn, for they shall be comforted" (Matt. 5:4 NKJV). "Rejoice with those who rejoice, and weep with those who weep" (Rom. 12:15 NKJV). "Grieve, mourn and wail. Change your laughter to mourning and your joy to gloom. Humble yourselves before the Lord, and he will lift you up" (James 4:9–10 NIV). Because we live in a broken world, we have to learn to cry. This grieving can take many forms but all are filled with cleansing, healing tears. It may be tears over a deep loss, as we work through those grieving stages of denial, anger, and hurt. It may be tears of remorse as we humble ourselves before God and seek His forgiveness.

Feelings somehow touch a deeper part of our being, that part in us which was made in God's image. They also communicate to us in a three-dimensional way: body, soul, and spirit. Short-term feelings often signal the need to deal with something in our lives. Anger signals something is wrong that needs to be addressed, and jealousy shows something important to us is being threatened. Grieving deals with a loss or mistake or woundedness. By contrast, long-term feelings like love, contentment, and sexual pleasure in marriage actually give us joy as we cultivate these over the years of our lives.

Short-term feelings shouldn't be our focus for long periods of time, but are God's tools for mending losses in those broken places, as He moves us back into places of joy and peace. It is so comforting that God knew we would need to cry and heal our souls in this broken world; He promised that we will be comforted. The victim of an affair or sexual trauma will find comfort and resolution on his or her journey back into sexual wholeness, and God will most often use other people to be the delivery system for such healing.

As a couple, help each other recognize and work through a myriad of feelings as you rebuild love. Help each other grieve over losses and work through hurt and anger. Grieving is not a process that can be worked through totally alone. We need others to share the process with us.

Time Out: What secret hurt haven't you faced and grieved over? Allow yourself to go there and feel sad. Share this with someone this week.

FORGIVENESS

We are told, "Judge not . . . Condemn not . . . Forgive, and you will be forgiven" (Luke 6:37 NKJV); and "Bearing with one another, and forgiving one another if anyone has a complaint against another; even as Christ forgave you, so you also must do" (Col. 3:13 NKJV). Sexuality is so full of mistakes, both sinful and immature, that we have to master forgiveness as one of God's healing arts. The ER won't function without it. It is a *process of letting go* of resentment and shame towards self and others.

I like to use the word *pardon* for forgiveness. It is reconciling the ledger even though justice has not been satisfied. This skill of forgiving separates sin from sinner and frees up emotional energy from shame, hurt, and resentment, directing it into deepening and rebuilding love. It is a choice we make independent of the other person's actions. The other person does not have to be repentant for us to forgive. We do it so we don't get eaten up with the cancer of resentment and revenge, and block God's best for us.

Though forgiveness doesn't have to include the other's changing, reconciliation is another process and *does* require the other person's involvement. Remember, forgiveness does not condone what has happened, nor does it create instant trust. Pardoning does not mean justice has been served but that we choose to let go and heal. Trust, like love, will be built over time, if the other person is truly repentant and wants to become trustworthy.

Realize forgiveness is indeed a *process* that slowly unfolds over time as you remember, deal with issues, and heal. Memories of other incidents or old hurt will pop into our memory and we have to keep forgiving as we work through to greater healing. We have to work through the hurt and anger before we can truly let go. This may be especially true of the survivor of sexual abuse. Forgiveness will take time. But throughout this process, never are you condoning what has been done.

Forgiveness is an invaluable tool and character trait (see Chapter 2) for intimate sexual relationships. You will probably find that the hardest person to forgive is yourself. I remember one young woman who told me, "I am getting married in three weeks and I have ruined my honeymoon night. I have had sex with other men and I've stolen what was special from our sex life. It will be a miserable time." I asked her if her fiancé had forgiven her and she said, "Totally." I then commented that God wasn't as worried about the wedding night but was really concerned about the next fifty years. *She* was running the risk of destroying her wedding night—not her boyfriend or God—and the nights to come with her inability to forgive herself. There are indeed consequences to sin but there is also repentance and forgiveness and redemption. She was restored as a soul virgin, and God saw her as such on her wedding night.

Learn to forgive and help others practice this important mechanism for healing.

Time Out: What haven't you been able to forgive yourself for? Take it to God this week over and over again in prayer and then confess to someone, as you feel that person's love and acceptance.

MAKING AMENDS AND RESTITUTION

After repenting, Zacchaeus told Christ that he was going to make amends to those he had cheated as a tax collector: "If I have cheated anybody out of anything, I will pay back four times the amount" (Luke 19:8 NIV). Christ saw true repentance in this act and realized Zacchaeus needed to make amends in order to experience deeper healing.

Synonyms for making amends might be *restoration, restitution,* or *penance.* I'm not talking about penance as punishment but as a tool of *restitution* that encourages repentant changes and restores intimacy. The prophet Ezekiel recognized this healing for a person who "turns from his sin and does what is lawful and right . . . gives back what he has stolen, and walks in the statutes of life without committing iniquity" (33:14–15 NKJV).

Making amends restores trust and can make restitution for harmful behaviors, bringing resolution and reconnection into the marriage. As I have stated, it is not vengeance, but doing what the mate needs to restore intimacy. Restitution should be tailored to the offense. One mate wanted her husband, after an affair, to do the dishes for the rest of their married life. I encouraged that a more appropriate restitution might be counseling and his bending over backwards with phone calls and real efforts at pursuing her, to reestablish her trust.

Time Out: Be creative and make restitution to your mate today for a hurt you have caused, as you continue the mutual healing.

May God give you His wisdom and courage to run to His emergency room and use His tools for growth and correction when intimacy is threatened or damaged. Practice and learn to use God's mechanisms for healing in those broken and painful times. These skills aren't fun or easy, but they will help you build the passionately intimate marriage and sex life that you desire.

CHAPTER TWENTY-SEVEN

Extramarital Affairs

AN INTIMATE MARRIAGE thrives on commitment, honesty, trust, comfortable companionship, and sex that is safe and connecting. Satan could not have devised a better scheme for striking at the heart of a marriage than adultery. Affairs hit the very foundation of commitment and trust in this special God-designed union—polluting and weakening it, and sometimes destroying it all together.

This chapter on extramarital sexual affairs starts off with guidelines that can prevent you from falling into the trap of adultery. The second section explores the phases of an affair and the healing steps that are possible. The third section summarizes five commonsense but crucial ways to "affair-proof" your marriage.

PREVENTION: NO TRESPASSING ALLOWED

In adultery everyone eventually suffers. Even if the affair is only an emotional adultery and never culminates in physical sex, if it is lived out in the mind and never acted upon, or even if it is never discovered, the people involved and their marriages are damaged. Unless confessed and healed couples often live with a very poor excuse for what companionship is designed to be—a deep intimacy and powerful partnership. They also suffer spiritual deterioration with dishonesty and divided loyalty, sacrificing the love, joy and peace that God promises His children who walk within His economy.

Erecting Good Fences

The following ten behaviors and attitudes are vital for keeping other people from trespassing into your intimate companionship. They can help you prevent adultery so that you never have to deal with its demoralizing consequences. How may of these fences do you have in place in your marriage right now?

1. Make a decision and commit to the fact that you will never have an extramarital affair. No circumstance or need or rationalization will ever make adultery right. You have determined, "Never!" and not, "I don't think so." There is no waffling on this certainty; you have willfully made this decision. That door is shut and will never be opened, and your "No Trespassing" sign is always up as you seek to protect and nurture your marriage. You never romance adultery with your mind, your heart, or your body.

2. Do not keep secrets or allow sexual feelings and fantasies to go unaddressed. Anytime you keep a secret, especially of a sexual nature, you invite trouble. Secrets need to be shared to prevent them from gathering energy and destructive possibilities. You are responsible for building an accountability network in which you can share secrets. Your mate is important, and anytime you avoid telling your spouse something, take note and examine what is going on. A trustworthy same-sex friend or colleague who shares your values is also invaluable. Infidelity is based on secrecy and dishonesty.

3. Keep all sexual fantasies that you willfully (intentionally) create focused on your partner. It may seem like trite advice, but your sexual thought life needs to be carefully disciplined. Sinful lust and acting out sexually are encouraged by obsessively making people sexual objects or continually fantasizing about a person or situation outside your marriage. Christ said that if we continually lust after someone, sin will usually result.

4. Set limits. Do not share intimate details of your marriage with a person of the opposite sex. Never complain about your partner or air your dirty laundry—even to a stranger on an airplane. Be careful how you provide a listening ear even in a church group. Revealing pain and frustration is a bonding behavior and makes you vulnerable to seek comforting. Mentioning your mate and children positively, refraining from long eye contact, avoiding intimate settings (riding alone in a car), including the whole group rather than seeking intense personal interactions—all help set limits with casual contacts. Affairs often start and flourish from a casual friendship that grows.

5. Do not permit an intimate friendship with an opposite-sex person to grow without tight boundaries. Adultery occurs so easily among couples who have become good friends. Not only is the marriage damaged, but long-term friendships are lost forever. Some boundaries are including both mates in all activities, dealing with sexual attraction or ending the friendship, avoiding secret e-mails or phone calls, not playing therapist with bonding sessions over personal woes, controlling sexual talk and joking, and preserving modesty, especially on vacations. The most common and destructive affairs are built out of intimate friendships.

6. Do not spend unaccounted time together with opposite-sex colleagues, committee members, schoolmates, or exercise partners. Females and males enjoy interacting, and there will naturally be attraction—don't think you are invulnerable. That late-night run or cup of coffee after the committee meeting, that study group meeting on Sunday afternoon or Saturday in the office can be dangerous. One-on-one interaction is intimate and increases temptation.

7. Be explicit with your mate about what is and is not appropriate behavior. One wife said that she knew her husband ate lunch with his secretary and they occasionally went shopping afterward, but she never thought they would go to a movie together. Never let your marital rules on fidelity be unspoken. Discuss openly what you think is and is not appropriate behavior. One saleswoman never sees clients on the road after 8:00 P.M. and limits herself to one drink with business dinners. A homemaker never allows her male neighbors in the house unless her husband is home, and vice versa. Don't assume you know how your mate thinks; discuss possible situations and talk to each other.

8. Pay attention to your guilty feelings. Guilt is a God-given, specific feeling that a particular value has been violated and there is a need for recognition and change (the process of confession and repentance). A Christian trains the conscience so it is in accord with God's Word and values. If you are feeling guilty about something, especially if you are being tempted to keep it a secret, take notice and stop doing it. When guilt flags a behavior or thought pattern as being inappropriate or dangerous, you should not engage in rationalizing. Examine what is happening and make changes.

9. Build an accountability network. You will not always recognize your rationalizations and errors in judgment. You need people in your life who know you well enough to indicate the times your attitudes and behaviors may be straying outside God's wisdom and economy. You can create structure in your life that keeps accountability and boundaries in place. For example, a certain pastor never counsels someone of the opposite sex without his secretary in the outer office, and he never chauffeurs women around town. God gives the wisdom for you to protect yourself from your sinful propensities with an appropriate accountability structure and network.

10. Never think that you are invulnerable. This may seem to contradict the first fence of never entertaining the possibility of an affair. But this fence is about avoiding cockiness. According to the Bible, pride comes before a fall (Prov. 16:18). Resting in our strong character and good past choices can make us very vulnerable. Many people have told me, "This is the last thing I thought would happen to me." I personally pray so often, "Lord, please shine Your truth and light into my life and keep me from sin and stupidity." Being humble, constantly repairing your fences, maintaining close friendships with people of the same sex and couples who also value fidelity, never keeping secrets, disciplining your sexual thought life, and growing ever closer to Christ and His wisdom are invaluable if you don't want someone trespassing into your intimate companionship. Think through what might be the chink in your armor that Satan could exploit. What type of person and situation would be most seductive to you?

The old saying that "an ounce of prevention is worth a pound of cure" certainly applies to adultery. How many of these "No Trespassing" guidelines are you violating? How vulnerable are you? If you are ignoring some of these wise boundaries, please don't think that you are the one person in the world who can spit in the wind without it coming back to hit you in the face. Start making some changes today. Others of you are reading this chapter, unfortunately, after the fact, and you need to understand how to work your way through the affair and be able to heal your marriages.

PHASES OF AN AFFAIR

There are five common phases of an affair: (1) inception, (2) prediscovery, (3) discovery, (4) recovery, and (5) resolution. Many affairs go undiscovered and never get to the discovery and resolution stages. In some marriages, the undiscovered adultery and the problems that created it are resolved and the intimacy is restored. Unfortunately, that is usually not the case, and two things happen. First, the individual issues and flaws in the marriage are never dealt with, and often there is another affair, or the partners settle for an unsatisfying relationship. Second, mistrust and dishonesty linger because the mate suspected the affair, or the partner who had the affair lives as an impostor fearing his or her mate could never forgive this dark secret. A deeper intimacy never blossoms.

Confession and the discovery phase are vital for healing infidelity and its damage to honesty and the committed companionship. All marriages do not make it to a recovery phase. Although Christ permits divorce because of adultery, He does not mandate it. Most marriages in which both partners are committed to making the partnership work and go through the confession and repentance process usually survive and often become even more intimate.

1. The Inception Phase

How do affairs get started? Whose fault are they? Are the causes usually sexual in nature? Can they occur even in a reasonably good marriage?

Yes, affairs can happen in a fairly intimate and committed marriage. Affairs do not always signal that the one cheating has no love for the spouse. Quite often I hear in counseling, "If he loved me he wouldn't have had the affair." I sadly respond, "He loves you and he had an affair." The reasons are more complex and may have nothing to do with the mate, as in a close friendship in which poor boundaries were set, sexual curiosity, acquaintance with a former sweetheart, or following in Dad's footsteps.

Adultery is often not centered on sex. Sex becomes a part of it, but it may have begun as a supportive friendship or an office flirtation that guaranteed ego strokes. For some, it is the thrill of the illicit and a sense of adventure. Often after the chase is over, the excitement and attraction are gone. Sexual curiosity and frustration initiate some extramarital liaisons, but sex is just one of many reasons affairs occur.

The offending spouse sometimes blames the mate or a deteriorating marriage for the affair. Poor companionship and a lack of lovemaking make a couple more vulnerable, but there is still a *choice*. If you leave the keys in your car and someone steals it, it is still the thief's fault. The adulterer chose to have the affair. Many deeper issues also launch affairs: a midlife crisis, spiritual poverty, a poor sex life, unchecked sexual fantasy, family scars and adulterous parents, or falling in love with someone else. These problems must be resolved, but the ultimate cause of infidelity is a series of poor choices. Adultery seldom begins by being blindsided.

I remember the salesman who said he was blindsided by a seductive woman and was sure it would never happen again. I replied, "You were in the hotel bar at 11:00 at night, you struck up a conversation, you got on the elevator with her, you chose to go back to her room—these are too many choices to be blindsided. I disagree with you, and unless there are many changes it will happen again."

2. The Prediscovery Phase

As the adulterous relationship comes into full bloom, there is a lot of guilt, excitement, stolen pleasures, much phone time, dishonesty and webs of deceit, and often not that much sex. The rendezvous take planning and deception, and there is more carelessness over time.

Some adultery involves a one-night stand, and there isn't a prediscovery phase. This is not to say that this type of affair is not destructive. It breaks the bonds of trust and faithfulness and love. Long-term infidelity can take an even greater toll on the marital relationship, and the cheated-on mate feels more deeply betrayed and blind for not discovering what was going on.

The one cheated on often knows something is not quite right but can't put a finger on it. The one in the affair is often oblivious to the changes taking place: the different behavior patterns, the irritability or indifference toward the mate and the marriage, and distorted thinking along these lines: the partner is becoming less attractive, the tension is somehow the mate's fault, the partner is no longer understanding, and the marriage was never that good anyway.

Tremendous rationalizing and compartmentalizing occur in the mind of the unfaithful partner. One mate stated he didn't think he was that dishonest because he left his wedding ring on the whole time. A wife told her husband she had never taken all of her clothes off during the affair. (Trust me; that wasn't very comforting to her husband.) The two worlds become more difficult to balance and keep separate, but the dishonesty gets easier.

The prediscovery phase creates growing anger, frustration, and distance. Something is gravely wrong, but no one is talking about it and denial reigns. Both mates are unsettled. Feelings oscillate from guilty excitement to self-loathing in the cheating partner, and from confused hope to fearful desperation in the one cheated on.

Not every affair is discovered or confessed and worked through. An issue most people struggle with is the advisability of confessing undiscovered affairs, both past and present.

Confession is vital in restoring honesty and rebuilding trust. It acknowledges that the adultery was destructive (and sinful) and brings it to the light of day so the power of secrecy and guilt can be broken. Confession helps the guilty one feel accepted and forgiven despite the sinful actions. As James encourages, "Confess your trespasses to one another, and pray for one another, that you may be healed" (5:16 NKJV). An ongoing or recent affair usually demands confession to one's mate as well as to God for healing to begin to take place.

Until this contrite spirit has been demonstrated and a recommitment to the marriage affirmed, it is impossible to create a true partnership again in which each has died to self and is unconditionally committed to the other's well-being. Trust takes time to rebuild, but with confession and reconciliation, the mates are back on the road to create a one-flesh union again.

The confession of past affairs is more difficult to determine. Treating your mate as fragile or fearing conflict are inadequate reasons for not confessing. If the confession is just to share the guilt and the issues of the adultery have already been resolved, a better confessor may be your pastor or counselor. The past affair may have been suspected and is still creating mistrust. It may demand confession to clear the air. A good rule of thumb is to talk over the possible confession with a trusted adviser before proceeding.

3. The Discovery Phase

A profusion of feelings, issues, and reactions must be worked through during this time of discovery. How the affair was discovered doesn't seem to cushion the shock from the partner. It is devastating whether it is confessed or discovered via taped phone conversations, a private detective, or a growing collection of evidence and a confrontation. It is all so tawdry and gut-wrenching and throws both mates into pain, guilt, betrayal, and deep loss. Choices have to be made, and both enter into a grieving process.

Adultery is like a funeral, and you need to view the body. Mates need a thorough, honest confession (viewing the body) to validate that a real loss has taken place. Then they can slowly grieve and reclaim the marriage. If confession comes out in dribbles then trust continues to be broken.

In Alcoholics Anonymous, recovering alcoholics go through twelve steps to promote healing. The fourth step is a very searching and fearless moral inventory in which they courageously write down all their past transgressions and then confess them to at least one person. You need one thorough confession with details that will help the mate heal: When did it start? How long? How sexual? In our house and bed? Was it protected sex? Did you go to our favorite restaurant? Who knows about it? and so on.

After this confession, encourage process questions and not detail questions. The couple needs to view the body, but eventually, it can become ineffective if they keep digging it up and do an endless autopsy with detail questions. Process questions deal with what was missing from the person's life and the relationship to cause the affair. How did the love for someone else grow? What needs to change? How could one help the other trust more? Detail questions—How may times and where? What positions? How much did you love him?—create vivid nightmares and are counterproductive as the imagination runs wild. Don't ask questions that you will have trouble handling and do not really need the answers to.

A betrayed mate feels the need for this interrogation. The one who has committed adultery will grow weary, but it is important for the cheated-on spouse to:

- break through the shock and denial and ventilate feelings as the grieving process is worked through.
- prevent, with enough questions and knowledge, another affair from happening.
- completely reclaim the mate by destroying all secrets and having everything in the relationship be mutually shared knowledge.
- exact some penance and perhaps some vengeance as the partner squirms and atones for the feelings of pain and being duped that the one cheated on experiences.

After the denial stage of grieving is broken through, intense anger will surface. The interrogation is a part of this, but it is also the feeling of being duped and wondering how foolish the individual must seem to others. Trust and fidelity, very special and important qualities, have been lost and violated. Healing is a tortuous process for both mates at this stage.

4. The Recovery Phase

In the recovery phase, the interrogation can continue. New outbursts of feelings and questions are occasionally triggered, and the adulterer is awakened in the middle of the night or receives a barrage over the phone while at work. A wrong number, a new sexual technique, twenty extra minutes getting home at night, and the angry attacking begins all over again. The one cheated on needs to remember to keep the questions more process, and not detail, in nature. Sometimes the one who cheated needs to make a simple answer to a detail question to lay an issue to rest. The one who cheated wonders if it will ever stop and if trust will ever be rebuilt. This is part of the penance and price paid to restore intimacy and heal the damage done.

An adulterer has stolen intimacy and commitment from the partner. Restitution in kind seems appropriate, not only to heal what has been damaged but also to help that person grow through penitence and to make some real changes. Time, money, and energy should be invested in rebuilding the marital intimacy that has been so damaged by the adultery.

In recovery, the one involved in the affair is ready to move on long before the wounded partner is able. Both can grow weary in the processes of grieving, rebuilding intimacy, and forgiving. The initial choice of forgiveness on both partners' parts may be done quickly, but the process of forgiving and letting go and rebuilding respect and trust takes time. Forgiving is not condoning what has been done or instantly forgetting. Partners don't forgive and immediately forget—they slowly let go as trust is earned.

New bubbles of resentment and hurt will pop to the surface as recovery goes on, and forgiveness will have to be an ongoing process. The recovery stage can be very different for various couples. Certain factors complicate the restoration process and demand more work for healing to take place:

- The length and intensity of the affair, especially feelings of love and friendship, relapses or making contact with the person again
- The state of the marital intimacy before, during, and after the affair—the depth of dishonesty, broken commitment, and disrespect, and the breakdown of one-flesh bonding
- The level of individual scars and immaturity and the amount of environmental pressures (finances, children, illness, work) that are present in addition to the stress of the affair

Even with all of these complex factors, God's healing grace abounds. If both partners are committed to restoring the marriage, they almost always succeed. The trauma often creates a deeper and more realistic intimacy with better boundaries in place. Greater maturity grows out of the crisis they have weathered.

Not everyone in the recovery phase chooses to stay married, however. The adultery may have tapped a deep, core fear within the soul of the one who was betrayed. Trust may be irreparably shattered as the couple tries to pick up the pieces but cannot. Sometimes the affair has pointed out deep flaws in their relationship, which they don't think they have the energy or respectful desire to repair. A tragic fact is that adultery can result in divorce.

After evaluating the marriage, the one in the affair may decide to get a divorce and marry the person involved in the affair. It is easy to be deceived into compounding the initial mistake. Affairs are very idealistic and are not the best perspective from which to choose a life partner.

If you have fallen in love with someone else but decide to honor your marital commitment, be aware of how difficult it can be to break that other bond. There is no good way to end it other than to stop it cold turkey. You will be vulnerable. Get an accountability network in place to support you in resisting temptation.

See your spouse as an apple and your former lover as an orange. Focus on apples. The issue is not that you could not be married to an orange and it would be its own happy, unique relationship, but that God has given you an apple. One husband put an index card in his wallet and reviewed it daily for a while. On one side were all the wonderful qualities of his wife. On the other side were the flaws in the adulterous relationship and what he stood to lose. Another husband insisted he had found true chemistry with his orange (mistress) and an apple (his wife) would never appeal again. In frustration I finally told him with a note of sarcasm that I would dump both women because he had never experienced mangoes, and that would make oranges pale in comparison.

Some couples experience a second honeymoon as a part of the recovery phase. This response is understandable and can help to heal wounds. The one involved in the affair is relieved to be beyond the secrecy and guilt and is rediscovering some of the reasons for the original attraction to the partner. The one cheated on, after dealing with anger and betrayal, is excited not to have lost a mate. After their marriage had such a close call, both have their adrenaline flowing and deeply appreciate that the disaster was averted. Sex has been forced out into the open with romantic activity and libidos running high. The problem with the honeymoon is that it can sweep issues under the rug, which can later come back to haunt the marriage. Individual and relational problems may not be uncovered and resolved.

5. The Resolution Phase

The couple working on recovery slowly reestablishes the equilibrium and deepens the intimacy of the partnership. Now comes a crucial time in the marriage—the final resolution phase of an affair as the healing process merges back into the humdrum of routine existence. The angry questioning is largely gone, and the grief and causes of the adultery have been worked through. The marriage now continues to grow stronger from the base of recovery and all the changes that have been made—or it settles back into the same routines and is prone to future affairs, sometimes with mates changing roles.

Changing personal and relational patterns in a permanent manner is not easy. The emotional and spiritual growth will come slowly as you continually resist sliding back into old patterns. The scars of the affair may still haunt you occasionally. Do not try to avoid the flashbacks, but talk through them. Keep strengthening and protecting your intimate companionship.

RELAPSE PREVENTION AND AFFAIR-PROOFING

You have already considered ten different behaviors and attitudes that can keep other people from trespassing into your sacred partnership. The ten behaviors that set solid fences in place to keep out trespassers are vital. Here are five other protective and growth-producing suggestions that you need to have in place as you affair-proof your marriage and prevent relapse.

Protecting Your Fences

1. Flag some behaviors to warn that the partnership is losing some of its intimacy and you are becoming vulnerable. Set in place some warning signals that you as mates will notice and act upon to make changes. Here are various behaviors that other couples have found helpful to flag:

- Making love infrequently and falling short of their sexual goals
- Avoiding conflict and suppressing anger
- Neglecting spirituality: no prayer, poor church attendance, and so on
- Keeping any secrets or tiptoeing around an issue
- Canceling date nights and spending little time alone together

2. Love and affirm the beauty of your mate and marriage. Resist the "greener grass" syndrome. If you focus on your mate's flaws and stay dissatisfied with your partnership—rather than make needed changes or affirm strengths—you adulterate your one-flesh union and invite trespassing. Focus your energy and attention on your garden instead of noticing every beautiful plant and the green grass outside your fence. I had a Snoopy poster that read: "The other man's grass is always greener, until you get there and find out it's artificial turf."

3. Learn the biblical and relational skills of confrontation, repentance, confession, grieving and expressing feelings, forgiveness, and making amends. These are vital processes when sin has damaged your partnership. (Be sure to read Chapter 26, in which these are discussed.)

4. Get your act together—personally and maritally! Remember that problems often precipitate affairs. Do whatever you need to do: Learn communication skills, deal with addiction or anger or some other personal problems, overcome your fear of conflict, get some therapy, take action—or the problems may manifest themselves through adultery.

5. Build an intimate marriage and learn to truly make love to your mate. Mates who are creating the one-flesh partnership that God designed and are falling more deeply in love are much less vulnerable to temptation. They are more aware of the damage infidelity would do to the beautiful, trusting companionship that they have worked so hard to build and nurture. This is also true of a fulfilling sex life. Affairs are often not sexual in nature, but making love frequently and passionately is a great prevention of adultery. Don't just have sex, but truly learn to make love to your partner and "know" your partner inside and out. Be tender, excited, nurturing, communicative, and loving. The "No Trespass" signs seem to be obvious to all who look in on a truly intimate marriage.

CHAPTER TWENTY-EIGHT

Sexual Integrity or Sexual Addiction

OUR SOCIETY SO BOMBARDS us with sex. It is easy to empathize with the early church father Origen, who made himself a eunuch in a desperate step to achieve greater purity and not be a stumbling block to the Christian sisters he was teaching. But God has also given us a wonderful gift in being sexually alive with exciting potential for deep, passionate intimacy. So much of whether our sexuality is a gift or a curse depends on our self-discipline.

CREATING SEXUAL INTEGRITY

The following are practical skills, actually disciplines, that men and women need to practice as they grow up into sexual maturity and intimacy. "For God did not give us a spirit of timidity, but a spirit of power, of love and of self-discipline" (2 Tim. 1:7 NIV). I have aimed these sexual integrity skills especially at men, with their greater fascination for specific visual stimulation and stronger testosterone surges at times. I know that women can profit from and utilize them too, as they tailor them to their own unique situations.

Access the Power of Your Position and Hate Evil

Recently one of my clients was real enough to admit, "The reason I haven't stopped looking at cybersex is that it is too exciting and I don't think I want to give it up yet." Lack of sexual integrity can be a sin problem, plain and simple, and this man couldn't see what sugar-coated poison he was eating. "The mind of the sinful man is death, but the mind controlled by the Spirit is life and peace" (Rom. 8:6 NIV). God has broken the power of sin in the lives of those who have a personal relationship with Him through Jesus Christ.

The Holy Spirit is in each of us to grow us up into sexual maturity, but we have to choose to access His power. Keeping infused with God's energy takes bravery and daily choice. "Submit yourselves, then, to God. Resist the devil, and he will flee from you. Come near to God and he will come near to you" (James 4:7–8 NIV). It may be hourly that we have to take up the Christian armor (Eph. 6:10–18) and resist sexual sin and immaturity.

It is also critical to remember the importance of breaking Satan's sexual strongholds and bondage in our lives. Accessing the power of our position in Christ may take strong prayers of deliverance from Satan's power. We have past relationships and fantasies that have bound us to evil and distortion. We have become "one flesh" with women other than our wife (1 Cor. 6:16 NIV), and God's power must be accessed to break this hold.

We will make better choices as God helps us become appalled at how shallow, ugly, stupid, and tragically destructive sexual sins are. Psalm 97:10 exhorts us to "let those who love the Lord hate evil" (NIV). When we lust after another woman or are tempted to have an affair, we can better understand the damage by switching to an evil we could never imagine ourselves doing—like taking a tire iron from our car and bashing our wife with it. We each need to recognize how cruel and mean God views our sinful fantasies and actions to be.

Practice Three-Dimensional Sexuality

God teaches us that sexuality is three-dimensional. It can never be just a body thing (1 Cor. 6:13–19) but naturally involves our soul and spirit. Three-D sexuality is a marvelous tool for achieving integrity. When you are at the mall and notice an attractive woman, look at her face and notice if she is tired. Observe the packages she is carrying and think, *I bet she's a great mom.* Make the woman a person and give her a life.

Body. Observe the eyes, which are the windows to the soul—Is she happy, sad, tired? Look at less common but very feminine features like hands, smile, and ways of gesturing. Let her body communicate her feminine heart, not just female parts.

Soul. Be aware of feelings and how she enjoys life and people. Honor the needs of her mind and heart for respect and affirmation, not lust. She is very precious to God. Would you want someone looking at your daughter or your wife the way you are looking at her?

Spirit. Remember that she wants someone special in her life and biblically this cannot be you. Think of her need for intimate connecting—Has she allowed God to meet those deep inner desires? Pray that God will bring that soul mate into her life to complete her.

One of my clients, after seeing a great body and struggling with lust, asks himself, "I wonder if she knows Jesus?" Giving her a spirit and praying for her gets him back on track. He laughs and tells me I have spoiled his lusting. Three-D women are easier to see as people and sisters, and harder to view as only sex objects.

Enjoy Daughters, Mothers, and Sisters and Quit Window-Shopping

God created sexuality to give us beautiful insights (windows) into His own image and His deep, loving desire for intimate relationships. God has this two-part sexual economy that works. One way of revealing His image to us through sexual relating is the family or gender connection: men as fathers, sons, and brothers and women as moms, daughters, and sisters.

The second type of sexual intimacy is romantic and reflects Christ and the Bride. All of erotic sexuality relates to the covenant of marriage, and making love is intended for that union only.

We can summarize God's plan quite simply: Every Adam courageously waits for and erotically connects only with his Eve—all other women are his sisters. A female client of mine recently asked why Christian men do so much window-shopping of women. She said, "If they are godly men, why are they sizing up women for mental or physical sexual relationships? Aren't we sisters?" Wow, that sure hits us where we live.

The last, and perhaps the summary, of the Ten Commandments is "You shall not covet" (Ex. 20:17 NKJV). The heart of coveting is not being content with what we have—ungratefully dumping on the rich gifts God has given us. It also includes spitefully stealing something that has been given to someone else. God did not create all women for us to participate with erotically. We have our Eve and the other "sisters" belong to their special Adams.

Quit coveting! I fondly think of a pastor friend of mine who, upon seeing an attractive woman, says to himself, "Thank you, Lord, for this woman." And then he adds, "But this isn't my woman, Lord. Thank you for mine." His wife was erotic to him and other women were his mothers, sisters, and daughters. "[Treat] older women as mothers, and younger women as sisters, with absolute purity" (1 Tim. 5:2 NIV).

Meet Nonsexual Needs Nonsexually

I recently asked my men's group, "It's Friday afternoon and you got off work early. The wife and kids are not home and you have time to relax and enjoy. How many of you might think of something sexual as a part of that recreation?" All of them admitted that it would cross their minds.

We brainstormed on what they were really desiring at the end of an exhausting week: diversion, a chance to let down and play, and maybe some adventure and excitement. Sex can accomplish this, but we started listing alternatives: wandering around Home Depot, competing on a computer game, biking, or a ball game.

Men long for connection, meaningful physical touch, and consolation when stressed—women aren't any different. False sexual intimacy can seem helpful, but this shallow substitute can never become the real thing. One of my friends, Mark Laaser, keeps saying that the antidote to lust is good male friendships. His excellent workbook, *Faithful and True*, helps men learn, in a support-group setting, how to help each other meet nonsexual needs non-sexually.

Letting God help us meet our needs, sexual and nonsexual, with wisdom and appropriateness, is a critical discipline for sexual integrity. I appreciate Ecclesiates 3:1: "There is a time for everything, and a season for every activity under heaven" (NIV). We often think that we need sex, when we are really searching for excitement, recreation, consolation, a compliment, or a hug.

Go to the Heart of Issues and Work Inside Out

Do you sometimes believe God doesn't hold up His part of the bargain with changing our sexual behaviors? You try so desperately to do the right behaviors sexually and yet always seem to slip.

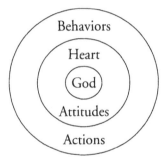

Quit trying to work outside in, instead of starting with God working His deeper changes in your hearts and creating true freedom and redemption. Real sexual integrity is not about what you *aren't* doing; it's about what you *are* doing. You may have stopped masturbation but haven't dealt with the deeper heart lust issues.

Go deeper than the behavior. How is masturbation affecting you and your relationships? What are the deeper God and heart issues? Are you lusting, lazy, avoiding intimacy, feeding an addiction? Go deep into God's character and to the heart of issues and work inside out.

I appreciate the recovery movements within Alcoholics Anonymous and Sex Addicts Anonymous that stress the difference between being dry and being sober. Dry is simply white-knuckling and not acting out, while sober is growing up and making deeper changes in honesty, healing hurts, and creating intimacy. Let God work inside out to change these behaviors and attitudes.

Discipline Fantasies and Sexual Surges

Men usually think they are more highly sexed than their wives are. It is true that most men think about sex more and are more visually specific as they zoom in on female bodies. But I don't think it is higher testosterone or our sexual natures that always make us more sexually aroused. Rather, it is our poor self-discipline of the environmental sexual cues.

Controlling sexual cues is an interesting discipline. It involves several ways of applying the wisdom to "take captive every thought" (2 Cor. 10:5 NIV) and considering that "the eye is the lamp of the body. If your eyes are good, your whole body will be full of light" (Matt. 6:22 NIV). Practicing the following really helps:

1. *Don't close your eyes or give "free rent."* When hearing or seeing a sexual cue (for example, a friend talking about making love with his attractive wife), keep from closing your eyes and visualizing/fantasizing the sexual image. You can't always avoid the sexual stimulation, but when a thought/visual cue comes into your mind you can choose not to give it rent-free lodging. God gives us the ability to switch topics in our minds.

2. *Direct your vision and practice the "one second" rule.* Try to discipline your vision to look at women's faces or see their bodies in a more general way—don't do the elevator routine as your eyes roam up and down, stopping at favorite floors. When seeing specific visual cues (a tight sweater, for example), do not allow your gaze to linger and further sexualize the cue. Move your mind and eyes on.

3. *Do not run with cues.* Noticing the cute runner may be natural. Following up that cue by almost driving off the road trying to see what her breasts look like in the rearview mirror is a step into dangerous territory. Now you're thinking, *Wow, great build, and a blonde!* You are off and running in your mind, as you take one cue and build it into seven. Choose to stop at one.

Practice Pre-Zone Choices

In sexual addiction there is an interesting concept of being in "the zone." This is when sexual temptation and lustful desire have headed down the slippery slope and have already given birth to sinfully following through on a behavior. It would take a team of wild horses to stop you once you reach the acting-out zone. "But each one is tempted when, by his own evil desire, he is dragged away and enticed. Then, after [evil] desire has conceived, it gives birth to sin" (James 1:14–15 NIV).

Carl claimed his car had a mind of its own and turned into the parking lot of the convenience store. However, Carl was already in the sinning *zone* by the time he got near the store, which had pornographic magazines for sale. The time for easier decisions was much earlier. That morning he could have called a friend for help. He could have exercised over lunch to relieve stress. He could have called his wife before he left work. He failed to make any of these pre-zone choices to preserve his sexual integrity.

Christian men often get angry at God and complain that He allowed sexual temptation that they couldn't stand up under. No, we simply did not make a series of healthy choices until it was too late. God didn't fail us (1 Cor. 10:13). We failed to take the first four choices He gave to keep us from sinning. The quicker you begin making decisions about sexual temptation, the easier it will be to choose God's intervention.

Bring Sexual Secrets into the Light

Mike met Linda on the job when both were mutually working on a stressful project. Six months later they were having an affair, mostly because Mike had never told anyone about Linda. He had never told his wife about the developing friendship; he never shared about the relationship with his best Christian buddy, Stan, whom he saw regularly; he never brought it to God. There were so many opportunities that developed over those six months. But instead, the guilt built to the point that he eventually was forced to share it with his wife, Stacy, and then Stan and then his pastor. Of course, God knew all along.

Wow! Isn't it amazing how Satan's system thrives in darkness and secrecy. It is exciting to practice the discipline of bringing a secret into the light of day and to actually experience its power disappearing. "Have nothing to do with the fruitless deeds of darkness, but rather expose them. For it is shameful even to mention what the disobedient do in secret. But everything exposed by the light becomes visible" (Eph. 5:11–13 NIV).

What a dynamic concept God has created with His emphasis on confession and walking in the light. An important part of this discipline is seeking out appropriate confessors, groups, and accountability buddies. Wives cannot be in that role alone. Men need a male buddy to help us bring our secrets into the light.

Time Out: From the skills discussed for sexual integrity, where do you need the most work? Which one do you violate the most? Choose two behaviors you will start practicing. For example: I will not run with visual cues or I will consciously see that a woman has a soul. Be specific and tell a same-sex friend and pray for God's wisdom to follow through on these actions.

Godly disciplines are not easy or natural. Keep practicing, because it's a no-brainer choice. Do we want pain, guilt, and failed intimacy, or the fruit of the Spirit with love, joy, and peace? "No discipline seems pleasant at the time, but painful. Later on, however, it produces a harvest of righteousness and peace for those who have been trained by it" (Heb. 12:11 NIV). Remember, you are God's courageous warrior, vigilantly protecting your sexual integrity. May He bless you with many wonderfully supportive brothers and a passionate intimacy with your wife.

UNDERSTANDING AND HEALING SEXUAL ADDICTION

In sexual addiction, sex is not joyful but filled with guilt, pain, wasted time, and self-loathing after a person has once again acted out. Lovemaking truly gets short-circuited in the world of sexual compulsions. The mate loses importance, and the person is guided more by the need to alter the mood than to playfully, passionately unite with his or her lover. The sex addict forfeits creativity, greater passion, and a lifetime of making love and enjoying sex with the mate. Sex addiction rapidly becomes a miserable, narrow, and sexually sterile existence.

For you who are struggling with this type of addiction, you are not alone or a terrible impostor, and there is hope for restoring a warm, intimate sex life with your mate. The steps will not be easy and the journey to healing will be time-consuming. It will necessitate giving up your will to God's will.

An important part of healing is breaking the conspiracy of silence for these secrets. Part of their power is that they probably have never been brought out to the light of day and been carefully addressed. I am sure you have tried to make changes and have vowed repeatedly that you will never engage in these behaviors again—only to relapse months, weeks, or even days later. You never seem to get to the root of the problem and achieve a depth of understanding so that you can make the deeper changes that are needed.

This section is also for the mates who have cried through years of deep frustration, suffering through a sex life that has never grown into intimacy. Making love has become confusing, hurtful, or perhaps nonexistent. One wife shared about her husband's sexual quest: "He is like a bucket with no bottom. Nothing sexual ever satisfies him or brings us closer together." Thank God, there is hope and healing for your relationship if your mate is willing to admit the problem and seek to make permanent changes. It will force some deep attitude changes concerning sexuality and intimacy.

Sex is a very powerful force, and pornography often gets hooked up with sexual compulsions and the false ways of trying to achieve intimate connection. Pornography makes persons into sexual objects and robs them of the three dimensions of being a real person of body, soul, and spirit. Oh, it includes the dimension of a body, but that is simply an imaginary sexual image in a secret world the user creates. There is a fear of truly going beneath the surface sexually and connecting with a real person, of allowing sex to have depth with strong connection to an intimate partnership.

Defining Sex Addiction

The essence of pornography and addiction is making a human being, created in God's image, into a depersonalized object for one's selfish sexual gratification. Addiction divorces sex from relationship. It distorts and shuns love, tenderness, and playful companionship. Sex becomes a commodity or an emotional buzz, a drug to create a high or to numb pain. This is far from God's design for a one-flesh sexual union.

Sex addiction therefore uses sex—either in numbing pain or seeking a pleasure high—to alter the mood in a one-dimensional, unfulfilling fashion. This acting out occurs in many ways. The husband sneaks to his stash of magazines and masturbates while viewing them. The youth pastor cruises to find a place to exhibit his genitals. The wife frequents the downtown hotels for quick, casual oral sex. The husband begs his wife to look at sexually explicit movies and to constantly try different and more sexually stimulating activities but is never satisfied. The deacon is arrested for shoplifting lingerie, or the newlywed calls phone-sex lines, running up an eight-hundred-dollar bill. The Sunday school teacher frequents prostitutes while maintaining a pious façade in front of his class. The husband sneaks out at night to look in windows, waiting hours for one brief glimpse of someone undressing; the mate engages in affair after affair and is constantly on the alert for sexual involvement; the husband visits the strip bars twice a week.

When the addiction is discovered, the partner often wonders why the addict doesn't use willpower and make better choices if the marriage is really valued. The addict must not really love the partner, or the addiction would have stopped. The partner is confused about why the addict keeps sinning and hurting the relationship without appropriating God's help. This is an addiction, and many factors have contributed to making the addict fall into sexually compulsive behaviors. It is not a simple matter of willpower, sin, repentance, and instant change. It is not that the addict doesn't really love the spouse. Deep-seated issues and long-term habits must be painfully worked through. It is a process, like so many other facets of becoming Christlike, as the person grows and renews the mind and heart.

Understanding the Addict

Here are eight factors that can contribute to someone's being prone to falling into sex addiction. These factors also contribute to the addict's staying stuck in the addictive behaviors—but these are not excuses for addictive behaviors. Showing causes or contributing factors for addiction helps the partner and the addict understand that the addiction is stronger than willpower. The addict is powerless without help. No one engages in dangerous affairs, drives miles on end to go to adult movies, spends countless hours viewing on-line pornography, shamefully hides pornographic magazines, or peeps in windows because it is fun and fulfilling. There is a compulsion fueled by many underlying problems.

1. Sexual abuse, early sexualization, and a dysfunctional family. The sex addict often was exposed to pornography or explicit sex early in life. Dad may have had his stashes of pornography or parents may have engaged openly in extramarital affairs. There may have been physical as well as psychological sexual abuse and the addict repeats the victimization, only now as the perpetrator. In victimization, sex is associated with power and intrusion into another's life in a one-dimensional fashion for personal sexual gratification. The addict repeats this intrusive sexuality. The family itself may have been rigid and very private, with an inability to demonstrate intimacy and playfulness. The child in growing up may have been starved for affirmation. In high school or late adolescence the destructive sexual patterns were further solidified with sexual acting out—continuing into the present.

2. Insecurity, lack of self-esteem, and loss of purpose. The addict often feels worthless and insecure. This feeling may be especially focused in the area of interpersonal relationships and interaction with the opposite sex but can extend into work and all areas of life. The person lacks self-assurance and the ability to confidently direct life. This, of course, is aggravated by the addiction and the shame and confusion that it produces. The person feels out of control and has strong fears about the future—what to expect from the marriage and what to be sure of spiritually. In the midst of fear and a poor self-image, it is difficult to love the Lord, feel in relationship with Him, and allow His truth to bring peace. It is almost impossible for addicts to love themselves and bring meaning to the injunction to "Love your neighbor as yourself." It is easy to act out to numb this pain.

3. Impostor phenomenon and dual lives with despair. The impostor phenomenon says that if others truly knew me, they would not accept and love me. The addict tries to compartmentalize and balance two separate lives. The first is the secret world of sexually compulsive behaviors, which can consume literally hours of time and demand a web of lies to conceal. The other is the public world of marriage, family, and job that would probably be forfeited if everything came out into the open. The person feels guilt and deep despair because often the addiction violates important values and beliefs. The Christian knows the acts go against God's truth, and the person often loves (as deeply as possible) the mate and family. Nevertheless, the person can't stop the addiction or admit the need to alter the mood. Addiction can produce real moral bankruptcy as the lies and sinful behaviors erode character and take so much time and energy to maintain—with a hopelessness permeating the core of life.

4. Isolated, socially shallow, and lonely. The addict often is socially isolated with no real, close friends. There may be comrades in the addiction as they try to hold off loneliness for each other, but the relationships are far from healthy. Because of dishonesty and lack of trust and intimacy, relationships, and even the marriage, stay casual and shallow. It is not surprising that the inability to relate goes hand in hand with the casual sexual objectifying and fear of intimacy. Addicts frequently hope that sex will drown out their pain and create instant intimacy, but that is not God's design for sex. Authentic lovemaking is deeply relational. Genuine connecting with others could bring so much healing, but it is impossible while walls and defenses stay rigidly in place. It can be very lonely behind those walls, and with such skill deficits you can't break through to intimacy.

5. Constant and intense guilt, shame, and pain. Shame both causes and is created by the addiction. It can be a vicious cycle. The addict feels intense shame and feelings of being unacceptable, and then acts out sexually to change and soothe these feelings. More intense feelings of shame and guilt occur, which then lead to more acting out. There is deep psychic pain and feelings of being unfulfilled, but the sexual fix does not relieve them except for a short time. Instead, it ultimately makes the shame and pain worse, as this negative cycle of acting out to numb pain has a downhill spiral. Some of this pain can be traced back to childhood and the confused and conditional love demonstrated in the family while growing up. The child needed acceptance, affirmation of worth, and a format to love and be loved. The child needed clear boundaries to guide life. In a shame-based dysfunctional family, none of that happened.

6. Stress and living on the edge with fear and adrenaline. An important part of acting out sexually is the risk that adds excitement and diverts attention from the current stressors and pain. The addict may be more likely to act out when there is a lot of stress. He or she will often have a ritual of preparing for the acting out. The ritual of cruising or fantasizing can be as exciting as the actual behavior.

The rituals and behaviors need to have illicitness and an emotional charge of fear to create the desired effect. Cruising bathhouses looking for an anonymous homosexual encounter, sneaking into a motel and watching videos all day, calling an escort service—all have a certain illicitness and excitement or they would not have appeal for the addict. The addict has a need to be outrageous and live on the edge. Often, to be peaceful feels abnormal and can be very uncomfortable at first. The addict needs that adrenaline rush of danger and excitement.

7. Obsession and objectification of sex with no fulfillment. Sex becomes the drug of the addict. It is used to relieve stress, to celebrate a significant accomplishment, or to overcome boredom; but it is not connected with intimacy, playfulness, relationship, satisfaction, or mutual enjoyment. Sex becomes objectifying use of others and results in tremendous guilt and dissatisfaction. The addict loses perspective and comes to feel that sex is the most important need in life. Sex has lost its true meaning of uniting the one-flesh companionship, and it is used for many other nonsexual and destructive purposes.

8. Personality propensities. As with many sexual problems, the personality of the addict can set him or her up. We have already mentioned several causes that can contribute to addiction. The addict's need to be outrageous and live on the edge and be an adrenaline junky propels him in the direction of acting out. Other factors like an introverted personality, shyness, and anxiety that comes out in social fears can get in the way of creating genuine, fulfilling companionship. Chemically, the addict's brain may have some anxiety, depression, or obsessive-compulsive difficulties that aggravate the addiction and actually can be helped with medication.

Recovering from Addiction

Recovery is multi-faceted and you must focus on each of the following areas if you wish to get beyond your addiction:

A support network. This network will need to include your mate, but your partner cannot be your therapist and group support, too. Part of healing will be working through your family issues, stress management, lack of intimacy, and shame. You will need the help of an individual who can counsel you and offer guidance as you sort through problems and make changes. A group of fellow addicts who are also working to recover can help you slice through the denial and support you through the grieving that will occur as you move beyond your addiction. You will need accountability and help, or the changes will not be deep and permanent.

You cannot change on your own! Don't procrastinate but seek out fellow recovering addicts who are working in a change program. This may be through a church program like Faithful and True groups, or a men's ministry that deals especially with lust and sexual addiction. A secular group could also be helpful, but be a good consumer and find one that meets your needs: S.A. (Sexaholics Anonymous), S.A.A. (Sex Addicts Anonymous), or S.L.A.A. (Sex & Love Addicts Anonymous). Often a contact number can be found through the yellow pages or on a Web site.

Sobriety. It may seem obvious, but the addict must stop the sexual self-destructive behaviors. This may require a time of complete sexual abstinence or at least completely limiting sex to mutual activity with your mate—no masturbation. With the help of your support network, you must resist engaging in any of the exciting but shameful activities. You will experience withdrawal and grief and there will be relapses. Relapse does not mean you are back to ground zero; make new resolutions and continue to grow and change.

Addicts often talk about being in the zone or in a trance, that place of compulsion when they know they are going to act out. Before they realize it, they are on their way to the bookstore, cruising the scene, or surfing porn sites. It is best to choose sobriety *before* you get into the zone. Call a friend or therapist or your mate. Let the person help restore sanity before you get fully into the zone. Remember, you will be prone to denial and some very slick thinking. Twelve-step communities affectionately refer to it as "stinking thinking."

One addict related that he was at a stoplight in front of the adult video store. At that point, he was so in the zone he couldn't stop himself from going in and renting a video. When asked what he was doing near the store, which is miles from his home, he said he was taking a shortcut home and happened upon the location. Rationalizations and distorted thinking will come like second nature to your mind as you work through withdrawal pains. Lean on your support network as you maintain sobriety.

Relentless honesty. In your secrets and dishonesty lies the power that perpetuates your addiction. You must become rigorously honest with yourself and others. You have lied so much as you have lived in your two worlds that truthfulness will not come naturally at first. Scripture stresses the importance of honesty. Read this message from Ephesians: "Having lost all sensitivity, they have given themselves over to sensuality so as to indulge in every kind of impurity, with a continual lust for more . . . Therefore each of you must put off falsehood and speak truthfully to his neighbor" (4:19, 25 NIV). Honesty will help break the chains of lust and give meaning back to your life and marriage.

Part of healing is a thorough confession in which you get honest with yourself and at least one other person—probably your therapist or pastor rather than your mate. Your mate will need honesty and confession, but you need others in your accountability network also. Confession helps break the impostor phenomenon, as someone knows all about you and still accepts and unconditionally loves you. Again, being honest will not come naturally, but it is irreplaceable for your recovery.

Intimate relating. Part of the pain and shame is generated by the desire to be close to people but a fear of what might happen if you were to become that vulnerable with them. Addiction is the opposite of intimate companionship: trusting, caring, playfulness, a positive sense of self, warmth, lightheartedness, comfort, and open communication. Sometimes addicts ask how they will be able to know the difference between creating intimate sex with their mates and sexually addictive behavior. I list the above characteristics of intimacy because healthy sex has less intensity and drivenness for the need to create sexual release. It is playful and tender and genuinely exciting, with much eye contact and physical affection.

You will need to provide opportunities that stretch you into relating on a deeper, more intimate level with your mate as well as with friends. Groups are great places to practice new relational skills and especially to find a same-sex friend. Talk and hug and learn to be openly self-aware and disclosing. Please remember that you won't change without the help of others.

You will not feel very comfortable with allowing yourself to be close to others, and getting close will produce real anxiety at first. Hang in there, and you will come to enjoy intimacy very much. The marriage companionship will require special work as you learn to communicate. Get some counseling, go to a marriage enrichment seminar together, read some good books on intimacy, and take vacations in which you play together. You will need to help your mate work through personal feelings, too—he or she will need to sort and grieve through the losses and hurt sustained from your addiction.

Sexual recovery. Sexual recovery has many dimensions to it. You are building an intimate marriage, perhaps for the first time. Sex is becoming a part of relating—not objectifying. This will mean building solid communication skills and learning to nurture your mate and yourself as Scripture exhorts. (Reread Chapters 1, 2, and 15.) A part of sexual recovery will be learning God's economy for great sexual relating. You will have to build the character traits of a mature and expert lover, and growing spiritually and allowing God into sex and the bedroom are also important. It will be a totally different experience as you bring God and His guidelines into your sex life rather than trying to hide and hope He is ignoring your secret world.

Another part of sexual recovery is utilizing good resources. There are excellent books and workbooks that can assist you on the journey. In the secular world, a person who has been an invaluable help is author Patrick Carnes, who has written many books on sexual addiction.

You can also visit a Christian bookstore and find real encouragement and insight in the books written on this topic. An excellent resource is Mark Laaser's *Faithful & True Workbook,* and Russell Willingham's *Breaking Free* can be helpful in understanding how God is there in the process to help assist change.

Never neglect growing spiritually and the importance of surrendering your will to the Lord, as He gives you His power to make needed changes. It will be a tough battle because Satan really uses the sexual to create bondage and distortion in our lives. You will need people to pray for and over you. Your freedom from addiction is tied so much into your spiritual growth and allowing a Power greater than yourself to guide you into needed changes. In sexual addiction, your life has become unmanageable and Jesus can make a difference.

Overcoming and recovering from addiction involve a process. This is also true of the Christian life in general, as you allow God to continually shine new truth into your life, helping you change areas of immaturity. No one ever gets it all together, but you can become more Christlike, with honesty, love, and intimacy permeating your life in wonderful ways that will revolutionize your sexuality and your lovemaking.

CHAPTER TWENTY-NINE

Homosexuality: Expanding Alternatives and Choices

(WITH MARK A. YARHOUSE, PSY.D.)

HOMOSEXUAL FEELINGS OR FEELINGS of same-sex attraction are reported by about 6 percent of men and 4 percent of women in the United States. Far fewer identify themselves as homosexual—only about 2 percent of men and 1 percent of women. So, although experiences of same-sex attraction are not a common experience, some couples do struggle in their marriages because one spouse contends with homosexual feelings. This chapter will be enlightening because it is difficult to find practical resources on the subject. When you are the one struggling with this issue you can feel so alone, ashamed, frustrated, and hopeless. There are also many myths about homosexuality, especially within the evangelical church, that need to be thoughtfully sorted through and dispelled.

The vast majority of people who experience same-sex attraction made no conscious effort to have these attractions. They simply find themselves attracted to members of the same sex. So people who struggle with same-sex attraction and those who love them will want to begin with a common understanding: the person did not do something that caused them to have homosexual attractions. What the person *does* with his or her homosexual attractions is a choice, but the fact that the attractions are there (in a vast majority of cases) is not.

Among those who experience same-sex attraction, some seem to have struggled for a life-time. They look back on their childhood and report always feeling "different" from their friends. Others can point to some specific relationship, trauma, or confusing experience that seemed to help them fall into this behavior that causes such internal conflict. So it is often difficult to point to any single "cause" of same-sex attraction, though there are many theories about why some people experience homosexual attractions. At the broadest level the theories revolve around nature or nurture; that is, that there was some kind of biological cause of homosexual feelings (nature) or some kind of environmental or relational cause of homosexual feelings (nurture). The research is mixed in both of these broad areas. Some research supports influences from biology that might be expressed as temperamental or personality differences; other studies do not support this view. Some research supports influences from the environment, such as parent-child relationships or early trauma; other studies discount these as critical. So it is difficult to say for certain why a specific person ultimately experiences homosexual attractions.

When people come in for counseling they often point to any number of factors they believe led to their experiences of same-sex attractions, including temperamental or personality differences, family relationships, difficulties in parent-child relationships (particularly with the parent of the same gender), emotional and sexual traumas, early sexualization, some masculine or feminine role confusion, and a breakdown in meeting affection needs (especially with the same sex, accompanied by feelings of rejection). Again, it is difficult to point to any one "cause" of homosexual attractions, and often a person does not know specifically why he or she experiences same-sex attraction. We believe that *a whole constellation of factors converges to create the struggle*, and that these factors vary from person to person.

UNDERSTANDING THE COMPLEXITY OF HOMOSEXUALITY

We are called to compassion and not to a fear or revulsion of homosexual behavior. The danger in taking a strong stance on any moral issue is that the persons do not feel we can empathetically listen and help them deal with their problem—they are unwilling to tell us the story of their tortuous journey for fear of rejection or pat advice. That does not have to be so. Christ carefully distinguished between sinner and sin, between the person and the actions. He associated with sinners and yet never compromised His values, loving and accepting the sinners into change. We as a church will have to do much better at lovingly working with those who are struggling with homosexual behavior and need our acceptance (of the person) and help. Like Christ, we will have to combine mercy and truth.

For you whose marriages have been distorted and damaged by homosexuality, there are no easy answers and there is no way to adequately understand the pain and suffering you have been through. Following initial reports of shock, anger, and grief, the spouse has often already traumatically worked through to a place of compassion and acceptance about the presence of homosexuality. A spouse is not homophobic with irrational fear of and disgust for the homosexual. He or she just wishes that there were some way to make the necessary changes and rid the marriage of this saboteur. The mate wants to reestablish trust and work toward greater intimacy and fulfillment.

Some spouses will, however, give serious consideration to a separation or divorce following the disclosure of homosexual behavior on the part of their partners. This is understandable, and we believe the scriptural allowance for divorce for unfaithfulness applies here. The matter is only made more complicated because it has involved same-sex behavior. In our experience, whether a spouse pursues divorce is not a reflection of his or her love for the spouse or a lack of courage; it is often a reflection of feeling like something is deeply broken and the options for pursuing intimacy, lovemaking, and delighting in one's marital covenant are too seriously compromised. We certainly sympathize with the dilemma the nonoffending spouse faces. We would like this chapter to give hope but recognize that any act of infidelity is such a threat to God's intention for marriage.

For those couples where both partners are willing to work on their marriage, we offer several suggestions throughout the remainder of this chapter in an attempt to support you down the rough road ahead. We would pray for God's grace and forgiveness, patience and stamina, and the ability to wisely accept the complexity of the situation while courageously persisting in creating alternative choices.

Some of the issues that need to be addressed revolve around simple education about homosexuality, same-sex attractions, and efforts at experiencing change. Other concerns revolve around what it means to live together, to love together, and to remain faithful to your vows *despite* the fact that one of you contends with same-sex attraction. Let's begin to unpack and increase awareness of several of the most important considerations.

Part of understanding and experiencing change is carefully exploring and understanding the evolution of the homosexual behavior and the personal issues behind the confusion and habit. Some people benefit from a careful consideration of the family background, especially the relationship with the same-sex parent. Often there are feelings of anger, rejection, and other unfinished business.

One perspective that resonates with many people who experience homosexual attractions is the common confusion that can occur to the extent that they try to meet nonsexual needs (companionship, affirmation) sexually. This can be true for anyone, but it is often noted among those who experience same-sex attraction. Another trap is the thinking that sexual behavior is the most and only truly intimate expression of affection. This is especially true for men who sexualize an important friendship without considering that the friendship will be forever changed. In a society of instant gratification, it is easy to hope that instant sex will create instant intimacy. It is also easy to hope that sex will meet deeper needs for closeness and connection with the same sex in ways that were never fulfilled by the same-sex parent.

A woman who contends with same-sex attraction often reports a different kind of experience. While a man's attraction may become sexualized, a woman's experience is often of desiring emotional closeness. She may feel a draw to or close connection with another woman that could then develop into overt sexual behavior. The behavior, however, is not the goal. More often than not, the drawing force is the actual process of connecting.

Some people who struggle with same-sex attraction identify rejection as an important issue to deal with in understanding the origins of homosexual behavior. It can be perceived rejection by the same-sex parent or actual acts of rejection experienced by the person in growing up. The anger and issues with parents must be resolved. Tied in with rejection are some of the same struggles of the sexual addict, with deep feelings of worthlessness and uneasy acceptance of masculinity or femininity. The tendency can be to isolate while desperately desiring to be close.

As with the sexual addict, there was sometimes early sexualization or abusive, confusing situations in sexual development. One client reported the confusion that came from sleeping in his mom's bed until he was eleven years old. He experienced the emotional incest of trying to fill Mom's friendship needs, though no physical boundaries were ever crossed. There may have been sexual repression and an absence of information regarding sexuality in general. Comfortable, appropriate sexual values and boundaries may not have been established. This confusion might have been further compounded in dating relationships—or a lack of such relationships. It is not that sexual abuse causes a person to experience same-sex attraction, but such abuse is often reported in a person's sexual or family history, and it may play a part amid a constellation of factors that contribute to same-sex attraction.

Sexual Identity

A place to begin is to set your experiences of same-sex attraction into a context for better understanding and acceptance of who you are as a person. One important consideration is how you think of yourself and your attractions. Some women may ask themselves, "Am I really a lesbian?" Some men may say to themselves, "Who am I trying to kid? I am and have always been gay." The language you use to think about and describe your experiences is of great importance as you seek to work on your marriage. The language of "gay" or "straight" is related to a person's *sexual identity*. This identity has to do with your gender as either male or female, the kinds of people you are attracted to, the behavior you engage in, and your personal and religious beliefs and values about sexual behavior. This can show the complexity of this issue, as some have a comfortable gender identity as male or female but struggle more with attraction.

We believe that sexual identity develops through five stages:[1] (1) experiences of confusion, (2) attributions about same-sex attractions, (3) foreclosing on your identity versus increasing your options, (4) reconsidering your identity, and (5) seamless sexual identity. It may be helpful for you to identify where you are in this process and where you can go from there.

1. Experiences of confusion. This is often the first experience of people who struggle with homosexual feelings. This could have happened at a very early age, perhaps as you were just beginning school, or it may have been your experience as you entered early or middle adolescence. You may remember feeling different from your peers. Possibly you felt confused. Others report a kind of crisis related to both feeling and having feelings so different from others. This may be more common during the teen years, when being "different" can be especially troubling. In some circles, however, identifying as "gay" may be met with greater acceptance. In this case, confusion and experience of crisis might be less prominent.

2. Attributions about same-sex attractions. People who experience homosexual attractions also make attributions about their homosexual attractions (*attribution* is a technical word for drawing conclusions, or explaining or accounting for something being a certain way). It is more common today than ever before for people who have same-sex attractions to say, "I must be gay," or "I guess that means I'm a lesbian." One young lady came in for counseling because she had experienced arousal when a female friend had tickled her and given her a backrub. She certainly fit the profile for confusion and drawing conclusions on identity, as she stated she was afraid she must be lesbian and she really did not want to be.

Perhaps this is something you say to yourself. Please know that ours is the first culture throughout history to have people identify themselves with their experiences of homosexual attraction. That is, there has never been a time or place when people have said of themselves, "I *am* gay," or "I *am* lesbian."

Rather than label yourself as the sum total of your experiences of homosexual attraction, we encourage you to be more descriptive as you think about yourself. For example, you might say, "I am a male who experiences same-sex attraction," or "I am a female who has occasional experiences of same-sex desire." This is not denial or minimization—we recognize that you experience homosexual attractions, and we're not suggesting you kid yourself about this or make it seem like you experience less of it than you do. Rather, we want you to accurately convey to yourself and to others your experiences of attraction while allowing God to convey to you His sense of your *identity*. We will discuss this further in the sections that follow.

3. Foreclosing on your identity versus increasing your options. This next stage is characterized by a decision people make to either foreclose on their sexual identity as "gay" or "lesbian" or to seek alternatives to that identity, as we mentioned before. When you seek an alternative identity you are essentially increasing your options (rather than limiting yourself to a "gay" identity). If you had at one time foreclosed on your sexual identity you probably identified yourself to others (and to yourself) as gay or lesbian. You thought this was who you were as a person. This is completely understandable. There are many sources in our society telling you that this must be who you are as a person. In fact, these same sources are subtly communicating to you that for you to be truly fulfilled, you should act on your desires, and if it costs you your marriage, so be it— you are being true to yourself and you are entitled to sexual self-actualization. But this is a remarkable distortion of what it means for God to have a call on your life and on your marriage, and we want you to at least explore other options before you make a decision about the direction and future of your marriage.

Of course, it is possible that you are not someone who had identified with your experiences of homosexual attractions. Perhaps you always resisted your attractions—not physical resistance of urges or desires, but perhaps you resisted identifying yourself by your homosexual attractions. In your own way maybe you have been seeking alternatives for your life. You do not deny that you have homosexual attractions, but you do not define who you are by these attractions, either. But you may be discouraged because you have asked God to remove your attractions, similar to the apostle Paul asking God to remove his "thorn in the flesh" (2 Cor. 12:7–9 NKJV), and you are disappointed because God has chosen, for reasons unclear to you, to allow your attractions to remain.

In either scenario, you may struggle with guilt and shame. You may feel guilty for specific instances of infidelity in your thought life or through sexual behavior. This is appropriate guilt. It should be distinguished from disabling shame, where you have come to hate who you are as a person because of your struggles with homosexual attractions. We want to say to you that this distorted shame is not God's intention for you. Though God may want you to experience guilt for specific instances of sin, we do not believe God wants you to despair of who you are and of who God has created you to be.

4. Reconsidering your identity. The next stage many people go through is a time of reflection upon the decisions they have made in their lives. This is a time when people reflect on their efforts at living one lifestyle or the other. For example, some people may have been trying to experience a change of sexual orientation. They may get very discouraged if there has not been as much of a change as they had hoped for in the amount of time they allowed for change to occur. This can and has led some people to give up on living a chaste life, and some have ended their marriages and pursued a gay lifestyle, identifying themselves with their homosexual attractions and pursuing a same-sex relationship. This can be a costly decision, of course, because it often means losing one's marriage, limited or no contact with one's children, and consequences in terms of family and social support.

Others may reconsider their experiences living the gay lifestyle. Perhaps they engaged in minor encounters with homosexuality or maybe they submerged themselves in gay culture. In any case, they may feel dissatisfied with their relationships or behavior and may reconsider the direction their lives have taken. Such an experience can lead people back to confusion about who they are and what they are all about.

5. Seamless sexual identity. Those who feel that they've made good decisions go on to synthesize their identities. What do we mean by this concept of "synthesis"? It is pulling together and creating a comfortable whole with your sexual identity. This is a kind of seamless, rather than patchwork, integration a person evolves of his or her experiences, values, and identity.

People who integrate their homosexual attractions into gay or lesbian identities do so in such a way that they feel this is consistent with their experiences, beliefs, and values.

If you have made a decision not to identify with your homosexual attractions, then a seamless sexual identity will be reflected in a sense of peace about living faithfully in your relationship with your spouse, and identifying with other aspects of who you are as a person. You may be asking yourself, *Does seamless sexual identity mean that I am free from all the pull of homosexual attraction?* Experiences of homosexual attractions may diminish, but even if they do not disappear they don't leave behind the same wake of destruction in your marriage. You have more seamlessly attributed yourself as a heterosexual mate who wants the marriage to work; you continue to make choices for those alternatives.

Recovering from Homosexual Confusion

Homosexual feelings and behaviors are so complex that hurting mates often ask, "Is there hope for change with such a deep-rooted problem?" We want to affirm that there certainly is hope for change. A person can change his or her thoughts and behaviors and remain faithful to a spouse. Someone may also experience a change in the intensity, frequency, and duration of same-sex attractions, though complete change of attractions is not the experience of most people who pursue change.

Those who report experiencing change of same-sex attraction and behavior generally say that it takes *time*. Some say that it took them as long as two years before they began to experience change, and that it took up to five years or more before they were at the end of their change experiences. Others continue to work toward change throughout their lifetimes. Obviously this has the potential to put great strain on a marriage. Presumably, the longer it takes the more a couple has to cope with issues of trust, intimacy, hope, and patient persistence.

We encourage you to look at five major areas of focus as you consider changing same-sex attractions and behavior: (1) making accurate attributions, (2) sobriety from the behaviors, (3) personal changes, (4) a renewed enjoyment of intimate companionship, both maritally and interpersonally, and (5) a reliance on and relationship with God.

1. Making accurate attributions. If you want to begin to make sense of your experiences of homosexual attraction, reflect how you attribute these attractions. Do you tend to think of these attractions as defining who you are as a person? As we mentioned earlier, there is a difference between saying to yourself, "I am a gay man trying to make my marriage work," and saying, "I am a married man who contends with same-sex attraction." The former self-statement identifies who you are with your homosexual attractions and places your marriage secondary to what you choose to make prominent in your life. The latter self-statement focuses on your marriage and your gender and places your attractions in the context of your prior commitments, beliefs, and values. So you may benefit from asking, What other parts of me would I like to move from the periphery of my experience to a place that is closer to the center of who I experience myself to be?

Begin by recognizing that there are other aspects of identity. We mentioned gender: Are you male or female? Then begin by identifying yourself with your gender. If you are having difficulty with this, this provides an important avenue for work with a professional counselor. There is also marital status: Are you a husband or a wife? Identify yourself with the covenant you have made with your partner. There is also your identity in Christ: Are you a Christian? Then consider thinking of yourself with Christ at the center of who you are as a person. This provides you with more of a sense of who you are than the fact that you also happen to experience same-sex attractions. The point is that attributions make a difference in how you see yourself. If you define who you are by your experiences of same-sex attraction, you may find yourself facing an uphill battle in your thought life about various struggles that may follow.

2. Sobriety. If spouses want to get beyond the effects of homosexuality and remain faithful to their marital vows, the individual struggling with these desires will need to believe it is wrong and truly want to change the behavior. If this is impossible, we believe Christ's allowance for divorce because of sexual immorality applies, and the mate is better off moving on rather than staying with the offending partner and risking further abuse. If the partner with homosexual confusion wants to change, a program of sobriety will have to be inaugurated, which applies to thoughts as well as actual behaviors. Active sexual fantasy should involve only your mate and heterosexuality. The goal is not to make you heterosexual but whole and able to enjoy intimacy with your mate.

A place to begin is in managing your environment. What do we mean here? Your environment includes your home, work (including travel), and leisure activities. Consider carefully examining each area for people, places, and items—such as gifts or souvenirs—that are in any way homosexually stimulating to you. You may need to carefully consider your work environment: With whom do you work? When you stop for coffee on the way to work, whom have you found attractive? When you travel, are you struggling with wandering eyes as you walk through the airport or check into your hotel? Are there places that are homosexually stimulating to you? Is it difficult for you to eat at certain restaurants for lunch or stop by a certain fitness center because of past experiences or current struggles with fantasies? Do you have items that you may need to get rid of? Sometimes people keep gifts or memorabilia from past relationships. These need to go. The bottom line is this: What are the people, places, and things that get in the way of what is in the best interest of your marriage? They will require changing.

Staying sober will probably be impossible without a support network. Build a strong friendship with a same-sex mentor who can set healthy boundaries on the friendship and model appropriate behaviors. Have an accountability group to help you work through the problems of making changes. Your mate, pastor, therapist, and other Christian friends can also encourage your staying sober from homosexually acting out. Please choose these friends carefully, as this is obviously a difficult area to discuss with even the closest of friends. But it is so important that you know and are known by trusted friends who can help to provide support and accountability. If you are starting from scratch, you might consider contacting a local Christian ministry group to see whether there is a support group in your area for you to meet with weekly for a period of time.[2]

3. *Personal growth.* An essential part of maintaining sobriety is growing into wholeness and healing the damaged areas of your life. You will need a counselor who can guide you through this process, someone who can help you explore your family background and find healing to the extent to which this is an area of concern for you. Your mate, your sponsor, and other friends can also be helpful in encouraging, confronting, and overcoming blind spots in your self-awareness. It is especially easy to rationalize exceptions to people, places, and items that may make sobriety difficult for you, particularly in your thought life, where fantasies are so difficult to manage. You will have to be ruthlessly honest and courageous as you grow personally in all areas, especially in the spiritual and relational aspects of your life.

Sort through the sexual distortions, bad habits, and attitudes. Set goals and structure a growth program in which you dispute ineffective attitudes (for example, "Sex is the primary way to experience intimacy," or "I am flawed and unable to create close friendships"). Create new attitudes and behaviors. Men and women alike will have to pair new behaviors with erotic excitement and allow them to gain momentum in producing arousal. Men may focus here more on actual sexual arousal and associated physical changes and sexual attractions with the opposite sex. Women may need to work on boundary setting in relationships, exploring this with a professional counselor if they are overreacting to setting limits by themselves or with others.

Both men and women who contend with homosexual feelings and behaviors will have to choose to let the opposite sex, and especially the mate, be the focus of sexual arousal and permit the homosexual preferences to slowly fade. It will take time and repeated conditioning before you have extinguished the old arousal patterns and established new ones with your mate. You may always have some attraction to the same sex, but you can choose to have sexual faithfulness and not feed those fantasies. Every covenant marriage has this task of disciplining thoughts and attractions.

Men, the goal is not to make you into a "breast man" so you can lust after feminine body parts. The goal is to allow you to become comfortable with and aroused by your wife in erotic closeness to *her*. Women who struggle in being attracted to masculinity, allow your heart to connect with your husband so the physical can flow out of that emotional intimacy. Mates, especially wives of those struggling, you will have to sort through (and grieve too) that attraction may be less about physical nudity and more about intimate touch and you as a person. This is perhaps the most difficult part of this journey. Don't become discouraged! You two can arrive at a truer and deeper sexual inimacy.

4. Renewed intimacy. Love and deeply intimate relationships will be the most effective agents of managing your sexual behavior and attractions. Your mate, your sponsor, your group, your growing network of friends, and your therapist will demonstrate affection and acceptance. They will help you to heal the wounds of the past and respond faithfully to the challenges in the present. To the extent that the past makes this area difficult for you, God's plan for healing the hurts of past negative relationship is to go through a healthy relationships and this time have your needs for intimacy and affirmation truly met. Some people refer to this as reparenting or refriending; we prefer to see this as simply unpacking the baggage from past relationships and reordering your life through close, healthy relationships with your mate, your friends, and possibly a counselor. These relationships essentially help you redo negative experiences in the parenting or friendship process, and real healing can result as your deeper needs for affirmation and intimacy are truly met.

Build intimate relationships with those people the Lord has placed in your life to love and accept you. Lean on them in overcoming temptations, and draw strength from them when the problems seem insurmountable. Work and play at sorting through your sexual attractions and allow your mate to become your lover in a bonding and exciting manner. You may also benefit from seeing a professional to help you through a brief course of sex counseling. Be prepared to be surprised on this journey—the changes you make you may never have thought possible.

You will also benefit from building deeply intimate, nonsexual same-sex friendships. Many people begin this process by working with a therapist of the same sex. The things that make connecting with the same sex difficult for you can be identified and worked through in that relationship, and then the insights and gains made in therapy can be generalized to other relationships with members of the same sex. Rather than these relationships becoming eroticized, you can learn to recognize that tendency and cultivate close, nonsexual relationships with the same sex. One man, struggling with these issues, related that it was a tremendously healing experience to have a male friend who was secure enough to hold him and let him cry through the pain he had bottled up so long.

5. Relationship with God. When one partner in a marriage struggles with homosexual attractions, the greatest resource for that person and for that marriage is each person's relationship with God. Only as you admit your powerlessness and trust Him to provide growth and opportunities to discern His will can you work through needed changes in your life. Draw closer to Christ daily and appropriate His power. Ask God what He wants for you and for your marriage in overcoming same-sex attractions. Admit to Him your frustration or anger for having this particular struggle in your life and in the life of your marriage. Ask God to help you find your calling; that is, how He wants you to serve Him in light of your struggles with same-sex attraction.

Give yourself up to His love and truth as you learn to trust and be intimate. Ask God what He wants for you in your relationships with others. Pray that God would help you see your spouse through His eyes, to love your spouse as He intends. Ask God for the strength to say no to some things in your life that, left to your own devices, you are drawn toward. Then you will be able to say yes to other aspects of who you are as a person. These are the aspects God wants to give you so you can relate to Him, your spouse, and to others more richly. It is through this process that you continue to allow God to make you more and more in the image and likeness of Christ, to be sanctified and made holy for His purposes.

Mark A. Yarhouse, Psy.D., is associate professor of psychology at Regent University in Virginia Beach, Virginia. He is the coauthor of Homosexuality: The Use of Scientific Research in the Church's Moral Debate (Intervarsity, 2000) *and author of* Expanding Alternatives to Same-Sex Attraction: Clinical Modules for Informed Consent, Assessment, and Intervention. *Dr. Yarhouse is also a professor in the Institute for Sexual Wholeness, training sex therapists.*

Sexually Transmitted Diseases

WE WILL FIRST CONSIDER SEVERAL of the most common sexually transmitted diseases (STDs). We will then explore some questions and fears that need confronting. (For further information, the Centers for Disease Control has an STD hotline: 1-800-227-8922.)

COMMON SEXUALLY TRANSMITTED DISEASES

One couple contracted herpes (simplex 2, a virus that in simplex 3 is a cold sore) after being married six months. Neither suspected the other was involved in an affair, but great doubts and distancing occurred. They learned from their physician that someone can be a carrier without having actual outbreaks of the disease and therefore not even know it is present. One of them had apparently acquired the disease in a previous sexual relationship and had given it to the partner after marriage. This is true of most STDs in a small percentage of people; a person can be a carrier and spread the infection without having active symptoms.

Bacteria and viruses of STDs can be spread without sexual contact, but it is a rather unlikely possibility. Catching a sexually transmitted disease from shaking hands or sitting on a toilet seat is statistically very remote, though it can be a common excuse of mates who have contracted an STD.

Don't avoid getting these diseases diagnosed and treated because you feel guilty or embarrassed. They won't go away, and ignoring them can have serious health consequences. With bacterial infections like gonorrhea, both mates will have to undergo treatment to be sure the bacteria are killed and aren't passed back and forth. There is no recourse but an honest disclosure to your (future) mate about any STD you might have.

Gonorrhea

Gonorrhea is the most common kind of STD, and it is a bacterial infection. With men, the symptoms are a yellowish discharge and burning with urination because the urethra gets infected. Many women have gonorrhea without noticeable symptoms, or very mild symptoms at first, and so go untreated. The noticeable symptoms are vaginal discharge, painful urination, irritation of external genitals, and abnormal menstrual bleeding. Untreated gonorrhea can cause pelvic inflammatory disease (PID), which is the most common cause of infertility. PID can cause scarring that blocks the fallopian tubes. The symptoms of PID are nausea, fever, lower abdominal pain, and perhaps pain with intercourse. Penicillin and other antibiotics can cure gonorrhea.

Genital Herpes

This STD is caused by a herpes virus that is in the same family as chicken pox and cold sores. Genital herpes can be spread by herpes simplex 1 and 2. The infection is usually contracted through intercourse or direct genital contact or oral sex with a partner who has an outbreak of the disease. Important to note is that cold sores (simplex 1) can create herpes breakouts on the genitals with oral to genital contact. Some mates falsely accuse their partners of an affair when they have transmitted the simplex 1. In rarer cases, genital herpes can be transmitted by a carrier without any symptomatic breakout of the skin. The symptoms of genital herpes are small, painful blisters on the pubic area, penis, vaginal opening, cervix, or rectum. The first episode of herpes is usually the most severe, with fever, headaches, and painful irritation at the site of the blisters and subsequent sores when the blisters burst. With some people there is never a second outbreak, but others experience a reoccurrence, often stress- or illness-induced.

Presently, there is no cure for genital herpes. The drug acyclovir (Zovirax) helps some people lessen the painfulness of the symptoms and shorten the healing time of the blisters, especially in the first occurrences. If taken on a long-term basis, it can reduce the rate and duration of recurrences. Women need to be conscious of two health hazards (which their physicians can monitor): (1) There is risk to the fetus at birth if there is a breakout, so a cesarean section may be required; and (2) added caution must be taken to watch out for cancer of the cervix and vulva.

It is very difficult to keep from infecting a mate, but refraining from intercourse during active recurrences and at least two days after an episode has healed will help. During this time, using separate washcloths and not having contact with the sores are essential. Use of a condom can prevent spreading infection, though sometimes all the area is not contained within the condom or other genital contact occurs before the condom is put on.

Genital Warts

Genital warts are transmitted by the human papilloma virus (HPV). These warts appear on the genitals and on the cervix in women. They can be removed with liquid nitrogen or laser treatment in an office procedure. Care must be taken to watch out for cervical and genital cancer.

Chlamydial Infections

These infections are caused by *Chlamydia trachomatis*. It may be the most common bacterial STD, though it has not received much attention until recently. In men, chlamydia bacteria can cause infection in the urethra and the epididymis. The damage is much more severe in women because the bacteria attack the reproductive tract and can cause pelvic inflammatory disease (PID), infections of the endometrium, and complications during pregnancy. Often there is an initial lack of symptoms until the infection has progressed, but testing for antibodies can detect the disease earlier. Penicillin will not cure chlamydial infection. Fortunately, various other antibiotics are effective.

Pubic Lice

Sometimes called crabs, the parasites attach themselves to pubic hair and can cause intense itching. They can be killed with a specially medicated shampoo or cream but not by simple washing.

AIDS

Acquired immune deficiency syndrome has become a horror that affects all our lives. It is caused by the human immunodeficienty virus (HIV).

Many people are very frightened and worry that AIDS can be contracted with casual contact. HIV is transmitted through sexual contact and the exchange of bodily fluids. HIV is present in saliva but in much lower concentration than in blood or sexual secretions.

Completely safe sex is possible only if there is no exchange of bodily fluids, though use of a latex condom lessens the risk. After infection, the HIV antibodies can be detected usually within two to three months—immediately going for an AIDS test is not always effective. Testing positive for HIV does not mean having AIDS; many people remain a carrier of the virus for three to five years without developing AIDS or AIDS-related symptoms. There is no cure for AIDS at present, and everyone who is HIV-positive will eventually contract AIDS. There is not enough research to definitely say how long this will take. Recent cocktails of medication can help reduce viral counts and prolong effective living. It is important to keep current with research and medications for treatment. These are constantly changing.

COPING WITH SEXUALLY TRANSMITTED DISEASES

Too often we as a Christian community are not on the vanguard of bringing hope and help to wounded souls who need our loving ministry. We sit in judgment rather than reach out. Each of us must become involved and learn more about AIDS. Persons living with AIDS need our understanding and tender care, and we can do this without endangering our health. We will have friends and relatives who need our hugs and support.

Because there is no cure for herpes, many individuals see it as a badge of shame. They fear Christian dating partners will immediately reject them if it becomes known. These people suffer intense emotional pain and worry as they wear a capital *H* as their own scarlet letter of guilt. Any sin is able to be forgiven, and we are much more than our sinful mistakes. Like any skeleton in the closet, it should not be revealed immediately in a dating situation. However, as trust and commitment build, you must disclose it and work through this with your partner. If the person cannot deal with this aspect of you, that is a commentary on the person's values and needs—not your worth and ability to be loved.

Herpes or other STDs need not destroy a potentially intimate marriage and a great sex life. Consult a physician, and get appropriate medical help immediately. It will take work to ensure that the wounds and emotional issues are healed and will not come back to haunt your companionship and lovemaking. You may be able to talk it through together, or you may need a wise counselor to assist you in this process. Persevere. God can help bring a gracious healing. Together you can help each other find wholeness and unconditional love and acceptance within your intimate partnership.

Notes

CHAPTER 10

1. Abridged from Desmond Morris, *Intimate Behaviour* (New York: Random House, 1971). Originally published in the UK by Jonathan Cape, an imprint of the Random House UK Group.

CHAPTER 16

1. Archibald Hart, Catherine Hart Weber, and Debra Taylor, *Secrets of Eve* (Nashville, Word Publishing, 1998).

CHAPTER 18

1. Hart, Hart, and Taylor, *Secrets of Eve.*
2. Theresa Crenshaw, *The Alchemy of Love and Lust* (Simon & Schuster, 1996) p. 96–98.

CHAPTER 20

1. M. Scott Peck, *The Road Less Traveled* (Simon & Schuster, 1978) p. 81.

CHAPTER 24

1. Wendy Maltz, *The Sexual Healing Journey* (Quill, 2001) p. 89–97.

CHAPTER 25

1. R. M. Sabatelli, R. L. Meth, and S. M. Gavazzi, "Factors mediating the adjustment to involuntary childlessness," *Family Relations* (1988), 37, 338–43.

CHAPTER 29

1. This model is from Mark A. Yarhouse, "Sexual identity development: The influence of valuative frameworks on identity synthesis," *Psychotherapy, 38* (3), 331–41.

The most developed application of this model for counseling practice is found in Mark A. Yarhouse, *Expanding alternatives to same-sex attraction and behavior: Clinical modules for informed consent, assess-*

ment, and intervention, self-published therapist workbook, Regent University, Virginia Beach, Va. Available from the author.

2. You might consider three such ministry organizations. Courage is a Catholic organization that can be reached through St. John the Baptist Church, 210 West 31st Street, New York, NY 10001; phone: (212) 268-1010; e-mail: NYCourage@aol.com; Internet: http://courageRC.org

Exodus International North America is a nondenominational, umbrella organization of Christian ministries. Exodus International North America's contact information is P.O. Box 540119, Orlando, FL; phone: (888) 264-0877; Internet: www.exodusnorthamerica.org.

Homosexuals Anonymous also offers ministries throughout the United States. For updates and information on on-line chapters, phone: (610) 376-1146; Internet: http://members.aol.com/ hawebpage.

Index

Finances, handling, xii–xiv
Foreplay. *See* Loveplay

G spot, 33, 141, 147, 160
Gender. *See also* Female; male
      characteristics, 3
      differences and similarities, 3,
39–41, 76–77, 214–15, 239–40
Genital herpes, 379
Genital warts, 380
Genitals
      female, 30–33
      male, 27–30
Goals, sexual, 66–72
Gonorrhea, 379,
Grafenberg, Ernst, 161
Grafenberg, the, 161
Grief, 220–21, 274, 298, 329–30
Guilt, 222, 274, 339, 346

Haykawa, 91
Health, 64–65
Herpes, 379
HIV (Human immunodeficiency virus),
380–81
Homosexuality, 367–77
Honesty, 16–17
Honeymoon disease, 244
Honeymoons, xii–xiii
Hormonal interventions, 56
Hormones, 23, 34, 217–20
HPV (human papilloma virus), 380
Human immunodeficienty virus (HIV),
380–81
Human papilloma virus (HPV), 380
Hygiene, 60–62
Hymen, 31
Hysterosalpingogram, 326–27

Illness (as diabetes), 307–08
Impotence, 273–78
Individuating, xi
Infertility, 321–36
      and adoption, 334–35
      and miscarriage, 329–32
      misconceptions about, 322–23
      testing for, 325–28
Infidelity. *See* Adultery
Injuries (as disability), 299, 30507
Intercourse, *See also* Sexual activity;
Lovemaking and aging,
      painful, 218, 245, 282–93
      positions of, 143–51
      crosswise, 146–47
      for disabilities, 143, 149–51
      face-to-face, 149
      husband-on-top, 145–46
      missionary, 145–46
      during pregnancy, 147–48
      with props, 150
      rear-entry, 147–48
      side-by-side, 144–45
      standing, 148
      wife-on-top, 143–44
Interstitial cystitis, 284
Intimacy, vii, xii–xvi, 118–19
Intrauterine device (IUD), 57
In vitro fertilization, 332–34
IUD (intrauterine device), 57

Jung, Carl, 2

Kegel, Dr. Arnold, 167
Kegel exercises, 167–68, 172, 204, 292–93
Kissing, 159–60
Kubler-Ross, Elisabeth, 298
K-Y Jelly, 58, 301

Acknowledgments

CATHERINE, WONDERFUL PARTNER, without your support and encouragement *A Celebration of Sex*, in its first or second edition, would never have been written. Thank you for sacrificing so much. You have taken down my walls and truly taught me the rich and deep concept of being in love and making love over all these years.

My special friends and fellow sex therapists in Sexual Wholeness, Inc. (Christopher McCluskey, Debra Taylor, Michael Sytsma) have helped me so much with their love, support and wisdom over the years. They have also added valuable information to this second edition. Thanks to some of the faculty of the Sexual Wholeness Institute, Mark Yarhouse, Bill Cutrer and Jim (and Carolyn) Childerston, for their crucial contributions. Several colleagues read over selected chapters and also made helpful suggestions: Todd Wilson, Vickie George, Debbie Neel, Susan Townsend, Debbie Born, Vilda Brannen, Ellen Fox, Hollis and Tanya Black.

I want to thank two wise teachers who have greatly increased my ability as a sex therapist: Domeena Renshaw, M.D., who started me on my journey and gave me the beginning skills; William Talmadge, Ph.D., who continues to be a thoughtful supervisor.

I appreciate my editors who made such crucial contributions to guiding, shaping, and polishing A *Celebration of Sex*: Victor Oliver, who took a chance on an unknown author and made many important changes in the original manuscript; Lila Empson, who wisely shaped and pushed through the first edition in 1994; and Elizabeth Kea, who used her editorial talent in 2002 with wise and skillful decisions.

Thanks, Al Tiegreen, for making changes in illustrations and helping me create the needed drawings for this book.

About the Author

DOUGLAS ROSENAU, ED.D., is a Licensed Psychologist, Marriage & Family Therapist, and Diplomate of the American Board of Sexology (ABS). A pioneer in Christian sex therapy, Dr. Rosenau has written numerous articles on healthy sexuality for such publications as *Christian Counseling Today* and *New Man*. He is a graduate of Dallas Theological Seminary (Th.M.) and received his doctorate (Ed.D.) in counseling from Northern Illinois University. He is also a full clinical member of the Society for Sex Therapy and Research (SSTAR) and an approved supervisor with the American Association of Marriage and Family Therapists. Dr. Rosenau teaches Human Sexuality as an adjunct professor at Reformed Theological Seminary and Psychological Studies Institute. As co-founder of the Christian organization Sexual Wholeness, Doug has helped to create the Institute for Sexual Wholeness that trains Christian sex therapists and creates teaching videos and materials.

Dr. Rosenau and his wife, Cathy, live in Atlanta, Georgia, and have a daughter, Merrill, son-in-law, Tom, and granddaughter, Caitlyn, who is the apple of his eye.

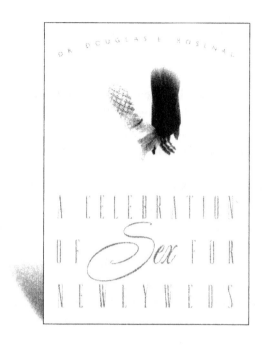

DRAWN FROM THE MATERIAL IN *A CELEBRATION OF SEX,*
A Celebration of Sex for Newlyweds answers specific, often unasked questions
about sexual topics, and presents newly-married couples with detailed techniques and behavioral skills for learning sexual pleasure and intimate companionship. An excellent tool for premarital counseling and a wonderful
gift for the newly-married, this book offers invaluable information in a professional yet sensitive style.

ISBN 0-7852-6523-6

$13.99 • 5x7 • 128 pages

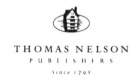

THOMAS NELSON
PUBLISHERS
Since 1798